OSHA Regulations
and Guidelines:
A Guide for
Health Care Providers

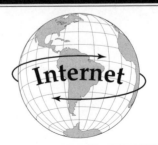

OSHA Regulations and Guidelines: A Guide for Health Care Providers

Ronald P. Nielsen, WSO-CSM

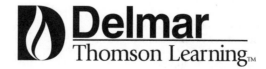

Africa • Australia • Canada • Denmark • Japan • Mexico
New Zealand • Phillipines • Puerto Rico • Singapore
Spain • United Kingdom • United States

NOTICE TO THE READER

Delmar Staff:

Director, Health Care Publishing: William Brottmiller
Executive Editor: Cathy L. Esperti
Executive Marketing Manager: Dawn F. Gerrain
Acquisitions Editor: Doris Smith

Developmental Editor: Marjorie A. Bruce
Production Coordinator: John Mickelbank
Production Editor: Mary C. Liburdi
Project Editor: Stacey Prus

Library of Congress Cataloging-in-Publication Data
Nielsen, Ronald P.
    OSHA regulations and guidelines : a guide for health care
    providers / by Ronald P. Nielsen.
        p.   cm.
    Includes bibliographical references and index.
    ISBN 0-7668-0478-X
    1. Health facilities—Law and legislation—United States.
    2. Industrial hygiene—Law and legislation—United States.
    3. Industrial safety—Law and legislation—United States.   4. Health
    facilities—United States—Safety measures.   I. Title.
    [DNLM: WA 400 N669o 1999.]
    KF3574.H66N54   1999
    344.73'0465—dc21
    DNLM/DLC   99-11382
    for Library of Congress   CIP

DEDICATION

To my wife Eleanor without whose help
this book might not have been written.

CONTENTS

The Occupational Safety and Health Act (OSH Act) was passed by the federal government in 1970 and marked the first time business and industry were covered by uniform safety and health laws. In the past, the various states had their own laws, and these varied as to strictness and coverage.

When OSHA was passed, it made it mandatory that every private sector employer of one or more workers maintain a workplace free of recognized hazards. Initially, OSHA did not cover state, county, and municipal employees, but the Act was later amended to allow states to form their own plans to include these workers. The state-adopted plans had to be approved by OSHA and equal or exceed the OSHA standards. OSHA does not cover self-employed persons, farms that employ only immediate family members, and employee situations regulated by other federal requirements.

The **Occupational Safety and Health Administration (OSHA)** is responsible for enforcing the OSHA standards and has the authority to assess fines for noncompliance. In several instances employers were not only fined, but had criminal charges brought against them because they did not correct violations that caused employee injuries or death. When a particular standard cannot be applied, OSHA can invoke the "general duty clause." This clause states that "the employer shall furnish to each of his/her employees employment and a place of employment which are free from recognized hazards that are causing or are likely to cause death or serious physical harm to his/her employees."

In order of frequency of citation, the following standards are the most often cited OSHA violations in the health care industry:

1. Bloodborne Pathogens
2. Hazard Communication
3. Personal Protective Equipment
4. Lockout/Tagout
5. Formaldehyde Standard
6. Eye Wash Protection
7. Respirator Standard
8. Maintenance of the Log for Injuries and Illnesses
9. Electrical Systems—Wiring
10. Electrical Systems—General

These topics, among others, are discussed in the guide.

Employee complaints are the main reason health care facilities receive visits from OSHA compliance health and safety officers (CHSO). This type of inspection occurs more frequently than programmed inspections where the compliance health and safety officer arrives at the worksite unannounced.

Comments are frequently made indicating that the OSHA standards are quite formidable and difficult to understand and follow. Finding a particular requirement can be difficult for those not used to the format and content. Employers who diligently want to comply with the safety and health standards find it difficult to find the information that applies to their particular situation.

The guide is designed to assist the health care provider in understanding and complying with the OSHA standards and guidelines so that he/she will be able to maintain a safe and healthy workplace. It will also help the employer when counseling employees who are concerned with safety and health conditions at their worksite.

The guide is organized into four main sections. Each section contains those standards and guidelines pertaining to a general category. The standards and guidelines are broken down into main headings and subheadings. They are written in an easy to follow format, which should help to comply with OSHA requirements. The subjects covered are not only the OSHA standards the health care industry is most involved with but also other federal mandates. Some of the standards and guidelines may not apply directly to allied health but are areas the reviewers felt should be included in the text.

Providers will find that the medical examination requirements described under specific standards will be easy to follow. Employees exposed to lead, asbestos, formaldehyde, ethylene oxide, and the like, require periodic medical examinations. It is important that physicians understand their responsibilities concerning the examining of employees, what the examination is to consist of, and the essential information to obtain. They must also know what information the employee and employer must be told and what cannot be divulged.

The health care provider must be aware of the methods used to protect employees. This may consist of ways to reduce contaminant exposure, advising on frequency of examinations, explaining how chemicals harm certain parts of the body, proper protective equipment to wear, engineering controls used, and so on. When employees are instructed in safe methods, employee illnesses and injuries will decrease, which results in a safer workplace with less violations and a decrease in compensation costs. Also, the provider's knowledge of biology, anatomy, and physiology will be extremely helpful in understanding chronic exposure. Exposure to low concentrations (below OSHA limits) of toxic substances over long periods (chronic) can be just as harmful as high exposures over short periods (acute).

It is important that the terms and definitions used when dealing with safety and health issues are understood. A glossary of safety and health definitions used in the text, as well as some not in the text, is included.

The material safety data sheet (MSDS) is described in the appropriate chapter. This document, in conjunction with worker consultation, is important in the control of employee exposure. When reading the MSDS, there should be an understanding of the various sections listed on the document that identifies the hazards of a particular substance and how to control exposure. Certainly, the section concerning first aid procedures to be used before medical help arrives should be reviewed and checked for accuracy.

Health care providers must be aware of the requirements for employee exposure and medical records. They should know what constitutes an exposure and medical record and what information can be divulged to the employer and employee without violating the standard and employee confidentiality.

The guide should assist the provider in his/her understanding of the health and safety issues in the health care workplace. Besides remuneration, employees who realize that their employer is concerned with their well-being have proven to be more loyal and cooperative.

I appreciated the comments concerning the book. These comments made me realize that there were topics the health care industry was concerned with that did not directly relate to the medical environment. The suggestions helped to strengthen the guide, and I would appreciate future comments from health care providers in what, I believe, is a dynamic profession.

ACKNOWLEDGMENTS

The author expresses his appreciation to the following professionals who shared their knowledge and experience through reviews of the manuscript during development.

Kate McNally, RN, BS, MS
Des Moines Area Community College, Ankeny, IA

Vincent C. Madama, M. Ed., RRT
Rock Valley College, Rockford, IL

Phyllis J. Nichols, RN
Tucson College, Tucson, AZ

Rosa Quintones, MA, MT (ASCP)
TBT Health Academy, Tampa, FL

Ann E. Sims, RN
Albuquerque Technical Vocational Institute, Albuquerque, NM

Michael L. Snapp, MS, CSP
Mayo Clinic, Jacksonville, FL

Mary Therriault, RN
Our Lady of Mercy Life Center, Albany, NY

SECTION I

Facility Standards and Guidelines

CHAPTER 1

Health Care Facility Safety Program

After studying this chapter, you should be able to

➤ Identify the elements of an effective health care facility safety program.
➤ Describe an effective safety and health plan.
➤ Explain the representation of a health care facility safety committee.
➤ Identify what areas or departments of the health care facility should be addressed concerning safety and health issues.
➤ Explain the importance of maintaining good communication with the worker.

MANAGEMENT COMMITMENT

No safety and health program will succeed if it does not have the commitment from management. The CEO should issue a signed statement to all employees that the program is fully supported, both from an administrative and financial standpoint and that it is the goal of the facility to ensure the safety and health of everyone, including employees and visitors.

The CEO or president should, as his/her schedule permits, speak directly to employees to reinforce this commitment. He/she should also speak with members of the safety committee and safety staff to reinforce this commitment.

The safety staff and/or safety and health committee should invite the president and other members of management to attend training sessions so that they can get an appreciation of what is required under federal and state training mandates.

Any safety manuals generated by the safety and health staff should include a statement signed by the president supporting the safety program.

Management should also be aware that any fines assessed because of violations of safety and health standards will impact the operating budget. If an employee is injured or killed when no attempt has been made to correct serious citations, the president and other members of management may have criminal charges brought against them by OSHA.

WRITTEN SAFETY AND HEALTH PROGRAM

Every health care facility should have a written safety and health plan that should state the facility's goals and how they will be achieved as well as who will have overall responsibility. The plan should contain procedures and policies that are expected to be followed by all employees from administrators to rank and file.

The following elements should be included in the safety and health plan:

• Safety and Health Inspections
• Safety Analyses
• Exposure Monitoring
• Recordkeeping
• Physical Plant
• Emergency Plans
• Employee Training
• Safety and Health Program Review

Safety and Health Inspections

Facility inspections should be conducted on a scheduled basis and whenever new operations or procedures are introduced. Employees who are trained in safety and health must be designated to conduct inspections and report to a team supervisor. The supervisor must have an understanding of the many safety and health hazards that can occur in a health care facility and be able to maintain an effective inspection program.

Prior to inspecting for hazards, the inspection team or inspector should discuss the reason for the inspection with the area supervisor(s). The supervisor(s) or employees in the area should be given the opportunity to discuss any safety concerns. These discussions can reveal situations that are not readily apparent by inspection.

Inspection checklists can be prepared that contain information unique to that department. Situations encountered that are not on the checklist should be added and included in future inspections.

Many hazardous conditions can be corrected by management and employees when there is cooperation between them.

Safety Analyses

An analysis locates and focuses on the more dangerous activities with the purpose of establishing effective control measures. Each stage of the activity is evaluated, and recommendations are then made to reduce or eliminate the hazard. The activity should be evaluated based on the frequency and severity of injuries and illnesses it has caused. The potential for injury and illness should also be evaluated.

Analyses should be reviewed and updated at least annually and whenever new processes or operations are introduced into the workplace.

Exposure Monitoring

Whenever employees are exposed to chemical or biological agents, monitoring should be done, by using appropriate instruments, to establish exposure levels. Monitoring should be conducted to

- Determine airborne levels of a specific substance in the general work area.

- Determine levels in an employee's work area.
- Determine levels in the employee's breathing zone.
- Assess exposure to any biological agents.

Recordkeeping

OSHA requires that accurate accident and illness records be maintained on the OSHA 101 log (or workers' compensation form) and 200 logs.

Medical and exposure records for employees that comply with OSHA requirements must also be kept.

OSHA recommends that accident and illness data be used to analyze injury and illness trends so that appropriate action can be taken to prevent future occurrences.

Physical Plant

Any effective safety and health program must have a good relationship with the physical plant department. This is essential if equipment is to be maintained to prevent hazardous situations and costly breakdowns. It is important that a strong preventative maintenance program include all critical equipment and systems.

Emergency Plans

Emergency plans that meet OSHA requirements must be established. This includes fire, chemical spill, airborne release of hazardous substances, and natural disaster emergencies. Drills should be conducted at prescribed intervals so that employees become aware of their responsibilities if the plan is activated.

Employee Training

Training requirements must be established and employees must receive the appropriate training as required by OSHA. Materials must be presented so that employees can understand the subject matter. The person doing the training must be competent.

After initial training of employees, there must be periodic training as mandated by OSHA.

Management and supervisors should be included in all training programs to make them aware of requirements. This also includes input from the safety and health committee and/or safety department concerning the training program and ways to make it more effective, if necessary.

Safety and Health Program Review

The facility safety and health program should be reviewed and evaluated by the safety and health committee in conjunction with the safety department, if the facility has one, at least annually or whenever major changes are made to facility operations.

Effectiveness of the program can be determined by comparing injury and illness trends, speaking with employees to see if they understand safety and health program policies and procedures, and by conducting walk-through inspections to determine if policies and procedures are being followed.

EMPLOYEE AWARENESS

The safety staff and/or committee should keep employees continually aware of the safety and health program. The primary concern is for their safety. An effective program must include employee contact where they work. The safety staff and committee should be available to all employees. Safety staff should not become bogged down in paperwork.

Talking to workers and finding out what they do and asking for their input can be very helpful. Many times employees will give information concerning how they think their job can be done more safely. This not only helps to correct hazardous conditions but also makes the employees feel that they are contributing, which makes for a stronger program that employees are more apt to fully support.

DEPARTMENT SAFETY REPRESENTATIVES

Large departments should have at least one employee acting as a coordinator responsible for reporting unsafe conditions and acts to the safety department or committee. Employees in the department should be able to voice their concerns to this representative.

The safety staff or committee should make sure these representatives are trained in basic safety and health principles. The training need not be involved, but it should develop the expertise to enable the employee to recognize unsafe conditions and acts so that they may be reported and corrected.

SAFETY AND HEALTH COMMITTEES

The committee should consist of representatives from each major department. The size is dictated by the number of departments and size of the health care operation. Overly large committees may become inefficient and sometimes stray from discussion topics. Always have an agenda before meeting.

A member of the safety staff should be an ad hoc member to keep current on safety and health problems discussed and to offer assistance when needed. The committee chairperson and department representatives should be rotated at selected intervals to keep a "fresh approach" and allow more employees to become involved in the program. Chairpersons and representatives, if on the committee too long, can become "stale."

Meetings should be held at least once a month. If an important issue must be resolved, a special meeting should be held between monthly meetings.

The safety meeting lets the various health care areas know what the safety and health concerns are in their departments. Often, the concerns are common to more than one department. Solutions to problems can be shared from departmental experiences.

The CEO or president of the health care facility or a member of management should be invited to these meetings, for input and to get an idea of the problems being discussed. The presence of the CEO also reinforces support for the program.

AREAS OF CONCERN

The safety staff and/or committee should be responsible for, but not limited to, the following areas:

- Training (fire, electrical, infection control, bloodborne pathogens, hazard communica-

tion, personal protective equipment [PPE], and emergency procedures)
- Control and removal of hazardous and medical waste
- Emergency procedures
- Periodic inspection and monitoring of toxic and bio-aerosol materials
- Immunization of exposed workers (infectious diseases)
- Electrical equipment and systems
- Bio-safety cabinets
- Floors
- Pharmacy
- Operating room
- Laboratories
- Hazardous drugs
- Radioactive areas
- Lasers
- X-ray machines
- Ventilation
- Maintenance schedules
- Signage
- Safe work practices
- Personal protective equipment (gowns, eye protection, and the like)
- Respirators
- Engineering controls

- Work practices and administrative controls
- Hazardous materials (flammables and combustibles)
- OSHA industrial standards requirements (where applicable)
- Ergonomics

The safety staff and/or committee should be involved in any plan reviews that affect facility operations. This includes making sure that any renovations or additions meet applicable safety and health laws. The staff or committee should make sure that any machinery purchased has proper guards, ventilation hoods are properly installed, ergonomic equipment is used where needed, and other safe practices are followed.

CONCLUSION

There is no such thing as "a perfect program." Once a program is supported and ongoing, the safety staff/safety committee must keep abreast of changes in the safety and health laws by attending seminars and dialoguing with peers. It is not enough to rest on laurels when everything seems to be going well. Keeping a strong program requires constant attention.

CHAPTER REVIEW

Multiple Choice
Select the best answer from the choices provided.

1. To succeed, a safety and health program must have a commitment from
   a. the safety committee
   b. the safety director
   c. management
   d. a, b, and c

2. A signed statement supporting the safety and health program should be made by the
   a. safety director
   b. safety inspector
   c. charge nurse
   d. president of the facility

3. Persons doing training must
   a. be strict
   b. be competent
   c. keep attendance records
   d. hand out course materials

4. Safety meetings should be held
   a. once a month
   b. once every two months
   c. once every three months
   d. once every six months

5. It is important that the safety staff/committee
    a. keep safety posters current
    b. keep updated on changes in safety and health laws
    c. conduct an effective prize incentive program
    d. project themselves as "nice guys or gals"

True/False

Indicate whether the statement is true or false by circling T or F.

6. T   F   A safety and health plan should contain procedures and policies to be followed by all employees.

7. T   F   Recordkeeping is not too important.

8. T   F   Employees should be given the option to attend or not attend training sessions.

9. T   F   The safety meeting is a good opportunity to discuss safety and health concerns.

10. T   F   Once a good safety and health program is in force, everyone can sit back and relax.

CHAPTER 2

Indoor Air Quality

OBJECTIVES

After studying this chapter, you should be able to

➤ Identify the types of indoor air quality (IAQ) problems a facility can experience.
➤ Discuss what OSHA intends to include in the proposed IAQ standard.
➤ Identify an IAQ compliance program.
➤ Identify facility IAQ problems.
➤ Explain the importance of addressing employee complaints.

INDOOR AIR QUALITY

Indoor air quality (IAQ) refers to the quality of indoor air as it relates to pollutants that may be airborne in the building. The pollutants may be brought into the building from outside or come from the building itself.

At the present time, OSHA does not have a standard that covers indoor air quality. This chapter discusses the proposed standard and what it will include for enforcement purposes. Presently, OSHA may invoke the **general duty clause** in certain cases where violations exist concerning employee health and indoor air. The general duty clause allows OSHA to give citations when a specific standard cannot be cited.

Indoor air quality can be a very complicated and vexing problem for those attempting to remedy various situations. It is usually not one factor causing poor indoor air quality, but several working in conjunction.

Safety and health professionals know what the various pollutants are in the indoor air, but sometimes identifying the specific contaminant(s) or problem(s) can challenge their expertise.

Often, in the past, when building occupants complained of distress, such as sore throats, tearing eyes, nasal irritation, headaches, and the like, they were looked on as "chronic complainers." It was particularly difficult for the lone employee who complained when no one else was suffering. It is only recently that sufficient studies have been done to address the problem, and scientists and engineers are paying more attention, particularly when designing new buildings.

TYPICAL BUILDING POLLUTANTS

Building pollutants may include any of the following (this is by no means a complete list):

• Pollen.
• **Dust**.
• Fungal spores.
• Vehicle or building exhaust getting into the building by **reentrainment**. Reentrainment occurs when exhausted materials get back into the building through air intakes or other openings.
• **Soil gas**. Gas found in the soil as a result of decaying matter, leakage, or spills.
• **Radon**. A colorless and odorless gas that is created when radium in soil and rock breaks down into smaller particles.
• Leakage from underground storage tanks.
• Landfill gas (if the building was built on or near an old landfill).
• Sewer gases.
• Standing water on roofs and in ducts that encourages microbial and fungal growth.

- Ozone from copy machines.
- **Volatile organic compounds (VOC)** from various toners, cements, markers, and glues. VOCs are organic liquids that have the ability to vaporize very rapidly. Examples are gasoline and alcohol.
- Tobacco smoke.
- Cooking.
- Cooling tower water that encourages microbial growth.
- Building vermin.
- Wet and damp areas, particularly in ductwork where ideal conditions cause pathogens to grow.
- Off-gassing of various building materials, such as the gases from chemicals found in carpets, paneling, and insulation (chief culprit is **formaldehyde**).

PROPOSED INDOOR AIR QUALITY STANDARD

The OSHA proposed standard will cover those employees in a nonindustrial work environment. This refers to employees working in offices, educational facilities, commercial establishments, health care facilities, cafeterias, and break rooms located in manufacturing or production facilities. Nonindustrial operations do not include manufacturing and production facilities, residences, vehicles, and agricultural activities. These operations are covered in other OSHA standards.

Designated Person

The employer must designate a responsible person to oversee the implementation of the IAQ compliance program.

Written Compliance Program

The **written compliance program** indicates the methods and procedures used to comply with certain OSHA standards. The proposed OSHA IAQ standard will require that the following be included:

1. A written narrative description of the facility building systems. This will include the **heating, ventilating, and air-conditioning (HVAC) system**. The HVAC system maintains building air quality and comfort.

2. A single line schematic or as-built construction document that locates major building system equipment and the areas they serve. If these documents are not on file in the building, they may be obtained from either the building architect or contractor.

3. Information for the daily operation and management of the building systems. This includes a description of normal operating procedures; special procedures (seasonal start-ups and shutdowns); and a list of operating criteria, such as minimum **outside air (OA)**, which is the air brought in from outside to mix with the recirculating air, ventilation rates, potable hot water storage and delivery temperatures, range of relative humidities, and any spaces that must be pressurized.

4. A general description of the building and its function, which includes work activity, number of employees and visitors, hours building is operated, weekend use, tenant requirements, and known air contaminants released into spaces.

5. A written maintenance program for the maintenance of building systems. This should be preventative in scope and reflect the manufacturer's recommendations and good practices as determined by the building systems maintenance industry. It should, as a minimum, describe the equipment to be maintained, establish procedures, and indicate the frequency of these procedures. Equipment maintenance manuals should be used that were issued upon building completion. Employers in buildings that are naturally ventilated should ensure that windows, doors, vents, stacks, and other openings designed for natural ventilation are in working order.

6. A checklist for visual inspection of building systems.

Additional Information

The following additional information, if available, must be retained by the employer to assist in IAQ evaluations:

- **As-built construction drawings**. These are the construction drawings revised and prepared that reflect all the changes made to the building and its systems.
- HVAC commissioning reports.
- HVAC system testing, adjusting, and balancing reports.
- Operations and maintenance manuals.
- Water treatment logs.
- Operator training materials.

EMPLOYEE COMPLAINTS

The employer must establish a written record of employee complaints of signs or symptoms that may be caused by building contaminants. The records must contain the nature of the illness reported, number of employees affected, date of complaint, and any remedial action taken to correct the problem.

COMPLIANCE PROGRAM IMPLEMENTATION

Employers must take at least the following actions when implementing the compliance program:

- Ensure that the HVAC system operates according to original design specifications and provides at least the minimum outside air (OA) ventilation rate, based on occupancy. This rate must conform to the requirements of the building code, mechanical code, or ventilation code applicable at the time the building was constructed, renovated, or remodeled, whichever is most recent.
- Conduct building systems inspections and maintenance in accordance with the written compliance program.
- Assure that the HVAC system is operating during all shifts, except during repairs and scheduled maintenance.

- Use **general** or **local exhaust ventilation** where housekeeping and maintenance activities involve operations that could release chemicals or **particulates** into other areas of the building. General ventilation or exhaust is an exhaust system that removes room air completely over a period of time by bringing in outside air to reduce contaminant levels. Local exhaust captures contaminant levels at their source and exhausts them outside through a hood, duct, fan, and air cleaner system.
- Maintain relative humidity below 60% in buildings with mechanical cooling systems. Minimum humidity levels would depend upon the air temperature and the type of activities in the building.
- Monitor carbon dioxide levels when routine maintenance of the HVAC system is done. When the carbon dioxide level reaches 800 ppm, the employer must check to make sure the HVAC system is operating properly. If it is not, the employer must take the necessary steps to correct any deficiencies.
- Assure that buildings with mechanical ventilation are maintained so that windows, doors, vents, stacks, and other openings designed or used for natural ventilation are operable.
- Assure that mechanical equipment rooms and any non-ducted air plenums or chases that carry air are kept in a clean condition. Make sure that hazardous substances are properly stored to prevent release, and that **asbestos**, if friable, is encapsulated or removed so that it does not enter the air distribution system.
- Assure that inspections and maintenance of building systems are done under the supervision of the designated responsible person.
- Establish a written record of building system inspections and maintenance.
- Assure that employees performing work on building systems are provided with appropriate **personal protective equipment** as required by OSHA. This is in compliance with 29 CFR 1926 subpart E, Personal Protective and Life Saving Equipment; 29 CFR 1926.52, Occupational Noise Exposure; 29 CFR 1910, subpart I, Personal

Protective Equipment; and 29 CFR 1910.95, Occupational Noise Exposure.

- Evaluate the need to make alterations to building systems when employees complain of building caused illnesses and take the necessary remedial action.

SPECIFIC CONTAMINANT SOURCE CONTROLS

Contaminants could be as varied as tobacco smoke, airborne microbes, chemicals, pesticides, and airborne contamination as a result of renovation and remodeling.

Tobacco Smoke

When the workplace allows smoking, the employer must set aside designated smoking areas and permit smoking only in those spaces. These areas must be enclosed and exhausted directly to the outside and maintained under negative pressure in relation to surrounding areas. The negative pressure must be sufficient to keep the tobacco smoke in the designated smoking area.

When cleaning and maintenance work are done in smoking areas, there must be no smoking during this operation. Employees cannot be required to enter smoking areas in the normal course of their duties.

Signs must be posted that clearly indicate to anyone entering the workplace that smoking is restricted to designated areas.

Smoking must be prohibited during times when the exhaust ventilation system serving that area is not operating properly.

Other Indoor Air Contaminants

If outdoor air contaminants can enter the building, the employer must determine where these areas are located and take measures to prevent re-entrainment. This may require relocating air intakes, keeping windows closed, adjusting roof intakes, or some similar repair. For instance, air intakes located in or near garages can cause problems.

If general ventilation is not sufficient to remove contaminants generated by point sources in spaces, local exhaust ventilation or substitution of a nontoxic material, if feasible, must be implemented.

Microbial Contamination

Microbial contamination must be controlled by routinely inspecting for water leaks that can encourage growth of pathogens. Leaks found must be promptly repaired, and wet or damp materials must be promptly dried, replaced, removed, or cleaned.

Any visible microbial contamination found in ductwork, humidifiers, other HVAC and building system components, or on building surfaces when found during regular or emergency maintenance activities, must be promptly removed.

Use of Hazardous Chemicals and Pesticides

The employer must ensure that these chemicals are applied according to manufacturer's recommendations. Employees working in areas to be treated must be informed, at least within twenty-four hours prior to application, of the type of chemicals to be applied. Distributing copies of the **material safety data sheets (MSDS)** for the chemicals to be applied is recommended. The MSDS is written or printed material concerning a hazardous chemical that presents information required by OSHA's hazard communication standard.

Air Quality During Renovation and Remodeling

During renovation or remodeling, the employer must make sure that proper measures are taken to avoid degradation of the air quality for employees doing the renovation or remodeling and for employees in other areas of the building. Duct returns may have to be sealed temporarily to avoid transportation of contaminants to other parts of the building, or temporary ventilation may have to be implemented to exhaust contaminants to the exterior or other safe area.

Developing a Work Plan. Before any renovation or remodeling is done, the employer must meet with the contractor or individual(s) doing the work to develop a work plan designed to control entry of air contaminants to other areas of the building. The work plan must consider the following, where appropriate:

- The maintaining of OSHA IAQ standard requirements
- The assurance that the HVAC systems continue to function properly
- The isolation or containment of work areas and negative pressure containment
- The use of air contaminant suppression controls or auxiliary air filtration and cleaning
- The prevention of contaminant entry into the HVAC system

Prior Notification of Employees Who Work in the Building

Employees must be notified at least twenty-four hours in advance, or promptly in emergency situations, of any work to be done that may introduce air contaminants into their areas.

The notification must include the expected adverse effects on air quality or workplace conditions.

INFORMATION AND TRAINING

Training must be provided for those employees who are involved in building system operation and maintenance. The training must include at least the following:

1. Use of personal protective equipment needed in operating and maintaining building systems
2. How to maintain adequate ventilation of air contaminants generated during building cleaning and maintenance
3. Training of maintenance personnel on how to minimize effects on indoor air quality when they use and dispose of chemicals and other harmful agents

Information Given to All Employees

All employees must be informed of the proposed OSHA IAQ standard and its appendices. They must also be informed of the signs and symptoms associated with building related illnesses and the requirement that the employer evaluate the system and take remedial action concerning the HVAC system when employees complain of building related illnesses.

Training Materials Availability

The employer must make IAQ training materials available, including the IAQ standard and its appendices, for inspection and copying. This material must be made available to employees, designated employee representatives, and OSHA.

RECORDKEEPING

Accurate inspection and maintenance records are essential if heating, ventilating, and air-conditioning (HVAC) systems are to be kept operating properly.

Maintenance Records

The employer must maintain inspection and maintenance records required by the proposed IAQ standard. It must include the specific remedial or maintenance actions taken, the name and affiliation of the person(s) doing the work, and the date of the inspection or maintenance.

Written IAQ Compliance Program

The written IAQ compliance program required under the standard must be maintained by the employer.

Employee Complaints

The employer has to keep records of employee complaints of signs or symptoms that may be caused by building related illness. These complaints must be relayed to the designated person for resolution.

Records Retention

Records must be retained for at least the previous three years, except for maintenance records and the written IAQ compliance program. They do not have to be retained for three years if they are replaced by more-recent records or become obsolete due to replacement or redesign of the HVAC system.

Records Availability

Records described under the IAQ standard must be available to employees, their designated representatives, and to OSHA.

Records Transfer

Whenever the employer ceases to do business, records required to be maintained under the standard must be given to and retained by the successor employer.

CHAPTER REVIEW

Multiple Choice

Select the best answer from the choices provided.

1. A written maintenance program should
   a. be preventative
   b. describe equipment to be maintained
   c. establish procedures
   d. a, b, and c

2. With mechanical cooling systems, relative humidity should be below
   a. 40%   c. 70%
   b. 60%   d. 75%

3. The employer should check the HVAC system when carbon dioxide levels reach
   a. 100 ppm   c. 800 ppm
   b. 300 ppm   d. 900 ppm

4. To develop a written compliance program is the responsibility of the
   a. maintenance supervisor
   b. employer
   c. line foreman
   d. complaining employee

5. Workers must be notified in advance of any work that could affect building air quality by at least
   a. seventy-two hours
   b. twenty-four hours
   c. thirty-six hours
   d. twelve hours

True/False

Indicate whether the statement is true or false by circling T or F.

6. T F Because there is no IAQ standard, OSHA cannot do anything concerning violations.

7. T F The proposed IAQ standard will cover employees in the industrial setting.

8. T F Gasoline and alcohol are examples of volatile organic compounds (VOCs).

9. T F The higher the carbon dioxide levels in the indoor air, the safer the air.

10. T F Smoking areas must be kept under positive pressure.

Short Answer

Briefly but thoroughly answer each statement.

11. Explain reentrainment and why it is important to prevent it.

12. Describe what is included in a written compliance program.

13. Discuss the causes of microbial contamination and how it can be prevented.

14. Discuss some ways toxic materials can be controlled.

15. Identify what must be included in the training of employees who operate HVAC systems.

CHAPTER 3

Recording and Reporting Occupational Injuries and Illnesses

After studying this chapter, you should be able to

> ➤ List the OSHA requirements for reporting injuries and illnesses (OSHA 29 CFR 1904).
> ➤ Explain how the required OSHA forms are to be completed.
> ➤ Identify what injuries and illnesses are recordable.

OSHA 29 CFR 1904 RECORDING AND REPORTING OCCUPATIONAL INJURIES AND ILLNESSES

The requirement for reporting injuries and illnesses is found in OSHA 29 CFR 1904. OSHA states that injury and illness reporting by the employer is necessary for enforcement of OSHA standards and for developing information regarding the causes and prevention of occupational accidents and illnesses. Reporting also helps maintain a program of collection, compilation, and analysis of occupational safety and health statistics.

OSHA requires that worker injuries and illnesses be reported so that the employer can see where the "problem" areas may exist and if the employer has an effective safety program. This information is also used by OSHA for evaluation purposes. Often, the first thing an OSHA inspector will want to see is the employer's **log of injury and illnesses.**

Log and Summary of Occupational Injuries and Illnesses

Each employer of eleven or more employees must maintain a log and summary of all recordable occupational injuries and illnesses. Each recordable injury and illness must be reported on the log and summary no later than six working days after receiving information that the injury or illness has occurred. The OSHA 200 Log "Summary of Occupational Injuries and Illnesses" or equivalent must be used for summary recording of injuries and illnesses. The OSHA 101 Log "Supplementary Record of Occupational Injuries and Illnesses" or equivalent must be used to record injuries and illnesses of each employee. The 101 log gives more specific information concerning the injury or illness than does the OSHA 200 log.

If the employer has multi-establishments, he/she may maintain the log through a data processing system or at another establishment or both, providing that

- There is sufficient information available at the establishment to complete the log within six working days after receiving the information that a recordable case has occurred.

- At each establishment there is a copy of the log that reflects the injury and illness records at that location and they are complete and current to a date within forty-five calendar days.

The OSHA 200 log indicates

- Whether the injury or illness was fatal
- The date of occurrence
- The employee involved
- Job title
- Department where regularly employed
- Whether it is an injury or illness
- The time lost as a result of the injury or illness

The OSHA 101 log gives more specific information about the injury or illness. It indicates the cause of the accident; the material/equipment or hazardous substances involved; the type of injury or illness; and what parts of the body were involved.

OSHA usually permits the Workers' Compensation form and other insurance forms to be used in place of the OSHA 101 log, providing these forms give the same information or more than the OSHA log.

OSHA Logs 200 and 101 Recordable Periods

The recordable injuries and illness are listed for the calendar year (January 1 to December 31).

Annual Summary

The **annual summary**, which is the calendar year's totals from the OSHA 200 log, must be posted by February 1 of the following year. The summary has to remain posted until at least March 1. The total of recordable cases is to be indicated at the bottom of the form on the totals line. The calendar year covered, establishment name, establishment address, signature of person certifying the data, person's title, and date have to be put on the form. The form requires posting even if there were no **recordable injuries or illnesses**. Zero would be indicated for the totals. A recordable injury or illness is one that must be reported on the OSHA 200 Log because it meets the reportable criteria.

Employees who do not report to or work at a single establishment or who do not report to any fixed establishment on a regular basis must be sent a copy of the summary during the month of February following the calendar year the cases were recorded.

Records Retention

Records must be maintained at the establishment for five years following the end of the year to which they relate. If the establishment comes under new ownership, the new owners must retain the records for the remainder of the five years. The new owners do not have to update any records that were established by the previous employer, but they are responsible for maintaining records during that part of the year they held ownership.

Recordable Cases

Recordable injuries and illnesses are as follows:

- Fatalities, regardless of the time between the injury and death or the length of the illness.
- Any case, other than a fatality, that resulted in lost workdays.
- Cases that did not have lost workdays but where the employee was transferred to another job or was terminated.
- Cases that required medical treatment other than first aid.
- Cases that involve loss of consciousness or restriction of work or motion (this includes any diagnosed occupational illnesses that are reported but not classified as fatalities or lost workdays).

Lost workdays are the number of days (excluding the day of the injury or illness) the employee would have worked but could not. This includes not being able to perform all or part of his/her normal assignment during all or any part of the workday or shift. Days the employee would normally be off are not counted as lost workdays.

Medical treatment includes treatment by a physician or by a registered professional under the standing orders of a physician. It does not include first aid treatment even if given by a physician or registered professional.

First aid treatment is not recordable. It is any one-time treatment and any follow-up visit for the purposes of observation of minor scratches, cuts, burns, splinters, and the like, which do not ordinarily require medical care. Such a follow-up visit for the purposes of observation is considered first aid even if it is performed by a physician or registered professional.

Availability of Records

The OSHA 200 log must be made available, upon request, to any employee, former employee, and to their representatives for examination and copying in a reasonable manner and time. These persons can have access to the log for any establishment in which the employee has been employed.

Employees and their representatives can also collective bargain to obtain access to information relating to occupational injuries and illnesses.

Reporting Fatalities or Multiple Hospitalization Cases

When there is a fatality to one or more employees or an accident or illness that results in the hospitalization of three or more employees as the result of a work-related accident, the employer must report the incident within eight hours. The report must be made in person to the OSHA regional office nearest the accident site or by calling the OSHA toll-free central telephone number at 1-800-321-6742. The report must establish name, location of incident, time of incident, number of fatalities or hospitalized employees, contact person, phone number, and a brief description of the incident.

APPENDIX

This appendix describes injuries and illnesses that are reportable and those that are not.

Injuries that must be reported include any work-related injury or illness that occurs on the employer's worksite or other employer locations where the employee is doing work for the employer (this includes areas where work is not normally done such as lunchrooms, rest rooms, and so forth); injuries that occur in the employer's parking lot if the employee was there because his/her duties required it; and injuries occurring while traveling for the employer (but not on personal business).

Injuries and illnesses that are not reportable include injuries occurring to the employee while visiting the employer's worksite (not working at the time); injuries occurring while the employee is traveling to and from work, including getting out of the car in the parking lot and walking into the building; and injuries occurring while the employee was doing personal business during a trip required by the employer. This includes injuries occurring while the employee was doing routine or normal activities while traveling for the employer.

Note: If you are not sure whether an illness or injury is reportable, contact the OSHA *consultation* office in your state.

CHAPTER REVIEW

Multiple Choice

Select the best answer from the choices provided.

1. The OSHA 101 Log records

   a. the illnesses and injuries of each employee
   b. a summary recording of employee illnesses and injuries
   c. only illnesses
   d. only injuries

2. An accident or illness must be reported to OSHA when it causes the hospitalization of the following minimum number of employees:

   a. three
   b. four
   c. five
   d. six

3. Medical treatment includes treatment by or under supervision of a

   a. nurse
   b. health technician
   c. physician
   d. licensed practical nurse

4. After the end of the year to which they relate, illness and injury records have to be retained for

    a. five years
    c. fifteen years
    b. ten years
    d. thirty years

True/False

Indicate whether the statement is true or false by circling T or F.

5. T F Workers' Compensation and insurance forms can be used in place of the OSHA 101 Log.

6. T F The OSHA 200 Log gives specific information about each accident or illness.

7. T F Even if an employee is injured on the premises as a visitor, it is reportable.

8. T F It is not reportable if the employee is injured while traveling for the employer.

9. T F One-time treatment for first aid is not recordable.

CHAPTER 4

Lifting and Ergonomic Guidelines

OBJECTIVES

After studying this chapter, you should be able to

➤ Identify OSHA's stand on ergonomics.
➤ Discuss the application of ergonomics in the workplace.
➤ Explain how OSHA cites for ergonomic injuries.
➤ State the OSHA proposed ergonomic standard.

WHAT IS ERGONOMICS?

Ergonomics is the process of dealing with the disciplines that involve the interaction between the worker and the total working environment. Its goal is to have the work environment adapt to the worker rather than the worker to the environment.

OSHA's Stand on Ergonomics

Presently, OSHA does not have a standard that covers ergonomics. The proposed standard is described in this chapter. Employers, in place of a standard, can be cited under the general duty clause. This clause states that "each employer must furnish to each of his/her employees employment, and a place of employment, which is free from recognized hazards that are causing, or are likely to cause, death, or serious physical harm to his/her employees."

The OSHA Compliance Health and Safety Officer (CHSO) will look at the employer's "OSHA 200 Log of Occupational Injuries and Illnesses." This is the log that must be maintained by the employer that lists all the recordable injuries and illnesses for the calendar year. If there is an above normal incidence of **musculoskeletal** injuries (this refers to injury to the muscle/skeletal system due to trauma), the CHSO will speak to employees concerning what the employer is doing or has done to reduce the incidence of these injuries. If it is determined that the employer is not training employees in proper lifting techniques, or using **work practices** (supervisory or administrative controls used to control or eliminate hazards), or using **engineering controls** (methods used to eliminate hazards by modifying the source of the hazard), the employer will be cited under the general duty clause.

Lifting Formula

The **National Institute for Occupational Safety and Health (NIOSH)**, the federal agency responsible for conducting research and making recommendations for the prevention of work-related injuries and illnesses, has a lifting formula that can be used to determine the safe two-hand lifting weight by one person. It calculates the **recommended weight limit (RWL)** and is defined as the weight of the load that nearly all healthy workers could lift over a substantial period of time without an increased risk of developing lifting-related low back pain. The equation is as follows:

$$RWL = LC \times HM \times VM \times DM \times AM \times FM \times CM$$

To obtain the RWL for a lifting task, the six task variable coefficients are multiplied. The variables are expressed as reduction coefficients obtained from tables in the "Revised NIOSH Lifting Equation" book.

LC is a load constant, which is the weight of the load.

HM is the horizontal multiplier obtained from Table 1. The multiplier is determined by the distance from the midpoint of the line joining the inner ankle bones to a point projected on the floor directly below the midpoint of the hand grasps.

VM is the vertical multiplier obtained from Table 2. The multiplier is determined by the vertical height of the hands above the floor.

DM is the distance multiplier obtained from Table 3. The multiplier is determined by the vertical travel distance of the hands between the origin and destination of the load.

AM is the asymmetric multiplier obtained from Table 4. The multiplier is determined when a lift begins or ends outside the mid-sagittal plane. The sagittal plane is the plane that goes through the midpoint of the body.

FM is the frequency multiplier obtained from Table 5. The multiplier is determined by the number of lifts per minute, the duration of the lifting activity, and the vertical height of the lift from the floor.

CM is the coupling multiplier obtained from Tables 6 and 7. The multiplier is determined by whether the coupling or grasping of the load is good, fair, or poor.

To obtain more details concerning the NIOSH revised lifting formula, the book can be purchased from:

U.S. Department of Commerce,
Technology Administration
National Technical Information Service (NTIS)
5285 Port Royal Road
Springfield, VA 22161

It is NTIS publication PB94-176930 and NIOSH publication 94-110.

Lifting Guidelines

The spine has twenty-six vertebrae. The vertebrae encase the spinal cord. Disks separate the vertebrae and protect the spine from stresses placed on it. Lower back pain is one of the most common back injuries suffered by employees. This is an injury to the lower spinal column or to the tendons or muscles.

Proper lifting procedures should be used when lifting loads. The same holds true when stretching to place a load and when lifting from awkward positions. Instead of stretching, employees should stand on a ladder or step stool. Bulky loads may require someone to help with the carry.

When carrying loads, vision should never be obstructed. When bringing down loads from shelves, test the load first by "jogging it" to make sure it's not too heavy. If it can be brought down by one person, slide it along the shelf before carrying it.

These types of lifting should be avoided whenever possible. If these lifts cannot be avoided, the employer must train employees in safe lifting procedures. Training is required regardless of the type of lifting that has to be done. Some loads may require assistance to help carry them or the use of materials-handling equipment or the use of lift-assisting devices in health care facilities. With proper training, lift-assisting devices such as mechanical hoists and other devices can be used effectively.

The standard lift procedure is as follows:

- Squat using the knees (don't bend over arching the back) and keep the back straight and head up.
- Don't keep the feet exactly opposite one another. One foot should be just in front of the other.
- Keep the load to be lifted close to the body.
- Get a secure hold on the load and keeping the back straight and head up, get up from the squat position with the load. Use the legs when straightening up. Don't bend over.
- Before traveling with the load, make sure that your path of travel is free of obstacles.
- When changing direction, move your whole body by pointing your feet in the direction you want to travel. Don't twist your body to change direction.

When putting the load down, reverse the procedure. Don't bend over. Place the load on the floor by squatting. Keep the load close to the body and the back straight. Try to place the load on a raised surface such as a table if it is going to be carried again.

This will eliminate the need to pick it up from the floor. Parts of the body can suffer **repetitive strain injuries (RSIs)**, which are injuries to the musculoskeletal system due to repeated trauma, **cumulative trauma disorders (CTDs)**, which are injuries to the musculoskeletal system due to repeated aggravation, and **carpal tunnel syndrome (CTS)**, which is an inflammation of the tendons in the carpal wrist tunnel.

People working in health care facilities, maintenance, offices, and other departments can suffer these injuries. Systems and procedures are available to reduce the incidence of this trauma. These include training, exercise, the proper use of ergonomically designed tools, worksite analysis, use of materials-handling equipment, lift-assisting devices, and properly designed workstations.

Using Back Belts

It has not been determined conclusively that back belts reduce back injuries. The back belt industry claims that studies show they reduce the chance of back injury, but a NIOSH study claims they do not.

If back belts are used, they should be used in coordination with an effective employer training program that involves proper lifting procedures.

PROPOSED OSHA ERGONOMICS STANDARD SUBPART U-ERGONOMICS 29 CFR 1910.500 TO 512

OSHA is proposing an ergonomics standard that would apply to the workplace. Presently, there is no ergonomics standard, but as mentioned before, OSHA can invoke the general duty clause and cite the employer for violations concerning employee injuries.

Standard Coverage

The standard is limited to workplaces in general industry. In these workplaces, the standard covers the employer if he/she has manufacturing operations or manual handling operations.

Purpose of the Standard

The purpose of the standard is to reduce the large number and severity of work-related musculoskeletal disorders employees have been experiencing. To accomplish this, employers will have to set up ergonomics programs in the workplace that identify and control hazards that are likely to cause musculoskeletal injuries.

Obligations of the Employer. The employer must set up an ergonomics program to control work-related musculoskeletal injuries.

The basic elements of the program are these:

- Management leadership and employee participation
- Hazard identification and information
- Job hazard analysis and control
- Training
- Medical management
- Program evaluation

If an ergonomics program already exists in the workplace, it may continue provided the employer can show the following:

- The existing program satisfies the obligation of the six basic elements just described.
- Any part of the program that differs from any of the rest of the requirements fulfills the intended purpose of each requirement.
- The employer has implemented and evaluated the program before the standard went into effect.
- The program is eliminating or controlling musculoskeletal injuries.

Management Leadership and Employee Participation. The employer must demonstrate management leadership of the program. Employees and their representatives must have ways to report problems, get responses, and be involved. The employer cannot have practices or policies that discourage employees from participating or making recommendations and reports in the program.

The employer must assign responsibilities for setting up and managing the program; provide those persons with authority, resources, training, and information; examine existing policies and practices; identify at least one person to receive and respond to reports of injuries and take action, when required to correct problems; and communicate regularly with employees about the program.

Employees and their representatives must have ways to report symptoms of injuries and hazards and to make recommendations for control, and they must get prompt responses to their reports and recommendations.

Ways for employees to become involved in developing, implementing, and evaluating the program include job analysis and control, training, and judging the effectiveness of the program and control measures.

Hazard Identification and Information. Musculoskeletal disorders and hazards must be identified to employees who are exposed to these injuries in manufacturing and manual handling operation jobs.

Employees must have a means to report signs, symptoms, and hazards and to make recommendations to control them. The report must be checked out to determine if medical management is necessary, and safety and health records must be reviewed to look for musculoskeletal injuries and hazards.

Employees must be provided with information on how to recognize signs and symptoms of musculoskeletal injuries; hazards that are likely to cause injuries; and how to report signs and symptoms, and make recommendations.

Job Hazard Analysis and Control. The employer must analyze problem jobs. If there are hazards, he/she must implement measures to eliminate or control them.

The analysis includes a representative sample of employees in the problem job and employees who perform the same physical work activities but in another job (similar job).

Employees must be asked whether they are experiencing signs or symptoms of injuries; whether they are having difficulty performing their work; and which physical work activities associate with the problem.

The employer must observe employees performing the job in order to identify job factors that need to be evaluated and evaluate those job factors to determine which are likely to cause or contribute to the problem.

When the problem is identified, the employer must identify, evaluate, and implement feasible control measures; track the progress in controlling injuries; communicate the results of the job hazard analysis to other areas in the workplace; and identify hazards when there is a change in design or purchased equipment, processes, and facilities.

Engineering and work practice controls and/or the use of personal protective equipment (PPE) can be used to control hazards.

If problems persist in spite of implementing controls, the employer must promptly check out employee reports of signs and symptoms of injury to determine if medical management must be provided; promptly identify and analyze musculoskeletal hazards and develop a control plan; track progress in implementing the plan; and continue to look for solutions for the problem job and implement feasible ones as soon as possible.

Training. Training must be provided to at least all employees in problem jobs and all employees in similar jobs that have been identified as problem jobs; their supervisors; and all persons involved in setting up and managing the ergonomics program.

Training for employees in problem jobs must include how to recognize musculoskeletal signs and symptoms and the importance of early reporting; how to report signs and symptoms and hazards and make recommendations; musculoskeletal hazards in their jobs and the measures they must follow for control; job-specific controls and practices that have been implemented in their jobs; the ergonomics program and their role in it; and the requirements of this standard.

Training for employees involved in setting up and managing the ergonomics program includes the ergonomics program and their role in it; how to identify and analyze work-related musculoskeletal hazards; how to identify, evaluate, and implement measures to control hazards; and how to evaluate the effectiveness of the ergonomics program.

Training must be provided for employees in problem jobs when the program is first set up in their jobs; when they are initially assigned to problem jobs; after control measures are implemented in their jobs; and periodically as needed and at least every three years.

Training must be provided for persons involved in setting up and managing the ergonomics program when they are initially assigned to setting up and managing the ergonomics program; and periodically as needed and at least every three years.

Medical Management. The employer must make medical management available whenever an employee has a musculoskeletal injury. He/she must provide medical management, including recommended work restrictions, at no cost to the employee.

The employee must be provided prompt access to health care professionals for effective evaluation, treatment, and follow-up; information must be provided to the health care professional by the employer to ensure effective medical management; and a written opinion must be obtained from the health care professional, which must also be given to the employee.

The employer must give the health care professional a description of the employee's job and hazards identified in the hazard analysis; descriptions of available changes to jobs or temporary alternative duty to fit the employee's capabilities during the recovery period; a copy of this standard; and opportunities to conduct workplace walk-throughs.

The health care professional's opinion must contain the work-related medical conditions related to the musculoskeletal disorder reported; recommended work restrictions, where necessary, and follow-up for the employee during the recovery period; a statement that the health care professional has informed the employee about results of the evaluation and any medical conditions resulting from exposure to musculoskeletal disorder hazards that require further evaluation or treatment; and a statement that the health care professional has informed the employee about other physical activities that could aggravate the musculoskeletal disorder during the recovery period.

If the health care professional recommends work restrictions, the employer must ensure that the work restrictions recommended for the employee are provided during the recovery period; maintain the employee's total normal earnings, seniority rights, and benefits when work restrictions are recommended by the health care professional or voluntarily provided by the employer. This must be continued until the first of these occurs:

- The employee is recovered and able to return to the job, or
- Effective measures are implemented that control the musculoskeletal disorder hazard to the extent the job does not pose a risk of harm to the employee even during the recovery period, or
- There is a final medical determination that the employee is permanently unable to return to the job, or
- Six months have passed.

The employer may reduce his/her obligation to maintain the employee's normal earnings, seniority, rights, and benefits by the amount the employee receives during the work restriction period from any of the following: worker's compensation payments for lost earnings; payments for lost earnings from a compensation or insurance program that is publicly funded or funded by the employer; and income from employment with another employer made possible by virtue of the work restrictions.

Program Evaluation. The employer must evaluate the ergonomics program and controls periodically, and at least every three years, to ensure that it is in compliance with the standard.

The employer must set up the following procedure to evaluate the effectiveness of the ergonomics program and control measures: the employer must monitor program activities to ensure that all the elements of the ergonomics program are functioning; effective measures must be selected for both activity and outcome measures, and they must be used to evaluate the program and its controls to ensure they are in compliance with the standard; and baseline measurements must be established so that there is a starting point for measuring the effectiveness of the program and controls.

If the evaluation indicates that the program is not controlling musculoskeletal disorder hazards in problem jobs, the deficiencies must be corrected promptly.

Recordkeeping. Written records of the program must be kept if the employer has more than one worksite or establishment in which this job is performed by employees; or the job involves more than one level of supervision; or the job involves shift work.

If the employer does not have ten or more full-time employees (including contingent and temporary employees) at any time during the preceding year, he/she is not required to keep written records of the ergonomics program.

Records must be retained as follows:

- Employee reports and responses are to be kept at least three years.
- Results of job hazard analysis plans for controlling musculoskeletal disorder hazards, and medical management records are to be kept at least three years or until replaced by an updated record.
- Medical management records must be kept for the duration of the injured employee's employment plus three years.

Key Terms Used in the Standard. The following are key definitions used in the standard.

Administrative controls are procedures and methods typically instituted by the employer that significantly reduce daily exposure to musculoskeletal disorder hazards by altering the way in which work is performed. Examples are employee rotation, job task enlargement, adjustment of work pace, redesign of work methods, alternative tasks, and rest breaks.

Engineering controls are physical changes to jobs that control exposure to muculoskeletal disorder hazards. Engineering controls act at the source of the hazard and control employee exposure to the hazard without relying on the employee to take self-protective action or intervention. Examples are changing, modifying, or redesigning workstations, tools, facilities, equipment, materials, and processes.

Ergonomics is the science of fitting jobs to people. Ergonomics encompasses the body of knowledge about physical abilities and limitations as well as other human characteristics that are relevant to job design.

Ergonomics program is a systematic process for anticipating, identifying, and controlling musculoskeletal disorder hazards.

Health care professionals are persons educated and trained in the delivery of health care services who are operating within the scope of their license, registration, certification, or legally authorized practice when they are performing the medical management requirements of this standard.

Job factors are workplace conditions and physical work activities that must be considered when conducting a job hazard analysis. These factors for physical demands are force, repetition, work postures, duration, and local contact stress. Factors for workstation layout and space are work reaches, work heights, seating, floor surfaces, and contact stress. Factors for equipment used and objects handled are size and shape, weight and weight distribution, handles and grasp surfaces, and vibration. Factors for environmental conditions are cold and heat, and glare. Factors for work organization are work-recovery cycles, work rate, and task variability.

Manual handling operations are physical work activities that involve lifting/lowering, pushing/pulling, or carrying; involve exertion of considerable force because the load is heavy; and when the work is a significant part of the employee's regular job duties.

Medical management is the employer's process for assuring that employees with musculoskeletal disorders are provided at no cost with the following: a means for early reporting of musculoskeletal disorders; early assessment of reports; access to prompt evaluation, treatment, and follow-up by health care professionals; and work restrictions recommended by health care professionals.

Musculoskeletal disorders (MSD) are injuries and disorders of the muscles, nerves, tendons, ligaments, joints, cartilage, and spinal disks. Examples are carpal tunnel syndrome, epicondylitis (pain in the elbow joint), synovitis (joint pain), muscle strains, Raynaud's syndrome (spasms of the blood vessels in the extremities), sciatica, tendinitis, rotator cuff tendinitis, De Quervain's disease, carpet layers knee, trigger finger, and low back pain.

Personal protective equipment (PPE) are interim control devices worn or used while working to protect employees from exposure to musculoskeletal disorder hazards. It includes gloves, knee pads, and so forth.

Safety and health records are information generated at or for the workplace. Records include OSHA 200 logs, worker's compensation claims, musculoskeletal related medical reports and infirmary logs, employee reports of musculoskeletal disorder hazards, and insurance or consultant reports prepared for the workplace,

Symptoms of musculoskeletal disorders are physical indications that the employee may be developing a musculoskeletal disorder. Examples are numbness, burning, pain, tinging, aching, and stiffness.

Work practice controls are controls that reduce the likelihood of exposure to musculoskeletal disorder hazards through alteration of the manner in which a job or physical work activities are performed. Examples are safe and proper work techniques and procedures that are understood and followed by managers, supervisors, and employees; conditioning period for new or reassigned employees; or training in the recognition of musculoskeletal disorder hazards and work techniques that can reduce exposure or ease task demands and burdens.

CHAPTER REVIEW

True/False

Indicate whether the statement is true or false by circling T or F.

1. T F Exercise is important in keeping a strong back.

2. T F Loads should be lifted by bending at the waist.

3. T F There are thirty-five vertebrae in the spine.

4. T F Ergonomics is fitting the job to the worker.

5. T F OSHA can cite for ergonomic violations under the general duty clause.

Matching

Match the terms in column 1 with the definitions in column 2.

Column 1
6. Musculoskeletal injury
7. Lifting formula
8. Cumulative trauma disorder
9. Carpal tunnel syndrome
10. Assisting device

Column 2
a. Added effect of repeated aggravation
b. Mechanical hoist
c. Tendon inflammation injury
d. Low back pain
e. Determines safe lifting weight

Short Answer

Briefly but thoroughly answer each statement.

11. Name some of the factors that might make a worker susceptible to back injury.

12. List the procedures for correct lifting.

13. Discuss the back belt controversy.

14. Discuss devices that assist in lifting.

15. Explain some of the objectives of the proposed OSHA ergonomics standard.

CHAPTER 5

Access to Employee Exposure and Medical Records

After studying this chapter, you should be able to

➤ Explain the OSHA requirements for employee access to exposure and medical records.
➤ Differentiate between exposure and medical records.
➤ State the retention periods for these records.
➤ Define authorized representative access.
➤ Explain the physician's requirements in the standard.

OSHA 29 CFR 1910.1020 ACCESS TO EMPLOYEE EXPOSURE AND MEDICAL RECORDS

This standard covers the requirements that allow employees and their designated representatives access to exposure and medical records. It also describes employer responsibilities.

Definitions

Exposure record is a record containing the following:

- Environmental (workplace) monitoring or measuring of a toxic substance or harmful physical agent, including personal area, area, grab, wipe, or other form of sampling, as well as related collection and analytical methodologies; and calculations and other background data relevant to interpretation of the results obtained

- Biological monitoring results that directly assess the absorption of a toxic substance or harmful physical agent by body systems (e.g., the level of a chemical in the blood, urine, breath, hair, fingernails, and so forth), but not including results that assess the biological effect of a substance or agent or that assess an employee's use of alcohol or drugs
- Material safety data sheets indicating that the material may pose a hazard to human health
- In the absence of the above, a chemical inventory or any other record that reveals where and when used and the identity (e.g., chemical, common, or trade name) of a substance or harmful physical agent

Medical record is a record containing the following:

- The health status of an employee, which is made or maintained by a physician, nurse, or other health care personnel, or technician, including medical and employment questionnaires or histories (including job description and occupational exposures)
- Results of medical examinations (pre-employment, pre-assignment, periodic, or episodic) and laboratory tests (including chest and other X-ray examinations taken for the purpose of establishing a baseline or detecting occupational illness, and all biological monitoring not defined as an "employee exposure record")
- Medical opinions, diagnoses, progress notes, and recommendations

- First aid records
- Descriptions of treatments and prescriptions
- Employee medical complaints

Employee medical records do not include medical information in the form of:

- Physical specimens (e.g., blood or urine samples), which are routinely discarded as a part of normal medical practice.
- Records concerning health insurance claims if maintained separately from the employer's medical program and its records, and is not accessible to the employer by employee name or other direct personal identifier (e.g., social security number, payroll number, and so forth).
- Records created solely in preparation for litigation, which are privileged from discovery under applicable rules of procedure or evidence.
- Records concerning voluntary employee assistance programs (alcohol, drug abuse, or personal counseling programs) if maintained separately from the employer's medical program and its records.

Specific written consent is a written authorization containing the following:

- The name and signature of the employee authorizing the release of medical information
- The date of the written authorization
- The name of the individual or organization that is authorized to release the medical information
- The name of the designated representative (individual or organization) that is authorized to receive the released information
- A general description of the medical information that is authorized to be released
- A general description of the purpose for the release of the medical information
- A date or condition upon which the written authorization will expire (if less than one year)

A written authorization does not operate to authorize the release of information not in existence on the date of the written authorization, unless the release of future information is expressly authorized, and does not operate for more than one year

from the date of the written authorization. A written authorization may be revoked prospectively at any time.

Toxic or harmful physical agent is any chemical substance, biological agent (bacteria, virus, fungus, and the like), or physical stress (noise, heat, cold, vibration, repetitive motion, ionizing and non-ionizing radiation, hypo- or hyperbaric pressure, and so forth) that

- Is listed in the latest edition of the National Institute for Occupational Safety and Health (NIOSH) Registry of Toxic Effects of Chemical Substances RTECS).
- Has yielded positive evidence of an acute or chronic health hazard in testing conducted by, or known to the employer.
- Is the subject of a material safety data sheet kept or known to the employer indicating that the material may pose a hazard to human health.

Designated representative is any individual or organization to whom the employee gives written authorization to exercise the right to access records.

Preservation of Records

Records preservation is required under the standard.

Medical Records. The medical record of each employee must be preserved and maintained for at least the duration of employment plus thirty years except that the following types of records need not be retained for any specific period:

- Health insurance records maintained separately from the employer's medical program and its records.
- First aid records (not including medical histories of one-time treatment and subsequent observation of minor scratches, cuts, burns, splinters, and the like that do not involve medical treatment, loss of consciousness, restriction of work, or motion, or transfer to another job, if made on site by a non-physician and if maintained separately from the employer's medical program and its record).

- The medical records of employees who have worked for less than one year for the employer need not be retained beyond the term of employment if they are provided to the employee upon termination of employment.

The exposure records of employees must be preserved and maintained for at least thirty years except that

- Background data to environmental (workplace) monitoring or measuring, such as laboratory reports and worksheets, need only be retained for one year so long as sampling results, the sampling plan, a description of the analytical and mathematical methods used, and a summary of other background data relevant to interpretation of results obtained, are retained for at least thirty years.
- Material safety data sheets and chemical inventories concerning identity of a substance or agent need not be retained for any specified period as long as some record of the identity of the substance or agent, where it was used, and when it was used is retained for at least thirty years.
- Biological monitoring results designated as exposure records by specific occupational safety and health standards shall be preserved and maintained as required by the specific standard.

Each analysis using exposure or medical records shall be preserved and maintained for at least thirty years.

X-ray films must be preserved in their original state.

Access to Records

Records access must be maintained.

General. Whenever an employee or designated representative requests access to a record, the employer shall assure that access is provided in a reasonable time, place, and manner. If the employer cannot reasonably provide access within fifteen working days, the employer shall apprise the employee or designated representative the reason for the delay

and the earliest date when the record can be made available.

The employer may require of the requester only such information as should be readily known to the requester and that will help locate or identify the records.

A copy of the record shall be provided at no cost to the employee or representative.

Copy facilities shall be made available to the requester.

In the case of an original X ray, the employer may restrict access to on-site examination or make suitable arrangements for the temporary loan of the X ray.

Whenever a record has been previously provided without cost to the employee or representative, the employer may charge reasonable, nondiscriminatory administrative costs for a request for additional copies.

An employer shall not charge for an initial request for a copy of new information that has been added to a record that was previously provided.

Employee and Designated Representative Access

Employees and their designated representatives must have access to records.

Employee Exposure Records. Each employer, except as noted in the standard, shall, upon request assure the access to each employee and designated representative to employee exposure records. This record consists of a record that measures or monitors the amount of a toxic substance or harmful physical agent to which the employee is or has been exposed.

In the absence of such a record, such records of other employees with past or present duties or working conditions related to or similar to those of the employee to the extent necessary to reasonably indicate the amount and nature of the toxic substance or harmful physical agents to which the employee is or has been subjected, shall be submitted.

Also, in the absence of the above record, exposure records to the extent necessary to reasonably indicate the amount and nature of the toxic substances or harmful physical agents at workplaces or under working conditions to which the employee is being assigned or transferred, shall be submitted.

Requests by designated representatives for unconsented access to employee exposure records shall be in writing and shall specify the following:

- The records requested to be disclosed
- The occupational health need for gaining access to the records

Employee Medical Records. Each employer shall, upon request, assure the access of each employee to employee medical records, except as provided in the standard.

Each employer shall, upon request, assure the access of each designated representative to the employee medical records of any employee who has given the designated representative specific written consent.

Whenever access to employee medical records is requested, a physician representing the employer may recommend that the employee or designated representative

- Consult with the physician for the purposes of reviewing and discussing the records requested.
- Accept a summary of material facts and opinions in lieu of the records requested.
- Accept release of the requested records only to a physician or other designated representative.

Whenever an employee requests access to his or her employee medical records and a physician representing the employer believes that direct access to the information obtained in the records regarding a specific diagnosis of a terminal illness or a psychiatric condition could be detrimental to the employee's health, the employer may inform the employee that access will only be provided to a designated representative having written consent, and deny the employee's request for access to this information only. This shall be done, even if it is known that the designated representative will give the information to the employee.

A physician, nurse, or other health care professional maintaining medical records may delete from requested medical records the identity of a family member, personal friend, or fellow employee who has provided confidential information concerning the employee's health status.

Each employer shall, upon request, assure the access of each employee and designated representative to each analysis using exposure or medical records concerning the employee's working conditions or workplace.

Trade Secrets

Except as provided, the employer may delete from records requested by a health professional, employee, or designated representative any trade secret data that discloses manufacturing processes, or discloses the percentage of a chemical substance in a mixture, as long as the health professional, employee, or designated representative is notified that the information has been deleted. Whenever deletion of the trade secret information substantially impairs evaluation of the place where or the time when exposure to a toxic substance or harmful physical agent has occurred, the employer shall provide alternative information that is sufficient to identify where and when exposure occurred.

The employer may withhold specific chemical identity, including the chemical name and other specific identification from a disclosable record, provided that

- The claim that the information withheld is a trade secret can be supported.
- All other available information on the properties and effects of the toxic substance is disclosed.
- The employer informs the requesting party that the specific chemical identity is being withheld as a trade secret.
- The specific chemical identity is made available to health professionals, employees, and designated representatives in accordance with provisions of the standard.

When a treating physician or nurse determines that a medical emergency exists and the specific identity of a toxic substance is necessary for emergency or first aid treatment, the employer shall immediately disclose the specific chemical identity of a trade secret chemical to the treating physician or nurse regardless of the existence of a written statement of need or a confidentiality agreement. The employer may require a written statement of need for confidentiality agreement as soon as circumstances permit.

In nonemergency situations, an employer shall, upon request, disclose a specific chemical identity if

- The request is in writing.
- The request describes in detail one or more of the following: assessment of hazards, assessment of the workplace atmosphere, conducting of pre-assignment or periodical medical surveillance, provision of medical treatment to exposed employees, selection and assessment of personal protective equipment, the design or assessment of engineering controls, and conducting of studies to determine health effects of exposure.

The request must contain in detail why disclosure of the specific chemical is essential and that no other information is available for the health professional, employee, or designated representative. The request must state the properties and effects of the chemical; measures for controlling worker's exposure to the chemical; methods of monitoring and analyzing worker exposure to the chemical; methods of diagnosing and treating harmful exposures to the chemical; a description of the procedures to be used to maintain the confidentiality of the disclosed information; and that the health professional, employee, or designated representative and the employer or contactor of the services of the health professional or designated representative agree in a written statement that they will not use the trade secret information for any reason other than for health needs.

If the employer denies a written request for disclosure of a specific chemical identity, the denial must be provided to the health professional, employee, or designated representative within thirty days of the request; be in writing; include evidence to support the claim that the specific chemical identity is a trade secret; state the specific reasons why the request is being denied; and explain in detail how alternative information may satisfy the specific need.

The health professional, employee, or designated representative may then refer the request and the written denial to OSHA. OSHA will then make a determination if the trade secret information must be disclosed.

Employee Information. Upon an employee's first entering into employment, and at least annually thereafter, each employer shall inform current employees of the following: the existence, location, and availability of any records; the person responsible for maintaining and providing access to records; and each employee's rights of access to these records.

Transfer of Records. Whenever an employer ceases to do business, the employer shall transfer all records to the successor employer. The successor employer shall receive and maintain these records.

Whenever an employer ceases to do business and there is no successor employer to receive and maintain the records, the employer shall notify employees of their right to access the records at least three months prior to cessation of the employer's business.

Whenever an employer either is ceasing to do business and there is no successor employer to receive and maintain the records, or intends to dispose of any records required to be preserved for at least thirty years, the employer shall transfer records to the director of the National Institute for Occupational Safety and Health (NIOSH) if so required by a particular standard or notify the Director of NIOSH in writing of the impending disposal of the records at least three months prior to disposal of the records.

Where an employer regularly disposes of records required to be preserved at least thirty years, the employer may, with at least three months' notice, notify the director of NIOSH on an annual basis of the records intended to be disposed of in the coming year.

CHAPTER REVIEW

Multiple Choice

Select the best answer from the choices provided.

1. A medical record does *not* include

    a. medical and employment questionnaires
    b. treatment and prescriptions
    c. privileged records used for litigation
    d. recommendations and diagnoses

2. An exposure record does *not* include

    a. first aid records
    b. a list of MSDSs
    c. chemical inventory
    d. noise and radiation level data

3. For OSHA to obtain exposure or medical records, they must

    a. ask for them
    b. just take them
    c. ask NIOSH to get them
    d. none of the above

True/False

Indicate whether the statement is true or false by circling T or F.

4. T F An employee need only ask the employer to see his/her exposure or medical records.

5. T F Material Safety Data Sheets can be used as exposure records.

6. T F Exposure monitoring is a medical record.

7. T F A physician may withhold medical information from an employee if the physician thinks that it could do harm.

8. T F Records deemed for disposal must first be sent to OSHA.

Matching

Match the terms in column 1 with the definitions in column 2.

Column 1	Column 2
9. Medical record	a. Fifteen days
10. Exposure record	b. Has right to access records
11. Access interval for records	c. Thirty years
12. Records retention	d. Methods and calculations to determine exposure
13. Designated representative	e. Biological monitoring results

CHAPTER 6

Employee Emergency and Fire Evacuation Plans

After studying this chapter, you should be able to

➤ Explain the requirements of the OSHA standard for employee emergency and fire evacuation plans (OSHA 29 CFR 1910.38).

➤ Identify the elements for both plans.

OSHA 29 CFR 1910.38 EMPLOYEE EMERGENCY PLAN

Employee emergency and fire evacuation plans are covered in OSHA 29 CFR 1910.38. These plans also apply to emergency and fire evacuation procedures to be followed when required by a particular OSHA standard.

The action plans must be in writing, unless otherwise indicated, and must cover designated actions employers and employees must take to ensure employee safety from fire and other emergencies. The plan must be kept at the worksite and made available for review by employees.

The evacuation plan must make provision for fire and other emergencies. The employer can design these plans to the particular operation at the facility.

Emergency Action Plan Information

The plan must include the following:

1. Emergency escape procedures and escape route assignments.
2. Procedures to be followed by employees who must remain to operate critical equipment before they evacuate.
3. Procedures that account for all employees after the evacuation.
4. Rescue and medical duties for those employees who will perform these duties.
5. The means of reporting fires and other emergencies.
6. Names or regular job titles of persons or departments to contact for further information or explanation of duties under the plan.

The employer must establish in the plan the types of evacuation to be used in emergency situations.

Alarm System

The employer must have an alarm system that provides warning when emergency action is indicated as described in the emergency action plan. The alarm must allow enough reaction time for safe escape of employees from the workplace or the immediate work area.

The alarm must be able to be heard and/or seen above ambient noise or light levels by all employees.

The alarm must be distinctive and recognizable as the means for reporting emergencies.

The employer must explain to each employee the selected means for reporting emergencies (e.g., manual pull boxes, public address systems, or radio or telephone). The emergency telephone number must be posted near telephones or on employee notice boards.

Installation and Restoration. The employer must make sure all alarm systems are operable. After testing, the employer must ensure that all alarm systems are put back on line. Parts must be available in sufficient quantities so that the system can be repaired as soon as possible when replacement is necessary.

Maintenance and Testing. A different alarm activating device (fire alarm station or detector) must be activated during each test. Backup means must be provided when the system is out of service.

Only trained persons can maintain and test alarm systems.

Training

The employer must designate and train a sufficient number of persons to assist in the safe and orderly emergency evacuation of employees.

The plan must be reviewed with each employee covered under the procedures when

- The plan is initially developed.
- Employee's responsibilities or actions change under the plan.
- The plan is changed.

OSHA 29 CFR 1910.38 EMPLOYEE FIRE EVACUATION PLAN

This plan must be designed to deal with fire emergencies. Employers must make sure that employees know how to protect themselves during this type of emergency.

Fire Prevention Plan Information

The plan must include the following:

1. A list of important workplace fire hazards.
2. Safe procedures for handling and storage.
3. Control measures for defined ignition sources.
4. Fire protection equipment and systems available to control ignition sources.
5. Names or regular job titles of personnel responsible for maintenance of equipment and systems installed to control fires.
6. Procedures and schedules for equipment maintenance.
7. Names or regular job titles of those personnel responsible for control of fuel hazard sources.

The plan must be written and kept at the workplace and be accessible to all employees.

Housekeeping

Employers must control accumulations of flammable and combustible waste materials and residues so that they don't fuel fires. Housekeeping procedures must be included in the written fire prevention plan.

Training

The employer must inform employees of the fire hazards of the materials and processes to which they are exposed.

The employer must also review with each employee upon initial assignment those parts of the fire prevention plan that the employee must know to protect himself/herself in the event of an emergency.

If there are ten or less employees, the plan can be communicated to the employees orally and need not be written.

Maintenance

The employer must, on a regular basis, maintain equipment and systems installed on heat-producing equipment so that accidental ignition of combustible materials is prevented. Maintenance of these systems must be in accordance with established procedures and the procedures incorporated in the fire prevention plan.

CHAPTER REVIEW

True/False

Indicate whether the statement is true or false by circling T or F.

1. T F Emergency plans do not have to be in writing.
2. T F Any alarm system will suffice for alerting employees in emergencies.
3. T F The same alarm activating device can be used each time the alarm is tested.
4. T F A fire evacuation plan can deal with other emergencies besides fire.
5. T F The testing and maintenance of alarm systems can be done by any designated employee.

CHAPTER 7

Means of Egress and Fire Protection

After studying this chapter, you should be able to

➤ Identify the OSHA basic requirements for fire prevention.
➤ Explain specific requirements as they relate to fire protection.
➤ Define worker training requirements and content of training.
➤ Identify the various devices used to protect against fires.
➤ List the various types of fires.

FIRE SAFETY

Fire safety is a very important part of any safety program. In most instances, safety professionals find that they devote more time to fire prevention and control than other aspects of health and safety. Also, the requirements for exiting a building safely are intertwined with the requirements for fire protection.

The regulations that cover fire safety and safe egress include OSHA 1910 Subpart E, Means of Egress and Subpart L, Fire Protection. Much of the OSHA fire regulations were adopted from the National Fire Protection Association (NFPA) consensus standards, particularly NFPA's **Life Safety Code (LSC) 101**. The LSC is a national consensus code of the NFPA that describes safety requirements in public buildings. The NFPA publishes over 250 standards that deal with all aspects of fire prevention and control.

This chapter describes the important OSHA regulations and NFPA recommendations as well as accepted safe practices.

OSHA SUBPART E MEANS OF EGRESS AND SUBPART L FIRE PROTECTION

OSHA has adopted the NFPA Life Safety Code (LSC) 101 for egress requirements and other NFPA codes that describe NFPA consensus standards for fire protection.

Means of Egress Requirements

Every building or structure, new or old and designed for human occupancy, must have sufficient exits to permit the prompt escape of occupants in case of fire or other emergency.

Buildings and structures must be constructed, arranged and equipped, and maintained, and operated to avoid danger to the lives and safety of the occupants from fire, fumes, smoke, or panic.

Exits must be provided in buildings and structures taking into consideration the type of occupancy, number of exposed persons, available fire protection, and the height and type of construction of the building.

Exits have to be arranged and maintained to provide free and unobstructed egress from all parts of the building. No lock or fastening device to prevent free escape can be installed except in penal or corrective institutions where supervisory personnel are continually on duty.

Exits and routes to exits must be clearly marked and visible so that occupants know where they are.

Buildings equipped with artificial illumination must have reliable illumination provided for all exits.

Exits cannot be blocked and there must be at least two exits from each floor.

Exits must be kept free of any obstructions and continuously maintained free of obstructions.

Fire detection and sprinkler equipment, fire doors, alarm systems, and exit lighting where provided must be kept in continuously operating condition.

Means of Egress, General

The exit must be protected and separated from other parts of the building by at least a one-hour **fire resistive rating** when the exit connects three stories or less. A fire resistive rating is the number of hours a building assembly can withstand a fire.

The exit must be protected and separated from other parts of the building with at least a two-hour fire resistive rating when the exit connects four or more stories.

Openings in exits must be protected by an approved self-closing fire door.

When more than one exit is required from a story, at least two exits must be provided that are as remote as possible from one another.

Doors from rooms to exits must be side-hinged, swinging type. When a room is occupied by more than fifty persons or is a high-hazard occupancy, the door must swing in the direction of exit travel. This is required so that the door opens easily when people egress the room.

Exits cannot go through rooms that lock.

Ways of exit must be recognizable. Hangings of draperies or other obstructions cannot be placed over exit doors or located so that the exit is obscured.

Minimum width of exits is 28 inches.

Exterior ways of exit access must have smooth solid floors.

Snow and ice must be cleared from exits or exits must be protected by roof covers.

Paths of exits must be as straight as possible.

Exterior exit ways of exit access cannot be so arranged that there are dead ends in excess of 20 feet.

All exits must discharge directly to the street, yard, court, or other open space that gives safe access to a public way. Streets, yards, courts, and so forth must be wide enough to accommodate all persons leaving the building.

Stairs that go beyond the floor of exit discharge must be separated at the floor of discharge by partitions, doors, or other effective means.

Furnishings and decorations cannot obstruct exits.

Automatic sprinkler systems must be continuously maintained.

Fire alarm systems must be maintained and tested.

Exits must be marked by visible signs and in all cases where the exit way is not readily visible.

Doors, passages, or stairways that are not exits or exit accesses must be identified by signs reading **"Not An Exit," "To Basement," "Storeroom," "Linen Closet"** or the like.

Exit signs must be distinctive in color.

When the direction of exit travel is not readily discernible, a sign reading **"Exit"** with directional arrow must be placed in the location where the direction to the nearest exit is not immediately apparent.

Exit signs must be illuminated by not less than 5 footcandles of light. The sign can be lighted externally or internally.

Exit signs shall have the word **"Exit"** in plainly legible letters not less than 6 inches high and not less than $3/4$ inch wide.

Fire Protection

Fire Brigades. Fire brigades are organized groups of employees who are knowledgeable, trained, and skilled in at least basic fire-fighting operations. If the employer establishes a fire brigade, he/she must have a written statement or written policy that establishes the existence of the brigade; the basic organizational structure; the type and amount of training; and what functions the brigade will perform in the workplace.

The employer must make sure that members of the brigade can perform their duties. An employee with a health condition such as heart disease, emphysema, or the like must have a physician's certificate if they are to be members.

Members of the brigade must be trained in their duties. Training must be done before they perform their duties. Training must be conducted at least annually.

The employer has to inform brigade members of any special hazards such as storage and use of flammable liquids, gases, toxic chemicals, radioactive sources, and the like. Procedures must be developed that describe actions to be taken in situations involving these special hazards.

Equipment must be maintained and inspected at least annually.

The employer must provide brigade members with protective clothing at no cost to the employees.

Respirators must be provided at no cost to employee members and the requirements of 29 CFR 1910.134 must be meet.

Portable Fire Extinguishers. Fire extinguishers are portable fire-fighting devices that are designed to put out small or incipient fires before the become major conflagrations.

Extinguishers must be mounted and located so that they are readily accessible.

They must be fully charged and operational at all times.

Extinguishers for Class A fires (fires that involve combustible materials such as rags, wood, cloth, and the like) have to be placed so that travel distance does not exceed 75 feet.

Extinguishers for Class B fires (fires that involve flammable materials such as flammable liquids and the like) have to be placed so that travel distance does not exceed 50 feet.

Extinguishers for Class C fires (fires that involve energized electrical equipment) must be placed based on the appropriate pattern for existing Class A and B hazards.

Extinguishers for Class D fires (fires that involve flammable metals such as sodium, potassium, and the like) have to be placed so that travel distance does not exceed 75 feet.

Portable fire extinguishers have to have an annual maintenance check. The maintenance date must be recorded.

Extinguishers must be hydrostatically tested (this is a test that determines if the extinguisher shell can still withstand internal pressure) at intervals established in accordance with Table 1 of 29 CFR 1910.157.

Employees must be trained in the use of extinguishers unless the employer determines that no employee is to use one, but instead evacuate the building.

Standpipe Hose Systems. Standpipe hose systems are systems installed in buildings to fight fires by either trained building personnel or by fire fighters.

The three classes of hose systems are class I for $2\frac{1}{2}$-inch hose, class II for $1\frac{1}{2}$-inch hose, and class III for $2\frac{1}{2}$- and $1\frac{1}{2}$-inch hose. These requirements apply to Class II and III systems.

Hoses must be used for only fire equipment.

Hoses must be rubber lined so that if there is leakage, the hose will not deteriorate.

Water supply must be sufficient to supply 100 gallons per minute.

Hoses must be hydrostatically tested to ensure that they will not burst under pressure.

Valves to hoses must be fully opened at all times.

Hose systems must be inspected at least annually. If a hose is found deficient, it must be replaced.

Trained persons must conduct inspections.

Automatic Sprinkler Systems. Automatic sprinkler systems are systems that activate sprinkler heads when the head is set off by the heat of the fire and water is sprayed to extinguish the flames.

Sprinkler systems must meet National Fire Protection Standards.

Sprinkler flow pipes must be prevented from freezing.

Sprinkler systems with more than twenty sprinklers must have a waterflow alarm that is audible throughout the premises.

Systems must be inspected and maintained to insure they are fully operational.

Fixed Extinguishing Systems. These are systems consisting of fixed pipes and compressed extinguishing tanks that flood the area with an extinguishing agent to put out fires.

They must be designed and approved for the specific fire they must extinguish.

If the system is inoperable, employees must be informed so that precautions can be taken.

They must have alarm systems that are distinctive and can be heard over ambient noise.

When discharge could affect employee health, effective safeguards must be installed.

Hazard warning signs must be posted if the extinguishing agent can affect employee health.

Systems must be inspected annually by persons knowledgeable in these systems. Weight and pressure of refillable containers must be checked annually. Nonrefillable containers must be checked semiannually. Inspection and maintenance dates must be recorded on a tag on the container.

The employer must train employees to inspect and maintain the systems.

At least one manual station must be provided for discharge.

Fixed Extinguishing Dry Chemical, Gaseous, and Water and Foam Systems. Dry chemical systems cannot be mixed with other systems.

Employees cannot be exposed to above-toxic levels in gaseous systems.

If a gaseous system can discharge gas above safe levels, it must have a pre-signal that alerts employees it is about to go off.

Water and foam systems must be sufficient to control the fire in the protected area or on the protected equipment.

Fire Detection Systems. After the system is tested, it must be restored to fully operational condition.

Systems must be maintained and tested as often as necessary to keep them in repair. Persons doing the repair must be knowledgeable.

Fire detectors must be kept free of corrosion and kept clean.

Fire detection equipment must be installed to provide a warning or emergency action so that employees can escape safely. No alarm detection can be longer than thirty minutes.

Employee Alarm Systems. All alarms must be capable of being heard above ambient noise levels.

The alarm must be distinctive from other alarms.

Employees must be told about the preferred method of reporting emergencies. Emergency numbers must be posted near telephones or on bulletin boards.

An alarm system with emergency back up must be installed in workplaces having more than ten employees.

After testing alarm systems, they must be put back in fully operational condition.

All alarm systems must be maintained in operating condition unless they are being repaired.

Alarm systems must be tested every two months using a different device each time.

Power supplies must be replaced as often as necessary to ensure that back up systems are operational.

Alarm systems installed after January 1, 1981, must be supervised so that if a trouble appears in the system, it will alert that fact. Supervisory systems must be tested at least annually.

Servicing and maintenance of alarm systems must be done by trained people.

APPENDIX

This appendix describes types of fire alarm systems, detection devices, fire extinguishers, and requirements for emergency lighting.

Local fire alarms sound only in the building. They do not report to an on- or off-the-premises receiving station. Proprietary alarms sound in the building and report to a supervised receiving station on the premises. Auxiliary alarms sound in the building and report to a fire alarm station or to a contracted agency that monitors alarms.

Depending upon their rating, fire detectors activate at fixed temperatures of 135°, 160°, 190°, or 212°F. Combination fixed temperature and rate of rise fire detectors activate at the fixed temperature or when the rise in temperature is more than 10°F in one minute.

Smoke detectors activate in the presence of smoke, infrared detectors to visible flame, and ionization detectors to products of combustion.

Pressurized water extinguishers are rated for class A fires (ordinary combustibles such as paper, cloth, rags, and the like). Carbon dioxide extinguishers are rated for BC fires (flammable liquids and energized electrical equipment fires). BC dry powder extinguishers are rated for flammable liquids and energized electrical equipment fires. ABC dry powder extinguishers are rated for ordinary combustibles, flammable liquids, and energized electrical equipment fires. Extinguishers that contain special extinguishing agents are rated for class D metals fires. Metals fires are fires involved with sodium, potassium, magnesium, and the like. Extinguishers are required to note on the shell the types of fires for which they are rated.

Emergency lighting should last for at least $1\frac{1}{2}$ hours. Battery systems should be maintained and inspected to make sure that after each outage they will still provide the $1\frac{1}{2}$ hours of essential lighting.

CHAPTER REVIEW

Multiple Choice

Select the best answer from the choices provided.

1. Employees must be trained to
    a. turn in an alarm
    b. store hazardous material safely
    c. safely evacuate a building
    d. a, b, and c

2. Stair fire doors can be left open providing they
    a. have latches and knobs
    b. are fire rated
    c. have magnetic holders tied into the fire alarm
    d. have sight glass

3. Standpipe hose must now be
    a. unlined linen
    b. installed in stairwells
    c. rubber lined
    d. installed in assembly occupancies

4. Alarm systems
    a. must be distinctive from other alarms
    b. can be the same as other alarms
    c. are not necessary
    d. should be ignored

5. Class A extinguishers must be placed so that travel distance does not exceed
    a. 50 feet
    c. 70 feet
    b. 60 feet
    d. 75 feet

True/False

Indicate whether the statement is true or false by circling T or F.

6. T F Each floor of a building must have at least three exits.

7. T F Alarm systems must be tested yearly.

8. T F Fire brigades are not required at worksites.

9. T F Class A fires are flammable liquid fires.

10. T F Stair doors must be fire rated.

11. T F Exits may go through rooms that lock.

12. T F The minimum width of doors is twenty-four inches.

13. T F Exit signs are not required when the door to exit is clearly visible.

14. T F Ionization smoke detectors respond to products of combustion.

15. T F Sprinkler systems should be flow tested at least annually.

Matching

Match the terms in column 1 with the definitions in column 2.

Column 1

16. Life Safety Code
17. Trained person
18. Fixed extinguishing system
19. Hydrostatic testing
20. A class of fire

Column 2

a. Pipes connected to extinguishing tanks
b. Energized electrical equipment
c. Test to make sure extinguisher is safe to use
d. Person allowed to maintain fire systems
e. National consensus standard

Short Answer

Briefly but thoroughly answer each statement.

21. Describe some of the requirements for fire alarm systems.

22. Explain how you would make provision for getting disabled persons out during a fire.

23. Identify some of the requirements to keep laboratories safe from fire.

24. List some of the recommendations needed to have a good housekeeping program.

25. Explain the emergency system used in your building.

CHAPTER 8

Electrical

After studying this chapter, you should be able to

➤ Identify the most frequently violated OSHA electrical standards.
➤ Identify the basic content of the electrical standard.
➤ List and identify electrical terms.
➤ Identify safe distances around electrical equipment.
➤ List grounding requirements.

OSHA 29 CFR SUBPART S ELECTRICAL

This subpart is extremely extensive, and some of it requires a technical understanding of electrical power. Described here are those requirements that the allied health professional can easily follow to ensure compliance.

Common Electrical Situations Cited by OSHA

These violations are most often cited by an OSHA inspector. They can be identified by the nontechnical person and, in most instances, are easily corrected.

Enclosing Electrical Installations. Electrical installations in a vault, room, closet, or in an area surrounded by a wall, screen, or fence, access to which is controlled by a lock and key or other approved means, are considered to be accessible to qualified persons only. The entrances to all buildings, rooms, or enclosures containing exposed live parts or exposed conductors operating at over 600 volts, shall be kept locked or shall be under the observation of qualified persons at all times. A sign must be posted that says **"Warning—High Voltage—Keep Out."**

Electrical installations having exposed live parts shall be accessible to qualified persons only.

Electrical installations that are open to unqualified persons shall be made with metal enclosed equipment or shall be enclosed in a vault or in an area to which access is controlled by a lock.

Guards shall be provided if the equipment is exposed to damage from vehicular traffic.

Identifying Electrical Disconnects and Circuits. Identification of switches and circuit breakers is required. This assists personnel in determining which device controls power to a particular circuit.

In times of emergency, it may be required to shut off power to particular circuits. This can only be done properly if equipment and circuits are identified with labels.

Switches, circuit breakers, and the like must be legibly marked to indicate their purpose. The labels shall be durable and able to withstand weathering.

Using Flexible Cords Correctly. Only approved flexible cords and cables shall be used. Flexible cords shall be used only for hanging lights, wiring of fixtures, portable lamps or appliances, appliances that have to be disconnected for repair, portable tools, and data processing cables. They must be equipped with approved plugs and the plug inserted in 3-wire grounded receptacle outlets. The plug should be either the polarized two-blade type or 3-wire grounded type.

Where Flexible Cords Are Not Permitted. Flexible cords must not be run through holes in walls, ceilings, floors, doorways, windows, or similar openings. They shall not be attached to building surfaces or concealed behind walls, ceilings, or floors.

Flexible cords must not be spliced or tapped except as noted in the standard.

They shall have strain relief so that when they are pulled, they will not be torn from the plug.

Fixed wiring must be installed whenever possible to avoid the use of flexible cords.

Preventing Pulls at Joints and Terminals. Only approved cords, plug caps, connector bodies, and lampholders that are substantial enough for the conditions, and have the provision to relieve the strain on connections and terminals, shall be used. All connections must be made to cords or devices inside enclosures. If any splices are made in cords, they must be made so that the pull on the cord will not apply tension to the conductor joints. Persons who assemble or repair cords must be trained to do it properly.

Grounding Electrical Devices. All electrical enclosures must be connected together to ensure grounding.

The equipment grounding conductor must be continuous between all enclosures and must be connected to the source of the electrical system, which is also grounded. Bonding is required to prevent arcing and sparking between enclosures. Proper grounding provides a ground fault path so that if an energized part is touched, the current follows to the ground and away from the person touching the energized part. Electrical equipment must be grounded if a person can touch that equipment and a grounded surface at the same time.

Systems that require grounding are 3-wire direct current systems, 2-wire direct current systems operating between 50 volts and 300 volts between conductors, fire alarm systems, overhead electrical wires outside of buildings, uninsulated wires and alternating current systems operating from 50 volts to 1,000 volts (except for certain conditions).

Grounding Equipment Connected by Cord and Plug. This refers to the grounding of appliances, hand tools, fans, and so forth. Proper **polarization** has to be observed. The "hot" conductor (conductor carrying the current) wire of the plug must connect up with the "hot" wire of the receptacle. The neutral wire of the plug (wire that is not energized) must connect up with the neutral of the receptacle. The ground wire of the plug must connect up with the ground wire of the receptacle. Whenever these wires are connected incorrectly, for instance a "hot" of a plug with the ground of the receptacle, it is called **reversed polarity**. This is a hazardous condition.

Cord and plug connected equipment that must be grounded includes refrigerators, freezers, air conditioners, clothes washing machines, clothes drying machines, dishwashing machines, sump pumps, electrical aquarium equipment, portable tools, hedge clippers, lawn mowers, snow blowers, wet scrubbers, equipment and tools used in damp or wet locations, portable and mobile X-ray equipment and EKG equipment and the like, and portable hand lamps.

Plugs should be either 2-blade polarized, or 3-wire grounding type.

Fixed electrical equipment must be properly grounded so that the current is directed away from energized surfaces and does not shock or electrocute the person touching the energized surface.

Locating Overcurrent Devices Safely. This refers to fuse boxes, panelboards, and the like. They must be located so that they can be accessed in case of emergency. These overcurrent devices cannot be located where they will be exposed to physical damage or in the vicinity of easily ignitable material.

Fuse boxes, circuit breakers, and the like must be located or shielded so that employees will not be burned or otherwise injured from arcing or sparking or by shock or electrocution.

Circuit breakers must be clearly marked to show whether they are in the off or on position.

Maintaining Sufficient Working Clearance. Working clearances must be kept around electrical equipment as noted in Tables 8-1 and 8-2.

The elevation of unguarded energized parts above working spaces is shown in Table 8-3.

TABLE 8-1	Working Clearances		
Nominal Voltage to Ground	Minimum Clear Distance for Condition in Feet		
	(a)	(b)	(c)
0–150	3[1]	3[1]	3
151–600	3[1]	3½	4

[1] Minimum clear distances may be 2 feet 6 inches for installations built prior to April 16, 1981.

Conditions (a), (b), and (c) are as follows:
   (a) Exposed live parts on one side and no live or grounded parts on the other side of the working space, or exposed live parts on both sides effectively guarded by suitable wood or other insulating material. Insulated wire or insulated busbars operating at not over 300 volts are not considered live parts.
   (b) Exposed live parts on one side and grounded parts on the other side. Concrete, brick, or tile walls will be considered ground surfaces.
   (c) Exposed live parts on both sides of the workspace [not guarded as provided in condition (a)] with the operator between.

Properly Splicing Flexible Cords. Flexible cords shall only be used in continuous lengths without a splice or a tap. A number 12 flexible cord (number 12 is an electrical designation) may be spliced if the splice retains the same insulation and properties of the original cord.

Making Proper Splices on Electrical Connections. Electrical wires must be spliced or joined with splicing devices that are proper for the use of the cords. The splicing must be done by brazing, welding, or soldering with a fusible metal or alloy. The splices must be electrically secure before being soldered. The splices and joints of the wires must be covered with an insulation equal to that of the original wire.

Marking Electrical Equipment. Electrical equipment must not be used unless the manufacturer's name, trademark, or other descriptive marking by which the manufacturer is identified is placed on the equipment. Other markings must include volt-

TABLE 8-2	Minimum Depth of Clear Working Space in Front of Electrical Equipment		
Nominal Voltage to Ground	Conditions in Feet		
	(a)	(b)	(c)
601–2500	3	4	5
2501–9000	4	5	6
9001–25000	5	6	9
25001–75 kV[1]	6	8	10
Above 75 kV[1]	8	10	12

[1] Minimum depth of clear working space in front of electric equipment with a nominal voltage to ground above 25,000 volts may be the same as for 25,000 volts under conditions (a), (b), and (c) for installations built prior to April 16, 1981.

Conditions (a), (b), and (c) are as follows:
   (a) Exposed live parts on one side and no live or grounded parts on the other side of the working space, or exposed live parts on both sides effectively guarded by suitable wood or other insulating material. Insulated wire or insulated busbars operating at not over 300 volts are not considered live parts.
   (b) Exposed live parts on one side and grounded parts on the other side. Concrete, brick, or tile walls will be considered ground surfaces.
   (c) Exposed live parts on both sides of the workspace [not guarded as provided in condition (a)] with the operator between.

TABLE 8-3	Elevation of Unguarded Energized Parts above Working Space
Nominal Voltage Between Phases	Minimum Elevation
601–7500	*8 feet 6 inches
7501–35000	9 feet
Over 35 kV	9 feet + 0.37 inch per kV above 35 kV

* Minimum elevation may be 8 feet 0 inches for installations built prior to April 16, 1981 if the nominal voltage between phases is in the range of 601–6,600 volts.

age, current, wattage, or other ratings as necessary. The markings must be durable and able to withstand weathering.

Electrical Information

The following are some helpful hints concerning electrical safety.

Things to Remember. Fuses should be sized properly for the circuits they protect. Household circuits take 15 and 20 ampere fuses. Improper fuse size can cause fires and shock.

Circuits must be **grounded**. Grounding ensures a path of current away from you if you touch an energized part. Grounding integrity should be checked by trained persons. The grounding must be continuous from the **service entrance panel (SEP)** to the branch circuit to the receptacle. The SEP is the panel to which the electrical service enters the building and then from which the building circuits branch out.

You should know how to properly use extension cords and other flexible cords.

You should know how to safely use 3-wire grounded plugs and 2-wire polarized plugs.

Polarization, which is the connecting of proper wires, is very important in maintaining electrical safety.

You should know not to overload receptacles and extension cords and the proper use of plug strips. This situation is called an **octopus connection**.

You should know when and how **ground fault circuit interrupters (GCFI)** are used. These are devices that cut off power in milliseconds when there is a ground fault in the circuit. This prevents shock or possible electrocution. They are designed to prevent shock or electrocution in wet and damp locations.

Hazardous Locations

OSHA and the National Electric Code (NEC) define hazardous areas as those where flammable gases, liquids, vapors, or combustible dusts are in sufficient quantity to cause an explosion if there is an arc or spark. These locations are subdivided as follows:

- Class I: Flammable and combustible gases, vapors and liquids
- Class II: Flammable and combustible dusts
- Class III: Flammable and combustible fibers and flyings (ignitable textiles and wood)

These classes are further subdivided into Division 1 and Division 2. Division 1 is where the hazardous material is normally present in explosive concentrations; Division 2 is where the material is not normally present in explosive concentrations, but can be if it is released accidentally.

OSHA requires that any electrical equipment located in Class I hazardous areas be explosion proof, in Class II areas be dust ignition proof, and in Class III areas be totally enclosed to prevent entry of fibers and flyings.

The reason the equipment must be enclosed is to protect against flammable and combustible substances in the air from contacting arcs or sparks. Devices that are installed in these areas must meet the OSHA and NEC requirements for the class and division that defines the hazard. This equipment must have the Underwriters Laboratory (UL) label affixed.

APPENDIX

It doesn't take much electrical current to shock and possibly kill. As little as one **milliampere** can shock a person. A milliampere is 1/1000 ampere. An ampere is a measure of the current that flows through a circuit. **Alternating current** is current that flows back and forth in a circuit 60 times a second. **Direct current** flows in one direction. The voltage, which is the electromotive force (EMF), causes the current to flow through the conductor.

CHAPTER REVIEW

True/False

Indicate whether the statement is true or false by circling T or F.

1. T F Ampere is a measure of voltage.

2. T F Grounding protects against shock.

3. T F Electrical equipment does not require guarding.

4. T F When a "hot" wire is connected to
another "hot" wire, polarity is correct.

5. T F Boxes can be placed in front of electrical panels as long as they can be
moved out of the way.

Matching

Match the terms in column 1 with the definitions in column 2.

Column 1

6. AC
7. GFCI
8. 15 and 20 amp
9. Reversed polarity
10. Octopus connection

Column 2

a. Household current
b. Connection of "hot" to "neutral" wire
c. Shock and electrocution protection
d. Overloaded receptacle or extension cord
e. Current that goes back and forth
    60 times a second

Fill-In

Fill in the word(s) that best complete the sentence.

11. Flexible cords are not considered _____
wiring.

12. Marking on electrical equipment must be
_____.

13. The three classes of hazardous locations are
(I) _____ (II) _____ and
(III) _____ .

14. Enclosures or cabinets containing voltages
over 600V must have signs that say
_____ .

15. The _____ is the point where
circuits that go throughout the facility start.

CHAPTER 9

Safety Color Code for Marking Physical Hazards and Specifications for Accident Prevention Signs and Tags

After studying this chapter, you should be able to

➤ Identify the OSHA requirements for accident prevention signs and tags.
➤ Explain the differences among the various signs and tags.
➤ Identify when tags can be used.

OSHA 29 CFR 1910.144 SAFETY COLOR CODE FOR MARKING PHYSICAL HAZARDS

Safety color coding for marking hazards is found under 29 CFR 1910.144. (Specifications for accident prevention signs and tags are found under 29 CFR 1910.145. Both standards dictate the color and specifications for various markings and signs that denote hazards.)

The color red is used to identify fire protection equipment and apparatus.

Safety cans or other portable containers that contain flammable liquids having flash points at or below 80°F must be painted red and have either the contents indicated on the container in yellow or have a painted yellow band around the container.

Red lights have to be provided at barricades and at temporary obstructions. Danger signs must be painted red.

The color yellow is used to designate caution for such hazards as striking against, stumbling, falling, tripping, and "caught between."

OSHA 29 CFR 1910.145 SPECIFICATIONS FOR ACCIDENT PREVENTION SIGNS AND TAGS

There are specific requirements for accident prevention signs and tags. This includes the colors and wording.

Danger Signs

Danger signs are used to warn of immediate danger and that special precautions are necessary. Employees must be instructed concerning what danger signs mean and what precautions to take. The color of danger signs must be red, black, and white.

Caution Signs

Caution signs are used only to warn against potential hazards or to caution against unsafe practices. Employees must be instructed what caution signs mean and what precautions to take. Standard color of caution signs has to be a yellow background and the panel black with yellow letters. Letters used against the yellow background must be black.

Safety Instruction Signs

Safety instruction signs are used when there is a need for general safety instructions and suggestions. Standard color of the background has to be white and the panel green with white letters. Letters used against the white background must be black.

Biological Hazard Signs

Biological hazard signs (biohazard) are used to identify actual or potential biohazards and to identify equipment, containers, rooms, materials, experimental animals, or combinations thereof, that contain, or are contaminated with, viable hazardous agents. These biohazards are to include those infectious agents that present a risk or potential risk to employee health.

Accident Prevention Tags

Accident prevention tags are considered by OSHA to be a temporary means of warning concerning hazardous conditions, defective equipment, and radiation hazards. They are not complete warning methods and are to be used for short periods until the condition is corrected.

The tag refers to a card, paper, pasteboard, or some temporary or nonpermanant material that contains letters and/or markings for cautioning or safety instruction. They are affixed by wire, string, or adhesive.

Accident prevention tags contain a signal word and a major message such as **"Danger," "Caution,"** or **"Biological Hazard"** or **"Biohazard,"** or the biological hazard symbol (Figure 9-1). The major mes-

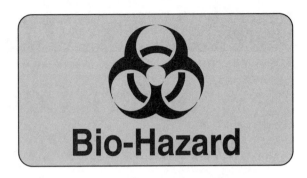

FIGURE 9-1 *Sign or label to warn of biohazardous material*

sage must indicate the specific hazardous condition or instruction.

The tag has to be readable at a minimum distance of 5 feet or at a greater distance if warranted by the hazard.

The tag's message can be in pictographs, written, or both, and the message must be understandable.

Employees are to be informed as to the meaning of the various tags and the special precautions that are necessary.

The tags must be secured as close as possible to the hazard by string, wire, or adhesive that prevents loss or unintentional removal.

Danger Tags. Danger tags are used only when an immediate hazard presents a threat of death or serious injury.

Caution Tags. Caution tags are used only when a nonimmediate or potential hazard, or unsafe practice, presents a lesser threat of injury.

Warning Tags. Warning tags are used to designate a hazard level between danger and caution, instead of the required caution tag, provided they have a signal word such as "Warning" and an appropriate major message.

Biological Hazard Tags (Biohazard). Biological hazard tags (biohazard) are used to identify the actual or potential presence of a biological hazard and to identify equipment, containers, rooms, experimental animals, or combinations thereof, that contain or are contaminated with hazardous biological agents. The standard biohazard symbol must be used if used on tags.

Sign Wording

Sign wording has to be concise and easily read. It has to contain sufficient information so that it is easily understood.

CHAPTER REVIEW

True/False

Indicate whether the statement is true or false by circling T or F.

1. T F The color red is used to designate caution.

2. T F Tags are temporary means of warning.

3. T F Biohazard signs can be used to warn of machine tool hazards.

4. T F Safety cans must be painted red.

5. T F Sign wording does not have to be concise.

CHAPTER 10

Abatement Verification

After studying this chapter, you should be able to

➤ Define the OSHA requirements for abatement verification.

➤ Explain when abatement documentation is required.

➤ Identify when abatement plans are required.

➤ Explain the importance of employee notification in the abatement process.

OSHA 29 CFR 1910.1903 ABATEMENT VERIFICATION

Verification of the abatement of cited safety violations is now required by OSHA. Employers must show that they take cited violations seriously. Failure to abate can bring on fines and in serious situations, criminal penalties.

Under OSHA 29 CFR 1910.1903, it is required that employers verify to OSHA that they have abated (corrected) safety and health violations that were cited by the OSHA inspector. The employer must also inform his/her affected employees or their authorized representatives of actions taken to correct the hazardous conditions that were cited.

Who Must Comply

This section of the OSHA law only pertains to those employers that were cited for workplace health and safety violations of the Occupational Safety and Health Act by an OSHA compliance officer. If an employer has not been cited for any violations, he/she does not have to comply with this section.

Employees Affected

Affected employees are those who are exposed to the health or safety hazard cited by the OSHA inspector. They are the employees who, because of their risk, must be informed by the employer of any abatement actions taken to correct the hazard.

Abatement Certification

Abatement certification is a certification to OSHA that must be sent within ten calendar days after completion of any abatement action indicating that the hazard has been eliminated. This ensures that abatement verification will be completed as quickly as possible.

If an employer abates a hazard immediately after it is cited by a compliance officer (such as during an inspection) or within twenty-four hours from the time the hazard was cited, the employer does not have to certify abatement to OSHA in a separate letter. The inspector will note in his/her records that there was immediate correction.

Abatement Documentation

Abatement documentation is submitted to OSHA by employers who have been cited for willful or repeat violations, or for specific serious violations. Employers must not only certify to any abatement actions but must also provide documentary evidence of these actions. Not all serious violations require documentation—only those that are considered hazards that have a high probability for an employee injury, illness, or death.

Acceptable documentation may include

• Invoices for equipment or supplies to abate the hazard.

- Photographs or videos that show the abated hazard.
- Reports by consultants describing actions taken or evaluations.
- Reports of analytical testing.
- A signed contract for personal protective equipment.
- Training records showing completed employee training (if the citation relates to training).
- Copy of program documents showing the missing required information (if the citation involved missing information such as in a respirator or hazard communication program).

Abatement Plans

OSHA may require employers to submit **abatement plans**. These are plans for abatements that have dates of ninety days or more. The exception is for other-than-serious violations. If it is required by OSHA, they (OSHA) must indicate in the citation which items require these plans. This requirement usually applies to the more serious, willful, or repeat violations that have been assigned dates of ninety days or more.

Abatement plans required by OSHA must be submitted within twenty-five calendar days of the final order date (date established by OSHA).

Progress Reports

Employers must submit periodic progress reports to OSHA in addition to abatement plans, for the more serious hazards that require long-term abatement (greater than ninety days) when the citation requires such a report.

OSHA must specify in the citation each item that requires a progress report and the dates for submission of the initial report. This date cannot be sooner than thirty calendar days after submission of an abatement plan.

The report must include a brief description of the action taken to abate each cited violation and the date the abatement activity was conducted.

If a violation requires a progress report or abatement plan and is abated prior to the submission date, the employer only has to submit the abatement certification and documentation required in the regulations.

Citation items may be combined in a single progress report if the items have the same abatement actions and proposed and actual completion dates.

Employee Notification

Employers must provide to those employees affected by the cited hazard and their authorized representatives, information concerning the abatement of the violations affecting them. This must be done by posting a copy or summary of each document submitted to OSHA near the place where the violation occurred.

For those employees who do not have a permanent workstation (such as those who work out of trucks), OSHA lets the employees determine the best way to notify them. This could be done in the employee's pay envelope or tool box, or some similar arrangement.

Affected employees and their designated representatives may request copies of all abatement documents for examining and copying. They must submit these requests to the employer within three working days from the time they are notified by the employer that these documents have been submitted to OSHA. The employer must respond to the request for this information within five working days of receipt of the request.

The employer must make sure that affected employees and their representatives are notified that the documents are available. This must be done at the same time or before the documents are transmitted to OSHA.

Employers must post abatement documents in a readily accessible place and also indicate in the posting that affected employees and their representatives have the right to examine and copy these documents.

Transmitting Abatement Documents

Abatement certification letters, abatement documentation, abatement plans, and progress reports must all contain the following information:

1. Employer's name and address
2. Inspection number
3. Citation number and citation item numbers

4. A statement that indicates that the provided information is accurate

5. Employer's or employer's designated representative's signature

The date of the postmark is used by OSHA as the date for mailed abatement verification.

Movable (Portable) Equipment

Movable (portable) equipment can take up floor space or be hand-held. Depending upon the circumstances and equipment, OSHA requires that cited movable equipment have a tag or affixed copy of the citation on the operating controls or hazardous components. The employer may determine whether to use a tag or a copy of the citation. If a tag is used, it must contain the information and design specifications required by OSHA (it must identify the equipment cited, indicate it was cited by OSHA, and specify where the citation is posted for employee review).

Tagging or Affixing Copy of Citation. Hand-held equipment (such as power tools) require immediate tagging. Other than hand-held equipment must be tagged only if the equipment is moved from the worksite where it was cited, or is moved to another worksite before the cited hazards are abated.

The tag or copy of the citation cannot be covered by other material, altered, or be illegible. The tag or copy of the citation can be removed when

- Abatement has been completed and any required abatement documents have been submitted to OSHA.
- The cited equipment has been permanently removed from the worksite.
- The cited equipment is no longer under the control of the employer.
- The Occupational Safety and Health Review Commission (OSHRC) has vacated (voided) the citation.

Other than serious violations do not require tagging or posting of the citation on the equipment. Other than serious violations do not expose affected employees to life-threatening or serious injury. They usually can be corrected on site or during short abatement periods. Tagging and posting of the citation is limited to serious, willful, and repeat violations and to conditions for which the employer has received a failure-to-abate notice.

CHAPTER REVIEW

True/False

Indicate whether the statement is true or false by circling T or F.

1. T F Abatement certification must be sent to OSHA within ten calendar days from abatement completion.

2. T F Abatement plans are required for abatement dates of thirty days or more.

3. T F An employer must notify all employees that a hazard has been abated.

4. T F Tags must be used on movable equipment indicating a citation.

5. T F Tags are limited to "other than serious" violations.

Matching

Match the terms in column 1 with the definitions in column 2.

Column 1

6. Abatement certification
7. Abatement documentation
8 Abatement plans
9. Acceptable documentation
10. When a tag can be removed

Column 2

a. Abatement dates of ninety days or more
b. Signed contract for personal protective equipment
c. Sent to OSHA within ten calendar days
d. Cited equipment removed from the worksite
e. Required for willful or repeat violations

CHAPTER 11

Health Care Security

OBJECTIVES

After studying this chapter, you should be able to

➤ Explain employee involvement in preventing workplace violence.

➤ Discuss the proposed OSHA workplace violence standard.

➤ Define correct responses to incidents of violence.

➤ List the various ways you can make your facility less prone to violence and vandalism.

➤ Explain an effective workplace violence plan.

FACILITY SECURITY

Violence in health care facilities is on the increase. Factors that encourage workplace violence include the following:

• Health care facilities have drugs that are sought after.

• Mental patients are being released without follow-up treatment.

• Insufficient staff.

• Patient and/or family buildup of anger while waiting to be seen by a provider.

• The increased use of weapons in society.

• The use of hospitals for mentally disturbed and violent criminals.

• Lack of training of staff in how to recognize signs of violent behavior.

• The fact that the public can wander unescorted in some facilities.

These are just some of the situations that help create "breeding grounds" for workplace violence.

Even though there is no OSHA standard that covers worksite violence, if there are a substantial number of injuries because of workplace violence, the employer can be cited under the general duty clause.

Employers should have programs in place to protect employees. Keeping them safe from molestation, harassment, and attack and other forms of violence is as important as protecting them against physical, chemical, and mechanical hazards.

The main factors of a good workplace security program include commitment and involvement by management and employees, worksite analysis, violence prevention and control, and training.

MANAGEMENT SUPPORT AND COMMITMENT

From the health care facility top administrator to the line employee, there should be a commitment to preventing workplace violence. This commitment should include the following:

• Demonstrated concern for employee emotional and physical safety.

• Commitment not only to employee safety, but safety of patients.

• Assigned duties to managers, supervisors, and employees involving a violence prevention program. These people must be given authority and the necessary resources to implement their part of the program.

• Accountability by managers, supervisors, and employees for actions occurring in their areas of responsibility.

- Programs that address medical and psychological counseling for employees who are victims of an assault or who witness a violent act.
- A promise by management to implement appropriate recommendations from worksite safety and health committees.

EMPLOYEE INVOLVEMENT

Employee involvement should include the following:

- An understanding of the program and compliance with established procedures.
- Making suggestions concerning the enhancement of facility security.
- Making prompt reports of assaults, regardless of whether it is actual, verbal, or threatening.
- Being members of safety and health committees that receive reports of violence or other security problems.
- Making facility inspections and recommendations concerning these inspections.
- Participating in ongoing educational programs to recognize when situations are becoming volatile, violent behavior, criminal intent, and discussing responses to these situations.

WRITTEN WORKPLACE VIOLENCE PROGRAM

The written program should be integrated into the facility safety and health program.

The following are guidelines for a written program:

- Establish a policy that workplace violence will not be tolerated, whether it is in the form of physical violence, verbal or nonverbal threats, or any other type of assault. All managers, supervisors, and other employees must be made aware of this policy.
- Reprisals will not be taken against employees who report or experience workplace violence.
- Encourage employees to report incidents and to make recommendations to prevent future occurrences.

- Require that all incidents, regardless of what form they take, be recorded.
- Describe a plan that involves a liaison with outside law enforcement and others who can assist in preventing workplace violence.
- Have certain people responsible for the program. These people should have the training and expertise to administer the program and the necessary resources for program implementation.
- Have procedures for post-incident response.

POST-INCIDENT RESPONSE

Proper response after an incident is essential to any worksite security program. This includes treatment for employees who were victims of violence or who may have been traumatized because they witnessed a violent incident. The employee should receive medical help and counseling. The injured employee should be transported to a medical facility if treatment is not available on-site.

When the employee returns to work, there should be follow-up to make sure he/she is not suffering from lingering medical or psychological problems. This helps him/her deal with problems and confront any future violence.

WORKSITE ANALYSIS

Worksite analysis includes looking at the procedures and activities that can precipitate workplace violence and the areas where it may happen.

The analysis team should include representatives from management, operations, employee assistance, security, safety and health, legal, and human resources.

Injury and illness and workers' compensation records should be reviewed by the team to determine where problem areas exist.

The team or team coordinator should do the following:

- Analyze incidences, including what, where, why, and how it happened.
- Identify jobs or locations that might have a high incidence of violence.

- Identify areas where there may be a lack of communication, employee isolation, or insufficient lighting.
- Determine the effectiveness of existing measures, including engineering or administrative controls.

EMPLOYEE SURVEYS

Employees should be surveyed so that they can tender their opinions on where and how violent incidents can occur in their areas. Surveys can also identify tasks that can cause employees to be put at increased risk of violence. These surveys should be conducted at least annually, or whenever workplace activities change, or when an incidence of violence occurs.

CONTROL AND PREVENTION OF VIOLENCE

When hazards have been identified, control measures such as specific engineering, administrative, or work practice controls should be put into effect.

Some controls that can be implemented include:

- Securing the building from the outside
- Keeping parking lots lit at night
- Having an employee escort service
- Encouraging the reporting of areas that might need increased security
- Ensuring employee communication from all facility areas
- Controlling entrances
- Installing building security devices
- Establishing an effective security program

These are just a few suggestions. The type of control you may wish to implement will depend upon your particular circumstances, which include the configuration of the facility, employee activities and operations, and existing controls.

TRAINING

Training is a very important aspect of workplace security. Training helps employees deal with violent situations more effectively.

Employee Training

Employers should train all employees on how to protect themselves at the worksite. This training should include the following (additional elements may be required depending upon work activities):

- Location of specific areas and types of activities that may encourage violent behavior.
- What the employee can do to control or prevent an incident.
- Where to get assistance when threatened.
- How to handle stressful situations.

Training should be done in the work area. Employees can familiarize themselves with the work area as it relates to violence prevention and be trained to use it to their advantage during an emergency. Floor layouts showing exits/entrances, and location of security control devices and equipment should be posted on all floors and employees made aware of these locations. Training should also include an explanation of the operation of these devices.

Training must be supported by management and be required of all employees. Training must be done at least annually and when methods and procedures change. Records of employee training should be maintained.

Management, Supervisory, and Security Training

Because managers and supervisors are responsible for employee security, they should have the same training as that of the employees. They should also have additional training so that they can establish an effective violence prevention program.

Security staff should have training in how to handle aggressive or abusive behavior. This should include ways of keeping situations from escalating.

Training for management, supervisory, and security staff should be conducted with the same frequency as that of other employees—at least annually or whenever activities and operations change that will require revised procedures.

RECORDKEEPING

Keeping records of incidences will help the employer in identifying problems and assist in developing solutions.

Essential records that should be maintained are as follows:

1. OSHA Log of Injury and Illness (OSHA 200).
2. Reports of assaults. The report should include type of attack, who was assaulted, location, cost, lost time, and nature of injuries.
3. Incidents of verbal abuse or threatening behavior that do not result in an injury.
4. Documentation of meetings, analyses of hazards, and corrective action taken to control or prevent incidents of violence.
5. Records of training, which include dates, names of employees who attended, and the qualifications of the trainer.

CHAPTER REVIEW

Multiple Choice

Select the best answer from the choices provided.

1. Involvement in the security program should include
   a. management
   b. employees
   c. patients
   d. a, b, and c

2. Employee training should include
   a. when to get assistance, if threatened
   b. keeping windows and doors locked
   c. doing surveys
   d. being trained individually

3. A security engineering control is
   a. employee training
   b. supervisor training
   c. a security device
   d. records of incidences

4. Training should be conducted at least
   a. weekly
   b. annually
   c. semiannually
   d. biweekly

5. A worksite analysis is important because it determines
   a. who smokes
   b. where the problem areas might be
   c. who is locking windows and doors
   d. who has weapons

Short Answer

Briefly but thoroughly answer each statement.

6. What position in the facility is needed for support if the security program is to succeed?

7. List some of the various ways employees can be involved in the security program.

8. What are the guidelines for a good security program?

9. List some of the areas that should be covered in a training program.

10. What are some of the essential records needed?

SECTION II

Health Standards and Guidelines

CHAPTER 12

Sanitation

After studying this chapter, you should be able to

➤ Explain the OSHA requirements for sanitation (OSHA 29 CFR 1910.141).

➤ Identify requirements for specific areas.

➤ Identify backflow and backsiphonage.

OSHA 29 CFR 1910.141 SANITATION

Sanitation is described under Subpart J, 29 CFR 1910.141 and applies to permanent places of employment.

Like all OSHA standards, the sanitation requirements are the minimum to be implemented. It is prudent to use the standards as a base to increase safeguards wherever necessary.

Housekeeping

Places of employment must be kept as clean as possible. Floors have to be kept as dry as possible, and if wet processes are used, drainage has to be maintained and false floors, platforms, mats, or other dry standing places must be provided. If this can't be done, waterproof footgear must be provided.

Floors, working places, and passageways have to be kept free from protruding nails, splinters, loose boards, and unnecessary holes and openings.

Waste Disposal

Receptacles used for putrescible solid or liquid waste or refuse must be constructed so that they do not leak. The receptacles must be thoroughly cleaned and maintained in a sanitary condition. Tight fitting covers have to be provided unless the receptacle can be kept sanitary without a cover.

All solid and liquid wastes, refuse, and garbage must be removed as often as necessary to maintain sanitary conditions.

Vermin Control

Workplaces, as much as possible, must prevent the entrance or harborage of rodents, insects, and other vermin. A continuing extermination program must be instituted when vermin are detected.

Water Supply

Potable (safe) drinking water must be provided for drinking, washing, cooking, washing of foods, utensils, food preparation areas, processing, and personal service rooms.

Dispensers must be designed so that sanitary conditions are maintained. They must be able to be closed and must be equipped with a tap.

Common drinking cups and utensils are prohibited.

Nonpotable Water

Nonpotable water outlets must be clearly marked to indicate that the water is unsafe and is not to be used for drinking, washing, cooking, washing of foods, utensils, food preparation areas, processing, and personal service rooms.

When nonpotable water systems are hooked into potable systems, they have to be equipped with **backflow** or **backsiphonage devices** to prevent flow back. Backflow and backsiphonage preventers consist of vacuum breakers, indirect drains, check valves, or other approved devices that guard against the contamination of potable water.

Toilet Facilities

Toilet facilities must be separate for each gender except if they are occupied by one person at a time and can be locked from the inside and contain at least one water closet.

Water closets are provided as follows:

Number of Employees	Minimum Number of Water Closets
1–15	1
16–35	2
36–55	3
56–80	4
81–110	5
111–150	6
Over 150	One additional fixture for each additional 40 employees

Sewage disposal methods cannot endanger employee health.

Toilet Room Construction

Water closets have to be in separate compartments with a door and walls for privacy.

Washing Facilities

Washing facilities must be kept in a sanitary condition. Lavatories must have hot and cold running water, and hand soap or similar cleanser has to be provided.

Towels. Cloth or paper hand towels must be provided. The toweling may be either individual or sectioned or continuous cloth.

Showers. If showers are provided, there has to be one for each ten employees of each gender, or numerical fraction thereof, if employees are required to shower during the same shift. Body soap or other cleansing agents have to be provided along with hot and cold water that feeds a common discharge line.

Employees who use showers must be provided with clean towels for each person.

Change Rooms

When employees are required to wear protective clothing because of the possibility of contamination with toxic materials, change rooms must be provided. These rooms have to be equipped with storage facilities for street clothes and separate storage facilities for the protective clothing.

Clothes Drying Facilities

Drying facilities must be provided when working clothes that are required to be worn by employees become wet or are washed between shifts.

Food and Beverage Consumption on the Premises

If employees are permitted to eat on the premises, they cannot be allowed to eat in toilet rooms or in areas exposed to toxic materials.

Waste Disposal Containers. Waste food must be disposed of in smooth, corrosion resistant, and easily cleanable containers. The number, size, and location of these containers must encourage use and not overfilling. They have to be emptied at least once every workday, unless not used, and must be maintained in a clean and sanitary condition. They have to be provided with solid tight fitting covers unless they can be maintained in a sanitary manner without the use of a cover.

Sanitary Storage. Food and beverages cannot be stored in toilet rooms or areas exposed to toxic materials.

Food Handling

Employee food service facilities and operations must be carried out using accepted hygienic principles. The food dispensed must be wholesome, free from spoilage, and must be processed, prepared, handled, and stored so that it is protected against contamination.

CHAPTER REVIEW

True/False
Indicate whether the statement is true or false by circling T or F.

1. T F Receptacles containing wet refuse may leak as long as it's cleaned up immediately.

2. T F Receptacles that contain food waste require covers unless they can be kept clean without them.

3. T F Potable water need not be supplied for washing clothes.

4. T F Change rooms must be provided for employees whose clothes may become contaminated.

5. T F Backflow and backsiphonage devices prevent contaminated water from getting into clean water.

CHAPTER 13

Medical Services and First Aid

After studying this chapter, you should be able to

➤ Explain the OSHA requirements for medical services and first aid.
➤ Identify the recommendations to ensure that water used in eye wash and drench showers is safe.

OSHA 29 CFR 1910.151 MEDICAL SERVICES AND FIRST AID

Medical and First Aid is described under Subpart K 1910.151 of the OSHA standard. It is a short standard and explains the general requirements for employee protection.

The standard describes the minimum requirements but should be used as a base to go above the minimum in furnishing first aid and medical services for employees.

Requirements

The employer must be sure there is ready availability of medical personnel for advice and consultation on matters of health pertaining to employees.

When there is no infirmary, clinic, or hospital within proximity of the workplace that is used for the treatment of injured employees, a person or persons must be adequately trained to give first aid. First aid supplies approved by the consulting physician must be readily available.

When the eyes or body of an employee may be exposed to injurious corrosive materials, there must be adequate facilities for emergency use for quick drenching or flushing of the eyes and body. These facilities must be located within the work area and accessible for immediate emergency use.

WATER RECOMMENDATIONS FOR EYE WASH STATIONS AND DRENCH SHOWERS

Eye wash stations and safety (drench) showers prevent damage to the skin by flushing away the contaminate before it has a chance to further eat into tissue. There are recommendations that should be followed to ensure that they will be readily available in case of emergency. The following are guidelines for eye wash stations and drench showers:

- Eye wash stations and drench showers should not be blocked so that they can be accessed immediately in case of an emergency.
- When flushing the eyes, they should be flushed for at least fifteen minutes. This will ensure the prompt removal of the contacted chemical.
- Potable (drinkable) water should be supplied to units that are connected to water pipes.
- The water supply should be free of bacteria and not contain high concentrations of disinfectants, especially chlorine, that can cause damage to skin or eyes.
- The temperature of the water should be maintained between 60° and 95°F. This temperature range is the most comfortable for the user.

- There should be a weekly inspection of eye wash stations and drench showers to make sure they are always operational. Records of these inspections should be kept on file.

- If the unit is a portable, self-contained unit (not connected to water pipes), follow the manufacturer's instructions when using it.

CHAPTER REVIEW

True/False

Indicate whether the statement is true or false by circling T or F.

1. T F Eyes should be flushed for at least fifteen minutes to remove corrosive materials.

2. T F If there is no health care facility near the workplace, an employee(s) must be trained to render first aid.

3. T F Flushing water need not be sanitary.

4. T F Eye wash stations and drench showers should be tested monthly.

5. T F Flushing water should be between 40° and 50°F.

CHAPTER 14

Tuberculosis Guidelines

After studying this chapter, you should be able to

➤ Discuss the relationship between the Centers for Disease Control and Prevention and OSHA in tuberculosis control.

➤ Define how OSHA cites for tuberculosis violations, in lieu of a standard.

➤ Explain the various methods used to protect against tuberculosis exposure.

➤ Discuss how general and local exhaust is used to protect against bacilli.

➤ State the use of personal protective equipment and how it is used in control.

CENTERS FOR DISEASE CONTROL AND PREVENTION GUIDELINES

Just when it was thought by the medical community that tuberculosis (TB) was pretty much eradicated, it raised its ugly head. Various socioeconomic factors came into play that encouraged its spread.

Because there is no specific standard that deals with tuberculosis, OSHA uses the general duty clause and the Centers for Disease Control and Prevention (CDC) guidelines to enforce safe practices to protect employees from TB.

The general duty clause mandates that the employer must maintain the workplace free from recognized hazards likely to cause death or serious injury. In order for the general duty clause to be invoked, the following requirements must be met:

1. The violation must be such that it can cause serious physical injury or illness.

2. It must be able to be abated by a feasible method.

3. An employee or employees are at risk.

TB infection meets the general duty clause criteria, which allows OSHA to give citations when OSHA and CDC guidelines are not met. This chapter describes those guidelines that must be followed by the health care industry to control the spread of TB to protect employees and to avoid costly citations.

The following guidelines are proposed by CDC to control the spread of TB in various settings.

Tuberculosis Control

The spread of TB in health care facilities has to be controlled by

1. Preventing the generation of infectious droplet nuclei.

2. Preventing droplet nuclei from contaminating the circulating clean air.

3. Keeping droplet nuclei to a minimum in air already contaminated with TB bacilli.

4. Following proper guidelines for cleaning, disinfecting, and sterilizing contaminated items.

5. Maintaining surveillance to ensure that employees are protected from TB bacilli.

Reducing the Risk of Transmission. To reduce the risk of tuberculosis transmission, the following steps should be taken:

• Screen patients and employees for both active tuberculosis and tuberculosis infection. Employees with positive skin tests should be evaluated for risk of HIV infection.

• Ensure that diagnoses are prompt.

• Prescribe curative and preventive therapy.

- Take physical measures, such as installing UV lamps and ventilation systems to eliminate or reduce microbial air infection.
- Provide negative pressure isolation rooms for persons with, or suspected of having, infectious tuberculosis.
- Investigate and control outbreaks promptly.
- Use NIOSH approved respirators.

Preventing Generation of Infectious Droplet Nuclei

These are the main points to consider in preventing the spread of TB:

- Early identification of persons with infectious TB.
- Early identification and treatment of persons with **active TB**.
- Determination of the degree of infection.

Early Identification of Persons with Tuberculosis Infection. The method available that is effective in determining tuberculosis infection is the mantoux tuberculin skin test when active tuberculosis is not evident. Skin tests should be conducted every three months for workers in a high-risk category and every six months for those in an intermediate risk category.

Early Identification and Treatment of Persons with Active Tuberculosis. Early diagnosis, isolation, and treatment of people with active TB is necessary to prevent the transmission of the disease.

Diagnosis may be difficult in persons with HIV infection or who have other pulmonary infections such as *pneumocystis carinii* pneumonia (PCP).

Diagnostic measures should include a history, physical examination, tuberculin skin test, chest X ray, microscopic examination and culture of sputum or other appropriate specimen, and bronchoscopy or biopsy.

Degree of Infection Determination. Persons with pulmonary, respiratory tract, or laryngeal tuberculosis are the most infectious. Extrapulmonary tuberculosis is usually not infectious except if it involves an open abscess or lesion.

Persons with a productive cough, pulmonary cavitation (as seen on chest X ray), and **acid fast bacilli (AFB)** on sputum smear, are highly communicable. Acid fast bacilli are microorganisms that retain certain stains or dyes when washed with acid and alcohol while the surrounding tissue becomes decolorized. Employees exposed to patients who have undiagnosed pulmonary tuberculosis or who are not receiving antituberculosis therapy can easily become infected. The patient may be refusing treatment, or the organism is drug resistant. Antituberculosis medication greatly reduces the infectiousness of persons with tuberculosis. Chemotherapy reduces the incidence of coughing, the amount of sputum, and the number of organisms in the sputum. Some patients will require medication for longer periods than others before they become noninfectious. Some may never become infectious, others may remain infectious for weeks or months.

Health care workers who have pulmonary or laryngeal tuberculosis are a risk to other employees as well as patients. It is necessary to establish work restrictions for these workers. They must be excluded from work until adequate treatment is started, cough is resolved, and sputum is free of bacilli on three consecutive smears taken at intervals determined by a physician. Health care employees with other forms of TB usually do not need to be excluded from work if pulmonary TB has not been diagnosed. Those workers who are otherwise healthy and are receiving treatment for TB infection can be allowed to perform their usual duties.

Persons suspected of or known to have active tuberculosis should be considered infectious if

- A cough is present.
- Cough-inducing procedures such as **sputum induction** are being performed. Sputum induction is the process of inducing a cough in order to expel sputum for evaluation of **microorganisms**.
- Sputum smears contain acid-fast bacilli.
- These patients are not on chemotherapy, have just started chemotherapy, or have poor response to chemotherapy.

Persons on chemotherapy for two to three weeks who have a reduction in cough, no fever, and a progressive decrease in quantity of bacilli on a smear are generally no longer infectious. When taken out of isolation, they should be monitored to ensure that they remain noninfectious, particularly if placed with a patient who has a suppressed immune system.

Preventing Spread of Infectious Droplet Nuclei at the Source

Local exhaust and respirator controls can be established to trap infectious nuclei as they are emitted by the patient. These controls can also be very effective in protecting against infectious droplet nuclei from aerosols generated by medical procedures.

Local Exhaust Ventilation. Local exhaust ventilation captures the contaminant near or at the source of generation. The main components of a local exhaust system are the following:

- The hood to capture the contaminant (booth).
- The duct to carry the contaminant to a safe location.
- The fan that creates static pressure to move the air through the duct.
- A filter or air cleaner that removes contaminants before they reach the outdoors or are recirculated.

All contaminated air that is transported through the duct that is exhausted to the outside must be kept under negative pressure until it is exhausted to the exterior. The exhausted air must be kept away from air intakes, pedestrian ways, and occupied areas.

An example of local exhaust ventilation used in health care facilities to trap infectious droplet nuclei at the source is a booth used for sputum induction or for the administration of **aerosolized treatment** medications. Aerosolized treatment is a therapy process for patients with pulmonary disorders that involves the use of aerosolized medications.

Booths used for source control should be equipped with fans that remove 99.9 percent of the airborne particles between the time when one patient leaves and the next enters. The efficiency of removal depends upon the number of air changes per hour (ACH) in the booth the exhaust fan is capable of producing and the rate of air intake (makeup) air into the booth. Exhaust and makeup air is measured in cubic feet per minute (cfm), and air volumes can be determined by using a velometer (airflow-measuring instrument).

The exhaust fan must maintain negative pressure in the booth. This means the pressure in the booth must be less than the pressure of the air outside the booth. This ensures that the infectious droplet nuclei will remain in the booth and not move into the adjacent room or corridors. Air that is exhausted from the booth to the outside must be kept away from air intakes, windows, people, and animals. If booth air cannot be safely exhausted because of reentrainment back into the building, the local exhaust system must be equipped with a **high-efficiency particulate air (HEPA)** filter. This filter is capable of filtering out 99.97 percent of particles with diameters of 0.3 **microns** or larger.

Use of Respirators for Source Control. HEPA air purifying filter particulate respirators (reusable type) can be effective in preventing infectious droplet nuclei from being inhaled by health care workers. These may be respirators with inhalation and exhalation valves with HEPA filters or the new NIOSH approved particulate respirator series that replaces the HEPA filter respirators. The new NIOSH approved series is described under "Respirators." Respirators must be worn during high-hazard procedures, when patients are transported, or when workers enter rooms of patients who are confirmed or suspected of having TB.

Respirators with inhalation and exhalation valves should *not* be worn by patients. They should wear respirators or ordinary face masks without valves, because the TB bacilli is in the respirator and must be prevented from becoming airborne.

When respirators are used, the OSHA respirator standard 29 CFR 1910.134 and 1910.139 must be followed.

Controlling Air Contamination

Infectious droplet nuclei that are released into a room can be controlled by

- Ventilation, supplemented by HEPA filters

- Germicidal ultraviolet (UV) irradiation
- Respirators
- A combination of the above.

Ventilation. The American Society of Heating, Refrigeration, and Air Conditioning Engineers (ASHRAE), has guidelines for controlling the emission of infectious droplet nuclei in health care settings. To obtain a copy of these guidelines, the address is:

ASHRAE
1791 Tullie Circle, NE
Atlanta, GA 30329

General exhaust ventilation. General exhaust ventilation systems reduce room contamination by introducing clean outside air into the room and exhausting the contaminated air safely to the exterior. Exhaust systems are considered **engineering controls**. Engineering controls either eliminate hazards by modifying the source of the hazard or by reducing the level of contaminants that become airborne.

General (dilution) ventilation introduces clean air from outside to dilute the contaminated air and exhausts the diluted contaminated air outside the building. This is known as the "push-pull effect." Unless it is impossible to exhaust contaminated air to the exterior, this air must always be exhausted safely outdoors. To be exhausted safely, the exhausted air should not come out where there are animals, pedestrian or vehicular traffic, or occupied areas. All attempts must be made to exhaust to the exterior and to a safe location. If it cannot be done, a system of HEPA filters must be installed in the building ventilation system to trap the microbes. These filters will require a scheduled monitoring program. The problem with recirculating this air is that eventually the infectious nuclei will concentrate in the duct.

The following rooms need air changes as indicated:

1. AFB isolation rooms require at least six complete **air changes per hour (ACH)** with at least two air changes per hour outside air (OA). ACH is the number of times per hour the air is completely changed in a room or space.
2. Treatment rooms require at least six ACH.

3. Intensive care units (ICU) require at least six ACH and at least two ACH of OA.
4. Emergency rooms and waiting areas require at least ten ACH.
5. Autopsy rooms require at least twelve ACH with good negative pressure in the room. The room air exhausted must be exhausted directly to the outside.

> *Note:* Six ACHs will remove 99.9% of TB bacilli in 69 minutes.
> Ten ACHs will remove 99.9% of TB bacilli in 41 minutes.
> Twelve ACHs will remove 99.9% of TB bacilli in 35 minutes.

Air mixing. For most of the microbes in a room to be exhausted, it is necessary to have efficient mixing of clean air with contaminated air. Mixing is more efficient when supply air ducts are located near the ceiling and the exhaust is near the floor.

Pressure differentials. Air flows from high-pressure to low-pressure areas. Therefore, it is important to have patient rooms and booths with air pressure less than the air pressure outside the room or booth.

The patient's room must always be under negative pressure. This will prevent contaminated air from getting into other areas of the building. Periodic checks with a smoke tube or smoke stick, will determine if proper airflow is being maintained. The smoke generated is harmless and will not affect the patient. Fans create **static pressure**, which is the air pressure in all directions as it moves in a room or in a duct. Likewise, ducts will convey air more efficiently if they are smooth and have a minimum of bends and transitions.

Opening and closing doors, movement of people, temperature, and stairwells and elevator shafts acting as plenums cause problems with maintaining negative pressure in the contaminated room. It is important to keep doors closed, particularly doors to contaminated areas. If a problem with maintaining pressure differential persists due to constant opening of doors, a pressurized anteroom may solve the problem.

Pressure differentials can also be upset when exhaust fans, ducts, or filters are not cleaned, when system components malfunction, when adjustments are made to the building ventilation system, or when the air intakes are closed during cold weather. Health care facilities should have employees knowledgeable in the proper maintenance of ventilation systems.

The OSHA guidelines for indoor air quality should be followed to ensure proper system operation. The section describing the OSHA guidelines should be reviewed.

HEPA Filters. High-efficiency particulate air (HEPA) filters should be used if air is recirculated in general use areas such as waiting or emergency rooms. As previously mentioned, HEPA filters are capable of filtering out 99.97 percent of particles 0.3 microns or larger. Infectious droplet nuclei (1.5-6 microns) fall within this size, so they should be effectively filtered out from recirculated air. It is *strongly* recommended that air from isolation rooms *not* be recirculated into the general building ventilation system even when HEPA filters are used.

HEPA filters have proven effective in centralized air-conditioning units as well as HEPA filtration systems with laminar airflow in isolation rooms. Portable units that filter room air rather than incoming air are also effective in filtering out the tuberculosis microbes. Portable units can be used as temporary controls when patients are housed in hospital areas that do not have recommended isolation controls. They can also be used in general use areas where other methods of control are inadequate.

Whenever HEPA filters are used, qualified personnel must assess and design the ventilation system to make sure there is adequate supply and exhaust air. It is essential that the HEPA system be properly maintained and tested on a regular basis, such as in a preventative maintenance program. Filters must be checked to make sure there are no gaps in the filter bed or gaps between the filter bed and frame that might allow passage of microbes. Filter inspections should be part of any preventative maintenance program.

A manometer to measure static pressure should be installed in the system to determine when filters need replacement. Filter removal, replacement, and disposal should be done by properly protected qualified personnel.

Germicidal Ultraviolet Lamps

Ultraviolet (UV) irradiation is recommended by the Centers for Disease Control and Prevention in controlling infectious droplet nuclei in patient rooms as long as proper safeguards are used to prevent short-term exposure. UV is a non-ionizing radiation that kills the TB bacilli with heat. Care must be taken that patients and workers are not over exposed to the UV radiation. UV is an effective supplement to the ventilation system when the risk of infection is high. It is recommended as a supplement in ICUs, emergency rooms, during bronchoscopy, and in waiting rooms when there is a high risk of infection. A negative aspect of UV lamp use is that it is less effective when the relative humidity in the room exceeds 70 percent.

UV lamps can be wall or ceiling mounted or installed in the ventilation system. Wall or ceiling units disinfect the air within the room. The effectiveness of these units depends upon the mixing of the air within the room. The organisms must be carried by air to within range of the UV units. Units installed in ducts disinfect the air ducts but will not protect persons in the isolation room. They are effective in general use areas such as waiting and emergency rooms.

UV irradiation *should not* be used to justify the recirculation of air from an isolation room into the building air system.

UV Health Hazards. The main drawback to using UV irradiation is that short-term exposure can cause inflammation of the cornea and conjunctiva of the eye, and skin redness, as is the case with other forms of non-ionizing radiation. Long-term exposure can cause basal cell carcinoma and cataracts. Over exposure to health care employees can be prevented if UV lamp configurations meet applicable safety guidelines and properly tinted eye or face protection is worn.

UV Warning Indicators. UV lamps installed in ducts should have warning signs placed on access doors leading to the lamps. This warning should indicate that it is a safety hazard to look at the lamps and that properly tinted glasses must be worn when accessing these lamps. The doors should also have a warning light that indicates when the lamps are on. UV lamps in the duct must be prevented from emitting radiation into occupied areas (lamps should not be placed near duct openings to rooms).

UV Installation and Maintenance. Only qualified persons should install UV lamps in ducts. After they are installed, they should be checked with a UV meter to determine their effectiveness.

Lamps must be periodically checked for dust buildup and cleaned as necessary. Cleaning personnel should be warned to shut off the lamps before servicing. It is recommended that a red warning light be on the lamp to indicate when the rated life of the lamp is nearing its end.

Respirators

Both the CDC and OSHA require that respirators be worn when the respiratory systems of employees are at risk because of exposure, or potential exposure, to tuberculosis pathogens.

The CDC guidelines require that these respirators be able to

1. Filter particles one micron in size in the unloaded state with a filter efficiency of equal to, or more than, 95%. This indicates filter leakage of no more than, or equal to, 5% when the flow rate is up to 50 liters per minute.
2. Be **qualitatively** or **quantitatively** fit tested to ensure face leakage of the face seal of equal to, or less than, 10%. These fit tests determine the adequacy of respirator fit by measuring the amount of contaminant in the facepiece to that outside the facepiece or by the wearer's reaction to a test material.
3. Make sure the different facial sizes of health care workers are accommodated by having the respirators available in a sufficient number of models and sizes.
4. Be checked for facepiece fit, in accordance with OSHA requirements and accepted industrial hygiene procedures, each time the respirator is donned by the worker. This must be done by either the negative or positive fit check.

The present HEPA filter respirators as well as the new NIOSH approved series of particulate respirators meet these specifications.

When HEPA Filter or NIOSH-Approved Particulate Respirators Are to Be Worn. The HEPA filter or NIOSH-approved particulate filter respirator must be worn

1. When entering rooms where the patient has, or may have, infectious TB.
2. During high-hazard procedures on patients who have suspected or confirmed infectious TB. This includes during the administering of **aerosolized pentamidine (AP)**[1], **bronchoscopy**[2], and **endotracheal intubation**[3] and suctioning.
3. When health care workers or emergency response personnel transport individuals who are suspected of having, or have, infectious TB.

Respirator replacement. If the health care facility elects to use disposable HEPA filter particulate respirators or the NIOSH-approved particulate respirators, they may be reused by the *same* health care worker providing the respirator maintains its structural and functional integrity and the filter material is not damaged or soiled. When resistance to breathing is encountered by the wearer, the respirator should be discarded and a new one worn. The facility is responsible for determining the circumstances in which the respirator is considered contaminated and not to be reused. How long it may be used will depend upon the frequency and circumstances of its use.

NIOSH-Approved Respirators. The National Institute for Occupational Safety and Health (NIOSH) has specified a series of respirators to replace the HEPA filter type. These respirators are tested at a flow rate of 85 liters per minute to determine the degree of penetration by particles with 0.3 micron diameter.

---

[1] Aerosolized pentamidine is a therapy process for TB patients that involves the use of AP.
[2] Bronchoscopy is the visual examination of the interior of the bronchos.
[3] Endotracheal intubation is the process of providing an airway through the trachea by inserting a tube.

If the respirator stops 99.97% of the particles, it will be rated as type 100; if it stops 99%, it is rated type 99; if it stops 95%, it is rated type 95. NIOSH indicates that all three types of these respirators effectively stop the tuberculosis pathogen. Therefore, the minimally accepted respirator that will protect against infectious droplet nuclei is the type 95.

Decontamination Procedures

Items requiring disinfection can be categorized as follows:

- Critical items: Needles (disposable needles should be used), surgical instruments, cardiac catheters, or implants introduced directly into the bloodstream, or into other normally sterile areas of the body.
- Semicritical items: Noninvasive flexible and rigid fibre optic endoscopes or bronchoscopes, endotracheal tubes, or anesthesia breathing circuits that may come in contact with mucous membranes but do not normally penetrate body surfaces.
- Noncritical items: Crutches, bedboards, blood pressure cuffs, and other medical accessories.

Critical items must be sterilized when they are used; semicritical items may be sterilized, but usually a high-level disinfection procedure that destroys microrganisms, fungal spores, tubercule bacilli, and small nonlipid viruses can be used. A good physical cleaning before high-level disinfection is important; noncritical items may be washed with a detergent.

The health care facility should determine when and which decontamination procedures must be implemented. Procedures followed should be based on the use of the item and not on the diagnosis of the patient. Selection of chemical disinfectants depends upon intended use, level of decontamination required, and the configuration and type of material to be disinfected.

Screening and Surveillance of Health Care Workers

Screening and surveillance of health care workers must include:

1. Employer offered TB skin testing (at no cost to employee) to all new employees and potentially exposed employees.
2. Periodic evaluations and TB skin testing every three months for workers in high-risk categories, every six months for workers in intermediate risk, annually for low-risk employees.
3. Reassessment when an employee has an exposure or change in health.

Emergency Transport Employees

When employees transport patients who have suspected or confirmed active TB, they must wear a HEPA filter respirator or NIOSH approved particulate respirator. It is recommended that they leave the rear windows of the vehicle open and the heating and air conditioning system set on a nonrecirculating cycle.

Home Health Services

Workers must wear a HEPA filter respirator or the NIOSH approved particulate filter respirator when they go to the home of a patient with suspected or confirmed active TB. Any cough-inducing procedures, such as aerosolized pentamidine (AP), must be done in a well-ventilated area away from other household members.

OSHA GUIDELINES

OSHA uses the CDC guidelines when enforcing procedures and scheduling for occupational exposure to tuberculosis.

When and Where OSHA Inspects

Evaluation of occupational exposure to TB will be conducted

- In response to employee complaints.
- In related fatalities.
- When catastrophes occur.
- As a part of industrial hygiene inspections in workplaces that the CDC has identified as those where workers have a greater risk of infection in relation to the general population.

Inspections will include a review of the employer's plan for TB control, respiratory protection program, skin testing, employee interviews, and site observations by the compliance health and safety officer (CHSO).

Inspection Procedures

The CHSO will request to see the infection control director, the employee responsible for occupational hazard control, records on training and exposure, and those employees who maintain them.

The CHSO will determine whether a facility had a suspected or confirmed case of TB within the past six months. If a determination is made, the CHSO will proceed with the TB portion of the inspection, which includes a review of emergency rooms, respiratory therapy areas, bronchoscopy suites, and morgue. Compliance will be determined by

- The facility plans for TB protection.
- Inspection of involved areas.
- Employee interviews.

Citation Policy

OSHA will cite the following standards when violations to the guidelines are noted:

- Section 5(a)(1): General Duty Clause.
- 29 CFR 1910.134 and 1910.139: Respiratory Protection.
- 29 CFR 1910.145: Accident Prevention Signs and Tags.
- 29 CFR 1910.1020: Access to Employee Exposure and Medical Records.
- 29 CFR 1904: Recording and Reporting Occupational Injuries and Illness.

The CHSO will address all of the above standards to ensure employee protection from TB infection. Violations are normally classified as serious.

Citations will be issued under the general duty clause as follows:

- When employees are exposed to the exhaled air of an individual with suspected or confirmed pulmonary TB.
- When employees are exposed without appropriate protection, to high-hazard procedures performed on patients with suspected or con-

firmed infectious TB, such as aerosolized medication treatment, bronchoscopy, sputum induction, endotracheal intubation and suctioning procedures, endoscopic procedures, emergency dental work, and hospital autopsies.

Feasible and Useful Abatement Methods

If OSHA determines that there are deficiencies in any of the following areas, citations may be issued under the general duty clause.

Early Identification of Patient or Client. The employer must develop a protocol for the identification of individuals with active TB. The CDC guidelines should be followed as described under the section "Degree of Infection Determination."

Medical Surveillance. Medical surveillance is very important in the control of TB. Examinations are mandatory for certain categories of employees.

Initial Examinations. The employer must offer the TB skin test, at no cost to employees, who are potentially exposed and to all new employees (prior to exposure). A two-step baseline must be used for new employees who have an initially negative PPD test result and who have not had a documented negative TB skin test result during the preceding twelve months. Tests are to be conducted at a time and place convenient to employees. Any follow-up and evaluations are to be offered at no cost to the workers.

Periodic Evaluations. TB skin tests must be done every three months for workers in high-risk situations, every six months for workers in intermediate risk situations, and annually for low-risk workers. CDC criteria must be used to determine high, intermediate, and low risk.

Workers with a documented positive TB skin test who have received treatment or preventative therapy for infection are exempt from the skin test. But they must be informed periodically by a physician or health care provider about the symptoms of TB, and the need for immediate evaluation of any signs suggestive of pulmonary TB. This will help the worker determine if symptoms have developed.

Reassessment Following Exposure or Health Change. Workers who have not been protected against TB transmission, who become exposed to an individual with suspected or confirmed infectious TB, must be managed according to CDC criteria. If an employee develops symptoms of active TB, he or she must be immediately evaluated according to CDC guidelines.

Management of Infected Employees. When an employee indicates a positive TB skin test, this must be followed as soon as possible by appropriate clinical, laboratory, and radiographic evaluations to determine whether the employee has infectious TB.

Depending upon the circumstances, work restrictions must be implemented, as appropriate.

Education and Training. All current employees and new employees upon hire, must be informed of:

1. The mode of TB transmission.
2. Its signs and symptoms.
3. The requirements for medical surveillance.
4. Therapeutic procedures to control the disease.
5. Site-specific protocols that include the purpose and proper use of controls.

Training should be repeated as the need arises.

Employees must also be trained to recognize, and report to a designated person, any individuals with symptoms suggestive of TB, and instructed on the post-exposure protocols to be followed if there is an exposure incident.

Engineering Controls. Persons with suspected or confirmed infectious TB must be placed in acid fast bacilli (AFB) isolation rooms. High-hazard procedures on persons suspected or confirmed to have infectious TB must be performed in AFB treatment rooms, AFB isolation rooms, or booths.

Isolation and treatment rooms must be kept under negative pressure. Air must flow from surrounding areas to the isolation or treatment room. The minimum check on airflow includes using a nonirritating smoke trail or similar indicator. If there is an anteroom, the direction of airflow is demonstrated at the inner door between the isolation or treatment room and the anteroom.

Exhaust air. The CDC guidelines concerning air exhausted from isolation and treatment rooms is mandated by OSHA. You should refer to the sections under CDC guidelines that describe local exhaust ventilation and general exhaust ventilation.

Recirculated contaminated air that goes back into the isolation or treatment room must be decontaminated by a recognized process, such as by a HEPA filter. UV radiation cannot be used as the only means of decontamination. UV is to be used only in waiting rooms, emergency rooms, corridors, and similar rooms where persons with undiagnosed TB could infect the air.

Opening and closing doors. When doors are opened and closed in an isolation or treatment room that does not have an anteroom, it compromises the negative pressure in the room. A combination of controls can be used to minimize pressure loss.

These controls include

- Restricting room entry.
- Adjusting the door closure to slow the door movement to reduce displacement effects.
- Having the doors swing into the room where fire codes permit.
- Avoiding placement of the room air intake near the door.

High-hazard procedures. If high-hazard procedures are used in AFB isolation or treatment rooms without benefit of source control ventilation, or local exhaust ventilation, and droplets are released into the air, then a purge time interval must be put into effect, during which time employees must wear a HEPA filter respirator or the new NIOSH approved particulate respirator before entering the room. In place of wearing a respirator, an interim supplemental ventilation unit (portable unit) equipped with HEPA filters is acceptable. The portable unit must effectively trap the TB bacilli.

Respirator Protection. Employer responsibilities include

- Establishing a respirator program that complies with OSHA 29 CFR 1910.134 and 1910.139.
- Providing respirators when it is necessary to protect the health of the employee.

- Making sure the respirators are adequate to protect for their intended purpose.

Minimal acceptable program. OSHA requires that the respirator meet the CDC specifications as described under the "Respirators" section and the section under "New NIOSH-Approved Respirators."

OSHA also requires respirators to be worn and replaced as described under the CDC section "When HEPA Filter or New NIOSH Approved Particulate Filter Respirators Are to Be Worn."

Access to Employee Exposure and Medical Records. A record of an employee exposed to TB is considered an exposure record and must be handled in accordance with OSHA 29 CFR 1910.1020.

Records of TB skin tests, medical evaluations, and treatment are employee medical records and must be handled in accordance with OSHA 29 CFR 1910.1020.

Accident Prevention Signs and Tags. Isolation and treatment rooms require that a sign stating **"Stop," "Halt,"** or **"No Admittance"** be posted outside the room. A sign showing the biological hazard symbol with appropriate message such as **"Special Respiratory Isolation," "Respiratory Isolation,"** or **"AFB Isolation,"** can also be posted in place of the signs.

A description of the necessary precautions must also be posted, such as **"Respirators Must Be Donned Before Entering."**

Signs are also required for respiratory isolation rooms in an emergency department or, if signs are not posted, a message must be posted that directs a person to a nursing station for instruction.

Biological hazard tags must be used on duct components of HVAC systems (e.g., fans, ducts, and filters) that carry contaminated air so that employees who may have to work on these systems are aware of TB hazard locations.

OSHA Form 200 Recordkeeping. Both the tuberculosis infections (as shown by a positive skin test) and active tuberculosis are recordable on the OSHA 200 log. A positive skin test on initial testing is recordable (except for preassignment screening) because there is a presumption of work-related infection unless it can be clearly shown that the infection was due to outside exposure.

If the employee's TB infection entered on the 200 log progresses to active TB during the five-year maintenance period, the log must be updated to show the new information.

The initial test must be conducted within the first two weeks of employment, prior to any exposure. A positive skin test result diagnosed within that time period does not have to be recorded on the OSHA 200 log.

CHAPTER REVIEW

Multiple Choice
Select the best answer from the choices provided.

1. In order for OSHA to use the general duty clause, the violation must
   a. be such that it can cause serious physical harm
   b. be able to be abated by a feasible method
   c. put an employee(s) at risk
   d. a, b, and c

2. Respiratory and laryngeal TB
   a. is not infectious if the patient is isolated
   b. is considered most infectious
   c. is not infectious if the patient doesn't cough
   d. cannot be treated with drug resistant medication

3. Patient rooms should be kept under

   a. positive pressure
   b. the same pressure as outside the room
   c. negative pressure
   d. same pressure as outside the building

4. OSHA will issue citations under the general duty clause when

   a. doors to isolation rooms are closed
   b. air from isolation rooms is not recirculated into the general building ventilation
   c. UV lamps are used to disinfect ducts
   d. employees are exposed to the exhaled breath of a patient with suspected or confirmed TB

5. For workers in high-risk situations, the TB skin test must be done

   a. every three months
   b. every six months
   c. annually
   d. every two years

True/False

Indicate whether the statement is true or false by circling T or F.

6. T F OSHA can use the general duty clause to cite for TB violations.

7. T F TB can be controlled by collecting the sputum of TB patients.

8. T F HEPA filters can capture 90 percent of particles 0.3 microns or larger.

9. T F UV lamps are most effective in waiting and emergency rooms.

10. T F Cars used to transport TB patients should have the windows closed.

Matching

Match the terms in column 1 with the definitions in column 2.

	Column 1		*Column 2*
11.	Local exhaust ventilation	a.	Administering AP
12.	Diagnostic measure	b.	Surgical instruments
13.	High-hazard procedure	c.	Booth
14.	Critical item	d.	Skin test for TB
15.	Mantoux	e.	Bronchoscopy or biopsy

Short Answer

Briefly but thoroughly answer each statement.

16. Explain some of the ways to control TB transmission in a health care facility.

17. What are some of the ways you would protect employees from getting TB from patients.

18. Why would you use respirators or engineering controls?

19. Why wouldn't you have patients wear respirators with valves?

20. Discuss the necessary records that are to be maintained.

CHAPTER 15

Bloodborne Pathogens

After studying this chapter, you should be able to

➤ State the OSHA requirements for bloodborne pathogens.
➤ Identify the requirements for an exposure control plan.
➤ List what are considered infectious materials.
➤ Explain the use of engineering and work practice controls.
➤ Define the term "universal precautions."

OSHA 29 CFR 1910.1030 BLOODBORNE PATHOGENS

The OSHA bloodborne pathogens standard is 29 CFR 1910.1030. The purpose of the standard is to limit exposure to bloodborne pathogens and other infectious materials that can lead to disease and death.

It covers all employees who are expected to come in contact with blood and other potentially infectious substances. This includes employees in the hospitals as well as those in doctors', dentists', and veterinary offices.

The important aspect of this standard for the employer is to ensure that employees, who come in contact with infectious materials, are trained to follow **universal precautions**. These precautions assume that *all* infectious materials are hazardous, unless proven otherwise.

Definitions

Blood means human blood, human blood components, and products made from human blood.

Bloodborne pathogen means pathogenic microorganisms that are present in human blood and can cause disease in humans.

Contaminated means the presence or the reasonably anticipated presence of blood or other potentially infectious materials on any item or surface.

Contaminated laundry means laundry that has been soiled with blood or other potentially infectious materials or may contain sharps.

Decontamination means the use of physical or chemical means to remove, inactivate, or destroy bloodborne pathogens on a surface or item.

Engineering controls means controls (e.g., sharps disposal containers, self-sheathing needles) that isolate or remove bloodborne pathogens.

Exposure incident means a specific eye, mouth, other mucous membrane, nonintact skin, or parenteral contact with blood or other potentially infectious materials.

HBV means hepatitis B virus.

HIV means human immunodeficiency virus.

Other potentially infectious materials means semen, vaginal secretions, cerebrospinal fluid, synovial fluid, pleural fluid, pericardial fluid, peritoneal fluid, amniotic fluid, saliva in dental procedures, any body fluid that is visibly contaminated with blood, and all body fluids in situations where it is difficult or impossible to differentiate between body fluids; any unfixed tissue or organ from a human (living or dead); and HIV-containing cell or tissue culture medium or other solutions from experimental animals infected with HBV or HIV.

Parenteral means piercing mucous membranes or the skin barrier through needlesticks, human bites, and abrasions.

Personal protective equipment (PPE) means

specialized clothing or equipment worn by the employee for protection against a hazard.

Regulated waste means liquid or semiliquid blood or other potentially infectious materials; contaminated items that would release blood or other potentially infectious materials in a liquid or semiliquid state if compressed; items that are caked with dried blood or other potentially infectious materials and are capable of releasing these materials during handling; contaminated sharps; and pathological and microbiological wastes containing blood or other potentially infectious materials.

Sterilize means the use of a physical or chemical procedure to destroy all microbial life including highly resistant bacterial spores.

Universal precautions is the concept that all human blood and certain human body fluids are treated as if known to be infectious for HIV, HBV, and other bloodborne pathogens.

Work practice controls means controls that reduce the likelihood of exposure by altering the manner in which a task is performed (e.g., prohibiting the recapping of needles by a two-handed technique).

Exposure Control Plan

Each employer having an employee(s) with occupational exposure to blood or other potentially infectious materials shall establish a written Exposure Control Plan designed to eliminate or minimize employee exposure.

The Exposure Control Plan shall contain at least the following elements:

- Those listed under Methods of Compliance
- Those listed under HIV and HBV Research Laboratories
- Those listed under Hepatitis B Vaccination and Post Exposure Evaluation and follow-up
- Those listed under Communication of Hazards to Employees
- Those listed under Recordkeeping

The employer shall ensure that a copy of the Exposure Control Plan is accessible to employees.

The Exposure Control Plan shall be reviewed and updated at least annually and whenever necessary to reflect new or modified tasks and proce-

dures that affect occupational exposure and to reflect new or revised employee positions with occupational exposure.

The Exposure Control Plan shall be made available to OSHA upon request.

Exposure Determination. The employer shall prepare an exposure determination, and it shall contain the following:

- A list of all job classifications in which all employees have exposure.
- A list of job classifications in which some employees have exposure.
- A list of tasks and procedures or groups of closely related tasks and procedures in which exposure occurs.

This exposure determination shall be made without regard to the use of personal protective equipment.

Methods of Compliance

Universal precautions shall be observed to prevent contact with blood or other potentially infectious materials. Under circumstances in which differentiation between body fluid types is difficult or impossible, all body fluids shall be considered potentially infectious materials.

Engineering and work practice controls shall be used to eliminate or minimize employee exposure. Where exposure remains after these controls are used, personal protective equipment shall also be used.

Engineering controls shall be examined and maintained or replaced on a regular schedule to ensure their effectiveness.

The employer shall provide handwashing facilities that are readily accessible.

Employers shall ensure that employees wash their hands and any other skin with soap and water, or flush mucous membranes with water immediately following contact with blood or other potentially infectious materials.

Contaminated needles and other contaminated sharps shall not be bent, recapped, or removed. Shearing or breaking of contaminated needles is prohibited. Bending, recapping, or removing of needles is permissible if the employer can show that there is no alternative and that it is done through the use of mechanical devices or a one-handed technique.

Immediately, or as soon as possible after use, contaminated reusable sharps shall be placed in appropriate containers until reprocessed. These containers shall be

- Puncture resistant
- Labeled or color-coded
- Leakproof on the sides and bottom
- Not processed or stored so that employees have to reach into them

Eating, drinking, smoking, applying cosmetics or lip balm, and handling contact lenses is prohibited in areas where there is the likelihood of exposure.

Food and drink shall not be kept in refrigerators, shelves, cabinets, or on countertops where blood or other potentially infectious materials are present.

All procedures involving blood or other potentially infectious materials shall be performed to minimize splashing, spraying, spattering, and generation of droplets.

Mouth pipetting, suctioning of blood or other potentially infectious materials, is prohibited.

Specimens of blood or other potentially infectious materials shall be placed in containers that prevent leakage during collection, handling, processing, storage, transport, or shipping. The container must be labeled or color-coded and closed.

If outside contamination of the container occurs, it must be put into a second container that prevents leakage.

If the specimen can puncture the container, the container must be put into a second container that is puncture resistant.

Equipment that may become contaminated with blood or other potentially infectious materials must be examined prior to servicing or shipping and must be decontaminated as necessary. A label must be attached to those portions of the equipment that could not be decontaminated.

Personal protective equipment must be provided to employees who are exposed. This includes gloves, gowns, laboratory coats, face shields or masks, eye protection, mouthpieces, resuscitation bags, pocket masks, or ventilation devices.

The employer shall ensure that employees use appropriate personal protective equipment and that such equipment is readily accessible.

The employer shall clean, launder, and dispose of personal protective equipment. Garments penetrated by blood or other potentially infectious materials must be removed as soon as possible.

All protective equipment shall be removed prior to leaving the work area. When it is removed, it must be placed in a designated area or container for storage, washing, decontamination, or disposal.

Gloves shall be worn if the employee may come in contact with potentially infectious materials, mucous membranes, and nonintact skin when performing vascular access procedures, and when handling or touching contaminated items. Disposal gloves must be replaced if they are torn or punctured.

Masks, eye protection, and face shields in combination with goggles or glasses shall be worn whenever splashes, spray, spatter, or droplets of blood or other potentially infectious materials may be generated that can get into the eyes, nose, or mouth.

Gowns, aprons, surgical caps, shoe covers, or boots shall be worn when the exposure dictates.

Employers shall ensure that the worksite is maintained in a clean and sanitary manner.

All equipment and working surfaces shall be cleaned and decontaminated after contact with blood and other potentially infectious materials. This must be done with an appropriate disinfectant.

All bins, pails, cans, and similar receptacles shall be inspected and decontaminated on a regular basis.

Broken glassware that may be contaminated must be cleaned up using a brush, dust pan, tongs, or forceps.

Reusable sharps that are contaminated must not be stored or processed in any manner that employees have to reach into them.

Regulated Waste. Contaminated sharps must be discarded immediately in containers that are closeable, puncture resistant, leakproof, and labeled or color-coded.

During use, sharps containers shall be easily accessible, be kept upright, and not be allowed to be overfilled.

When moving containers, they must be closed and placed in a second container if leakage is possible. The second container must be closed, leakproof, and labeled or color-coded.

Other regulated waste must be handled in a similar manner to that of the sharps.

Contaminated laundry must be handled as little as possible. The laundry must be placed in bags or containers that are labeled or color-coded.

Whenever contaminated laundry is wet, it must be placed in a second bag or container that is leakproof.

Employees who collect contaminated laundry must wear eye protection.

HIV and HBV Research Laboratories and Production Facilities

This section applies to facilities engaged in the culture, production, concentration, experimentation, and manipulation of HIV and HBV. It does not apply to clinical or diagnostic laboratories engaged solely in the analysis of blood, tissues, or organs.

All regulated waste must be either incinerated or decontaminated by autoclaving.

Access to work areas shall be limited to authorized persons.

Contaminated materials are to be placed in durable, leakproof containers that are closed before removing from the work area.

When infected materials or animals are in the work area, hazard warning signs shall be posted.

All activities involving infectious materials shall be done in biological safety cabinets or in similar containment devices.

Laboratory coats, gowns, smocks, and uniforms shall be used in work areas and animal rooms.

Gloves must be worn when handling animals or when coming in contact with infectious materials.

Before disposal, all waste from work areas and from animal rooms must be either incinerated or decontaminated by autoclaving.

Hypodermic needles and syringes must be used only for parenteral injection and aspiration of fluids from laboratory animals and diaphragm bottles. Only needle-locking syringes or disposable syringe-needle units must be used for injection or aspiration of other potentially infectious materials.

All spills must be immediately cleaned up by trained employees.

A spill or accident that results in an exposure must be reported immediately to the laboratory director or other authorized individual.

Biological safety cabinets and/or combinations of personal protective equipment must be used for all activities with other potentially infectious materials.

HBV and HIV laboratories must have handwashing and eyewash facilities and autoclave for decontamination.

Work areas must be separated from areas that are open to unrestricted traffic flow. Passage through two sets of doors is required to get to work areas. Surfaces of doors, walls, floors, and ceilings must be water-resistant.

Each work area must have a sink and eyewash facility.

Doors to work areas must be self-closing.

An autoclave must be located as near as possible to the work area.

A ducted ventilation system must be provided. The exhaust air cannot be recirculated to any other part of the building. It must be discharged outside and away from occupied areas and air intakes.

Hepatitis B Vaccination and Post-Exposure Follow-Up

The employer must make available the hepatitis B vaccine and vaccination series, and post-exposure follow-up to all employees who have exposure on the job.

Medical evaluations, vaccinations, and post-exposure follow-up must be at no cost to the employee. They must be at a reasonable time and place and performed by a licensed physician or under the supervision of a licensed health care professional.

All tests must be done by an accredited laboratory at no cost to the employee.

The hepatitis B vaccination must be made available to all exposed employees within ten working days of initial assignment unless the employee has previously received the vaccination series or is immune, or the vaccination is contraindicated for medical reasons.

If the employee declines the vaccination, but later decides to have it, the employer must make it available. If it is declined, the employer must have the employee sign a declination form.

Post-Exposure and Follow-Up. Following a report of an exposure incident, the employer shall make immediately available to the exposed employee a confidential medical evaluation and follow-up including at least the following elements:

- Documentation of the routes of exposure
- Identification and documentation of the source individual (unless required to be kept confidential)

The source individual's blood must be tested as soon as feasible and results of the test must be made available to the employee.

The health care professional responsible for the employee's hepatitis B vaccination must receive a copy of the bloodborne pathogens regulation, a description of the employee's duties, documentation of the route(s) of exposure, results of the individual's blood testing, and all medical records relevant to appropriate treatment.

The employer must obtain and provide the employee with a copy of the health care professional's written opinion within fifteen days of the completion of the evaluation.

The health care professional's written opinion for post-exposure evaluation and follow-up must be limited to the following information:

- That the employee has been informed of the results of the evaluation
- That the employee has been told about any medical condition resulting from exposure which requires further evaluation or treatment

All other findings must remain confidential.

Communication of Hazards to Employees

Warning labels must be affixed to containers of regulated waste, refrigerators and freezers containing infectious waste, and other containers used to store, transport, or ship infectious materials.

The label must include the standard biohazard legend with the word "Biohazard." These labels must be fluorescent orange-red with lettering or symbols in a contrasting color.

Red bags may be substituted for labels.

Regulated waste that has been decontaminated need not be labeled or color-coded.

The employer must post signs at the entrances to work areas in HIV and HBV Research Laboratory and Production Facilities. The sign must bear the biohazard sign with the word "Biohazard." It must also indicate the name of the infectious agent, special requirements when entering the area, and the name and telephone number of the laboratory director or other responsible person.

These signs shall be the same color as previously indicated.

Information and Training. All employees with exposure must be trained. Training must be provided as follows:

- At the time of initial assignment
- At least annually thereafter

Annual training must be provided within one year of the previous training.

Additional training must be provided when changes such as modification of tasks or procedures affect employee exposure.

Training must contain at least the following:

- A copy of this standard
- A general explanation of the epidemiology and symptoms of bloodborne diseases
- An explanation of the modes of transmission of bloodborne pathogens
- An explanation of the exposure control plan and where it is located
- An explanation of the methods for recognizing tasks that involve exposure to infectious materials
- An explanation of the use and limitations of methods that will prevent or reduce exposure (engineering and work practice controls, and PPE)

- Information on the types, use, removal, handling, decontamination, and disposal of PPE
- An explanation for the basis of selecting PPE
- Information on the hepatitis B vaccination
- Information on the action to take for emergencies involving infectious materials
- An explanation of the procedure to follow if an exposure occurs, including reporting and medical follow-up
- An explanation of the signs and labels required
- Question and answer period

Persons conducting the training must be knowledgeable.

Additional training (in addition to that just described) for employees in HIV and HBV laboratories and production facilities must include the following:

- The employer shall assure that employees demonstrate proficiency in standard microbiological practices and techniques.
- The employer shall assure that employees have had prior experience in handling human pathogens or tissue cultures.
- The employer must provide training to employees who have no prior experience in handling human pathogens.

Recordkeeping

Medical Records. The employer must establish and maintain an accurate record for each employee with occupational exposure. The records must include the name and social security number of the employee; a copy of the employee's hepatitis B vaccination status, including dates of vaccination and medical records relative to the vaccination; a copy of the results of examinations; the employer's copy of the health care professional's written opinion; and a copy of the information provided to the health care professional.

The contents of the record cannot be disclosed without the consent of the employee.

Training Records. Training records must include the dates of training, contents of the training, names and qualifications of trainers, and names and job titles of those attending.

Training records must be kept for three years from the date of training.

All records must be available to OSHA upon request.

Employee medical and training records must be made available to employees upon request.

CHAPTER REVIEW

True/False

Indicate whether the statement is true or false by indicating T or F.

1. T F Saliva generated in dental procedures is not considered potentially infectious.

2. T F The exposure control plan may be presented to employees verbally.

3. T F A method of compliance with the bloodborne pathogens standard is work practice controls.

4. T F Post-exposure follow-up includes employee counseling.

5. T F Health care providers treating employees must be given a sample of the fluid they were exposed to.

Matching

Match the terms in column 1 with the definitions in column 2.

Column 1		Column 2
6.	Universal precautions	a.	Making every attempt to identify source of fluids
7.	Infectious substance	b.	Assumption that all bodily fluids are hazardous
8.	Required in training	c.	How necessary records are kept
9.	Required in post-exposure follow-up	d.	Peritoneal fluid
10.	Required in exposure control plan	e.	A copy of the bloodborne pathogens standard

Short Answer

Briefly but thoroughly answer each statement.

11. Explain why post-exposure follow-up is important.

12. Discuss some engineering controls.

13. Discuss some work practice controls.

CHAPTER 16

Respirators

OBJECTIVES

After studying this chapter, you should be able to

➤ List the requirements for the OSHA respirator standard (OSHA 29 CFR 1910.134).
➤ Identify the various respirators and their limitations.
➤ State the situations when respirators are required.
➤ Identify the training requirements and content for employees who wear respirators.
➤ Explain written standard operating procedures for a respirator program.

OSHA 29 CFR 1910.134 RESPIRATORS

The OSHA respirator standard was extensively revised in April 1998. It was rewritten as a **performance standard**. A performance standard allows the employer flexibility in the methods he/she may use to conform to the standard.

The employer must determine first if contaminant levels can be brought below the **permissible exposure limits (PEL)** by substituting a less toxic material, using work practice controls or engineering controls. If these controls cannot be used, then respirators must be worn. The PEL is the limit of a toxic substance that a worker can be exposed to over a designated period. This should be determined by a qualified person (preferably an industrial hygienist) before a respirator is selected.

One of the important requirements for the employer is to ensure that the proper respirator is issued to the employee for the type and level of exposure and work conditions. Exposure levels must always be determined first before assigning a particular respirator.

If respirator use is not required by this standard, but the employee wishes to wear one, the employer may provide a respirator or permit the employee to use his/her own if the employer determines that its use will not in itself create a hazard. If the employer determines that voluntary use is permitted, the employer must provide the users with the information contained in Appendix D of the standard titled "Information for Employees Using Respirators When Not Required Under the Standard."

If voluntary use is permitted, the employer must include in the written respiratory program those elements necessary to ensure that the employee is medically able to use the respirator, and that the respirator is cleaned, stored, and maintained so that its use does not present a health hazard to the user.

Respiratory Protection Program

The OSHA standard requires employers to establish a written respiratory protection program. The program must contain worksite-specific procedures and be updated as necessary to reflect changes in workplace conditions that affect respirator use. The program has to be administered by a trained administrator and must consist of the following:

1. Procedures for selecting respirators to be used in the workplace
2. Medical evaluations of employees who must wear respirators
3. Fit testing procedures for tight fitting respirators
4. Procedures for proper respirator use for routine and emergency use situations

77

5. Procedures and schedules for cleaning, disinfecting, storing, inspecting, repairing, discarding, and maintaining respirators
6. Procedures to ensure that the air quality, quantity, and flow of breathing air for atmosphere supplying respirators is adequate
7. Training of employees who must wear respirators concerning the hazards to which they are potentially exposed during routine and emergency situations
8. Procedures used for evaluating the program on a regular basis

Procedures for Selecting Respirators to Be Used in the Workplace. The employer must select and provide a proper respirator based on the hazards to which the worker is exposed and factors in the workplace and use that affect respirator performance and reliability. Only NIOSH-certified respirators can be used and must be used in accordance with the conditions of their certification.

The identification and evaluation of respiratory hazards must include an estimate of the employee's exposure and an identification of the contaminant's chemical state and physical form. When the employer cannot identify or reasonably estimate the employee's exposure, the atmosphere must be considered **immediately dangerous to life or health (IDLH)**. IDLH atmospheres are atmospheres that pose an immediate threat to life, would cause irreversible adverse health effects, or would impair an individual's ability to escape from a dangerous atmosphere.

A respirator must be selected from a sufficient number of models and sizes to ensure that it will be acceptable to the employee and properly fit.

Respirators for IDLH atmospheres. Respirators approved for IDLH atmospheres include:

- Full face piece pressure demand **self-contained breathing apparatus (SCBA)** certified by NIOSH for a minimum service life of thirty minutes.
- Combination full face piece pressure demand supplied air respirator with auxiliary self-contained supply.

Respirators used for escape only from IDLH atmospheres must be NIOSH-certified for escape from the atmosphere in which they are used. Oxygen deficient atmospheres are considered IDLH.

Respirators for atmospheres that are not IDLH. The employer must provide a respirator that is adequate to protect the health of the employee and ensure compliance with other OSHA regulatory requirements. This includes compliance under routine use and under foreseeable emergency situations.

The respirator must be appropriate for the chemical and physical form of the contaminant.

Respirators approved for protection against gases and vapors include

- Atmosphere supplying.
- Air purifying, provided that the respirator is equipped with an end-of-service indicator certified by NIOSH for the contaminant. If there is no end-of-service indicator appropriate for worksite conditions, the employer must have a change schedule based upon objective information or data that ensures that canisters and cartridges are changed before the end of their service life. This procedure must be included in the respirator program.

Respirators approved for protection against particulates include

- Atmosphere supplying.
- Air purifying equipped with a NIOSH-certified filter under 30 CFR part 11 as a high-efficiency particulate (HEPA) filter, or an air purifying equipped with a filter certified by NIOSH under 42 CFR part 84.
- Air purifying for contaminants consisting primarily of particles with aerodynamic diameters of at least 2 micrometers.
- Air purifying equipped with any filter certified for particulates by NIOSH.

Medical Evaluations for Employees Who Must Wear Respirators. Employees who wear respirators can have physiological and medical problems placed on them. This can be due to the type of respirator worn, medical status, and worksite conditions.

The employer is required to determine the employee's ability to wear a respirator before any fit test or wearing of the respirator. The medical evaluation is not required when the employee no longer is required to wear a respirator.

Medical evaluation procedures. The employer must select a **physician or other licensed health care professional (PLHCP)** to conduct medical evaluations using a medical questionnaire or an initial medical examination that has the same information as the medical questionnaire. The medical evaluation must obtain the information indicated by the questionnaire in Sections 1 and 2, Part A of Appendix C of this standard. A PLHCP is a physician or other licensed health care professional whose legally permitted scope of work (that is, by license, registration, or certification) allows him or her to independently provide, or be delegated the responsibility to provide, some or all of the health care services required by this standard.

Follow-up medical examination. The follow-up medical examination has to include any medical tests, consultations, or diagnostic procedures that the PLHCP considers necessary to make a final determination.

Administration of the medical questionnaire and examinations. The medical questionnaire and examinations must be conducted during the employee's normal working hours or at a time and place convenient to the employee. The employee must understand the content of the medical questionnaire.

The employer must give the employee an opportunity to discuss the questionnaire and examination results with the PLHCP.

Information to be given to the PLHCP. The following information must be given to the PLHCP by the employer before the PLHCP makes a decision concerning an employee's ability to wear a respirator:

1. Type and weight of the respirator
2. Duration and frequency of use (including use for rescue and escape)
3. Expected physical work effort
4. Additional protective clothing and equipment to be worn
5. Temperature and humidity extremes that may be encountered

Any supplemental information previously provided to the PLHCP regarding an employee need not be provided for a subsequent medical evaluation if the information and the PLHCP remain the same.

The employer must provide the PLHCP with a copy of his/her written respiratory protection program and a copy of the medical evaluation section of the standard.

When the employer replaces the PLHCP, he/she must ensure that the new PLHCP obtains this information.

Medical determination. When determining the employee's ability to wear a respirator, the employer must obtain from the PLHCP a written recommendation concerning the employee's ability to wear a respirator. This recommendation must include the following information:

1. Any limitations on respirator use related to the medical condition of the employee, or relating to workplace conditions where it will be used, including whether the employee is medically able to use the respirator
2. The need for any follow-up medical evaluations
3. A statement that the PLHCP has provided the employee with a copy of the PLHCP's written recommendation

If the respirator is a negative pressure respirator and the PLHCP finds a medical condition that may place the employee's health at risk if the respirator is used, the employer must provide a powered air purifying respirator (PAPR) if the employee's medical evaluation finds that the employee can use this type of respirator. If a subsequent examination determines that the employee can wear a negative pressure type, then the employer no longer is required to provide a PAPR.

Additional medical examinations. Additional medical examinations are required if

- An employee reports medical signs or symptoms related to the ability to wear a respirator.
- A PLHCP, supervisor, or the respirator program administrator informs the employer that an employee needs reevaluation.
- Information from the respiratory protection program, including observations made during

fit testing and program evaluation, indicates a need for reevaluation.

- A change occurs in worksite conditions that may result in an increase in the physiological burden placed on an employee.

Fit Testing Procedures for Tight Fitting Respirators. The employer is required to ensure that all employees who must wear respirators pass a **qualitative fit test** or **quantitative fit test**. A qualitative fit test is a pass/fail fit test that assesses the adequacy of the respirator fit by observing the employee's response to a test agent, such as irritant smoke, banana oil, or sugar aerosol. A quantitative fit test assesses the adequacy of the respirator fit by measuring the amount of leakage in the respirator.

The fit test must be done before the respirator is worn by the employee, whenever a different respirator is used, and at least annually thereafter.

An additional fit test must be conducted whenever the employee reports, or the employer, PLHCP, supervisor, or program administrator makes visual observations of changes in the employee's physical condition that could affect respirator fit. This includes facial scarring, dental changes, cosmetic surgery, or change in body weight.

If, after passing the qualitative or quantitative fit test, the employee notifies the employer, program administrator, supervisor, or PLHCP that the fit of the respirator is not acceptable, the employee must be given reasonable opportunity to select a different respirator face piece and be retested.

Fit test criteria. The fit test protocol must follow procedures contained in Appendix A of this standard. The qualitative fit test can only be used to fit test negative pressure air purifying respirators that must achieve a **fit factor** of 100 or less. A fit factor is a quantitative estimate of the fit of a particular respirator to a specific individual. It estimates the ratio of the concentration of a substance in ambient air to its concentration inside the respirator when worn.

When quantitative fit testing, if the fit factor is equal to or greater than 100 for tight fitting half face pieces, or equal to or greater than 500 for tight fitting full face pieces, the respirator has passed the fit test.

Fit testing of atmosphere supplying and PAPR respirators. Fit testing of tight fitting atmosphere supplying respirators and tight fitting powered air purifying respirators must be done by performing quantitative or qualitative fit testing in the negative pressure mode, regardless of the mode of operation (negative or positive pressure in the face piece).

Qualitative fit testing of these respirators must be done by temporarily converting the face piece into a negative pressure respirator with appropriate filters, or by using an identical negative pressure air purifying respirator face piece with the same sealing surfaces as a surrogate for the atmosphere supplying or powered air purifying respirator face piece.

Quantitative fit testing of these respirators must be done by modifying the face piece to allow sampling inside the face piece breathing zone midway between the nose and the mouth. This is done by installing a permanent sampling probe onto a surrogate face piece, or by using a sampling adapter designed to temporarily provide a means of sampling air from inside the face piece.

Any modifications to the respirator face piece for fit testing must be completely removed and the face piece restored to NIOSH-approved configuration, before the face piece can be used in the workplace.

Procedures for Proper Respirator Use for Routine and Emergency Use Situations. Employers are required to implement procedures for the proper use of respirators. This includes prohibiting conditions that can result in face piece leakage, preventing employees from removing respirators in hazardous environments, taking actions to ensure continued effective respirator operation, and establishing procedures for use of respirators in IDLH atmospheres or in structural firefighting situations.

Face seal protection. Respirators with tight fitting face pieces cannot be worn when employees have facial hair that comes between the sealing surface of the face piece and the face or that interferes with valve function. This also includes any other condition that interferes with face-to-face piece seal or valve function.

The employer must ensure that if the employee wears corrective glasses or goggles or other personal protective equipment, that the equipment does not interfere with the face-to-face piece seal.

Each time an employee puts on a tight fitting respirator, the employer must require that he/she performs a negative or positive fit check. The procedures contained in Appendix B-1 of this standard or procedures recommended by the respirator manufacturer that are as effective as those in Appendix B-1 must be followed.

Continuing respirator effectiveness. Workplace surveillance of work area conditions and degree of employee exposure or stress must be maintained. If these conditions change that may affect respirator effectiveness, the employer has to reevaluate the continued effectiveness of the respirator.

The employer must allow employees to leave the respirator use area as follows:

1. To wash their faces and respirator face pieces as necessary to prevent eye or skin irritation associated with respirator use.
2. If they detect vapor or gas penetration, changes in breathing resistance, or leakage of the face piece.
3. To replace the respirator, filter, cartridge, or canister elements.

The respirator must be repaired or replaced before he/she may be allowed to return to the work area.

Procedures for IDLH atmospheres. For IDLH atmospheres, the employer must ensure the following:

1. That an employee or employees are located outside the IDLH atmosphere.
2. Visual, voice, or signal line communication is maintained between the employee(s) in the IDLH atmosphere and the employee(s) located outside.
3. The employee(s) located outside are equipped and trained to provide rescue.
4. The employer or designee is notified before the employee(s) located outside the IDLH atmosphere enter the IDLH atmosphere to provide emergency rescue.

5. After notification of the employer or designee, the employer or designee provides necessary assistance.
6. Employees located outside the IDLH are equipped with pressure demand or other positive pressure SCBAs, or a pressure demand or other positive pressure supplied air respirator with auxiliary SCBA, and either proper retrieval equipment, or equivalent means of rescue where retrieval equipment is not required as described in this paragraph.

Procedures and Schedules for Cleaning, Disinfecting, Storing, Inspecting, Repairing, Discarding, and Maintaining Respirators.
Employers are required to maintain and care for the respirators that employees use.

Cleaning and disinfecting. Respirators must be provided that are clean, sanitary, and in good working order. They must be cleaned and disinfected using procedures contained in Appendix B-2 of this standard or procedures recommended by the respirator manufacturer, provided that such procedures are equivalent in effectiveness.

Respirators must be cleaned and disinfected as follows:

1. Those used by the same employee must be cleaned and disinfected as often as necessary to maintain them in a sanitary condition.
2. Those issued to more than one employee must be cleaned and disinfected before being worn by different persons.
3. Those used for emergency use must be cleaned and disinfected after each use.
4. Those used in fit testing and training must be cleaned and disinfected after each use.

Storage. Respirators must be stored as follows:

1. Protected from damage, contamination, dust, sunlight, extreme temperatures, excessive moisture, and damaging chemicals. They also must be stored to prevent deformation of the face piece and exhalation valve.
2. Emergency respirators must be kept accessible, stored in compartments or covers that are clearly marked as containing emergency respi-

rators, and stored in accordance with manufacturer's instructions.

Inspection. Respirators must be inspected as follows:

1. Those used in routine situations must be inspected before each use and during cleaning.
2. Those used for emergencies must be inspected at least monthly and in accordance with manufacturer's recommendations, and checked for proper function before and after each use.
3. Those used for escape-only must be inspected before carried into the workplace for use.
4. Those that are self-contained breathing apparatuses must be inspected monthly.

Respirator inspections have to include the following:

1. A check of respirator function, tightness of connections, and the condition of the various parts, including the face piece, head straps, valves, connecting tube, cartridges, canisters, or filters.
2. A check of the elastomeric parts for pliability and signs of deterioration.
3. Self-contained breathing apparatuses must have the air and oxygen cylinders maintained in a fully charged state and must be recharged when the pressure falls to 90% of the manufacturer's recommended pressure level. The regulator and warning devices must function properly.
4. Respirators used for emergencies must have documentation showing the date of inspection, the name or signature of the inspecting person, the findings, required remedial action, and a serial number or other means of identifying the respirator. This information must be on a tag or label attached to the storage compartment, is kept with the respirator, or is included in inspection reports stored as paper electronic files. This information must be kept until replaced by a subsequent certification.

Repairs. The employer must assure that respirators that fail inspection or are found defective be removed from service and are discarded, repaired, or adjusted as follows:

1. Repairs or adjustments are to be made only by persons properly trained. Only those parts from the manufacturer that are NIOSH-approved and designed for the respirator can be used.
2. Repairs must be made according to the manufacturer's recommendations and specifications for the type and extent of repair.
3. Reducing and admission valves, regulators, and alarms, can only be adjusted or repaired by the manufacturer or a technician trained by the manufacturer.

Procedures to Ensure That the Air Quality, Quantity, and Flow of Breathing Air for Atmosphere Supplying Respirators Is Adequate. The employer has to ensure that compressed air, compressed oxygen, and liquid oxygen used for respiration is in accordance with the following:

1. Compressed and liquid oxygen must meet the United States Pharmacopoeia requirements for medical and breathing oxygen.
2. Compressed breathing air must meet the requirements for **Grade D breathing air** described in ANSI/Compressed Gas Association Commodity Specification for Air, G-7.1-1989. This includes

   a. Oxygen content (v/v) of 19.5–23.5%.
   b. Hydrocarbon (condensed) content of 5 milligrams per cubic meter of air or less.
   c. Carbon monoxide (CO) content of 10 ppm or less.
   d. Carbon dioxide (CO_2) content of 1,000 ppm or less.
   e. Lack of noticeable odor.

Compressed oxygen cannot be used in atmosphere supplying respirators that have previously used compressed air.

Oxygen concentrations greater than 23.5% can only be used in equipment designed for oxygen service and distribution.

Oxygen cylinders that are used to supply breathing air to respirators must meet the following requirements:

1. Cylinders must be tested and maintained as described in the Shipping Container Specifica-

tion Regulations of the Department of Transportation (49 CFR part 173 and part 178).

2. Cylinders purchased for breathing air must have a certificate of analysis from the supplier that certifies that the air meets the requirements for Grade D breathing air.

3. The moisture content in the cylinder cannot exceed a dew point of –50°F (–45°C) at one atmosphere pressure.

Compressors used to supply breathing air to respirators must

1. Prevent the entry of contaminated air into the air supply system.

2. Minimize moisture content so that the dew point at one atmosphere pressure is 10°F (5.56°C) below the ambient temperature.

3. Have in-line air purifying beds and filters to ensure breathing air quality. The beds and filters must be maintained and replaced following manufacturer's instructions.

4. Have a tag that contains the most recent bed or filter change date and signature of the person authorized to perform the change. This tag is to be maintained at the compressor.

For compressors that are not oil-lubricated, the employer must ensure that carbon monoxide levels in the breathing air do not exceed 10 ppm.

For oil-lubricated compressors, the employer must use a high-temperature or carbon monoxide alarm, or both, to monitor carbon monoxide levels. If only high-temperature alarms are used, the air supply must be monitored at intervals sufficient to prevent carbon monoxide in the breathing air from exceeding 10 ppm.

Breathing air couplings must be compatible with outlets for nonrespirable worksite air or other gas systems. Asphyxiating substances cannot be introduced into breathing air lines.

The employer must use breathing gas containers marked in accordance with the NIOSH respirator certification standard 42 CFR part 84.

All filters, cartridges, and canisters used in the workplace must be labeled and color coded with the NIOSH approval label. The label must not be removed and must remain legible.

Training of Employees Who Must Wear Respirators Concerning the Hazards to Which They Are Potentially Exposed during Routine and Emergency Situations. Training and information must be provided by the employer to all employees who are required to wear respirators. The training must be comprehensive, understandable, and done annually, and more often, if necessary. It is also required by the employer to provide basic information on respirators contained in Appendix D of this standard for those employees who wear respirators when not required by this standard or by the employer.

The employer must ensure that each employee can demonstrate the following:

1. Why the respirator is necessary and how proper fit, usage, or maintainance can compromise the protective effect of the respirator.

2. What the limitations and capabilities of the respirator are.

3. How to use the respirator effectively in emergency situations and those in which the respirator malfunctions.

4. How to inspect, put on, and remove, use, and check the respirator seals.

5. What procedures are used for maintenance and storage of the respirator.

6. How to recognize medical signs and symptoms that can limit the effective use of the respirator.

7. The general requirements of this standard.

Training must be conducted in a manner understandable to the employee and provided prior to requiring the employee to wear a respirator.

If an employer can show that a new employee received training within the last twelve months that covered the training elements, he/she is not required to repeat such training provided that the employee can demonstrate knowledge of the training elements. Previous training not repeated initially by the employer must be provided no later than twelve months from the date of the previous training.

Retraining must be conducted annually, and under the following conditions:

1. Changes in the workplace or type of respirator that make the previous training obsolete.
2. The employee does not demonstrate a knowledge in the use of respirators or has not retained the required understanding.
3. Any situation that makes retraining necessary to ensure safe respirator use.

Procedures Used for Evaluating the Program on a Regular Basis. The employer must conduct evaluations of the workplace to ensure that the written respiratory protection program is being properly implemented, and to consult with employees to make sure that they are using respirators properly.

The employer must consult with employees on a regular basis to assess the employee's views on program effectiveness and to identify any problems. Problems so identified must be corrected. Points to be assessed include:

- Respirator fit which includes use of the respirator without interfering with workplace performance.
- Respirator selection for the hazards to which the employee is exposed.
- Proper respirator use under the workplace conditions encountered.
- Respirator maintenance.

Recordkeeping. Records and written information must be kept concerning medical evaluations, fit testing, and the respirator program.

Records of medical evaluations required by this standard must be retained and made available in accordance with OSHA 29 CFR 1910.1020 (see Chapter 5).

Qualitative and quantitative fit testing records must be maintained. These records include:

1. The name or identification of the employee tested.
2. Type of fit test performed.
3. Specific make, model, style, and size of respirator tested.
4. Date of test.
5. The pass/fail results for the qualitative fit test or the fit factor and strip chart recording or

other recording of the test results for the quantitative fit test.

Fit test records must be retained for the respirator until the next fit test is conducted.

A written copy of the current respirator program must be retained by the employer.

Written materials required to be retained by this paragraph must be made available upon request to affected employees and to OSHA for examining and copying.

APPENDIX

This appendix describes the various types of respirators and their limitations.

Respirator Classes

Respirators are categorized into air purifying, atmosphere supplying, and combination air purifying and air supplying.

Air Purifying. *Negative pressure air purifying respirators* make use of filters that purify the air when it is inhaled through the face piece. The pressure in the face piece is negative as compared to outside air. Air is drawn into the face piece through inhalation valves and exhaled through exhalation valves. (See Figure 16-1.) The face piece can be quarter, half, or full size. Filters for particulates remove dusts, fumes, and mists. Particulate filter respirators are being replaced by the NIOSH-approved particulate filter respirators (see next paragraph). Organic vapor/acid gas filters remove gases and vapors. Combination filters remove all contaminants when a pre-filter is included with the filter.

NOISH-approved particulate filter respirators. Effective July 1995, the National Institute for Occupational Safety and Health (NIOSH) has put new regulations into effect concerning negative pressure air purifying respirators that use particulate filters. This is covered under 42 CFR 84, Code of Federal Regulations.

Under the old regulations, air purifying negative pressure particulate cartridge/filters were classified for "dust/mist," "dust/mist/fume," "paint spray,"

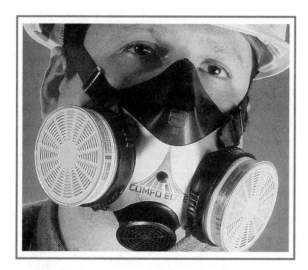

FIGURE 16-1 *Negative pressure air purifying respirator* (*Courtesy of* MSA [Mine Safety Appliances Company])

"pesticide," and "HEPA" applications. The new classifications will depend upon the ability of the filter to stop **oil-based aerosols**. The three new categories for particulate filters are:

1. *N* for Not Oil-Proof.
2. *R* for Oil-Resistant.
3. *P* for Oil-Proof.

N series filters can only be used in clean environments (where there are solids and no oil-containing particulates).

R series can be used in any environment, including where there are oil-containing particulates. If used where oil is present, the filter is limited to one eight-hour shift. Filters can be reused if there are no airborne oil particulates.

P series can be used for any particulate contaminant, which includes where oil-containing particulates are present. Filters may be used for more than one workshift.

Note: (1) An oil aerosol may include particles of a mineral, vegetable, synthetic material, animal or vegetable fat. It is a viscous liquid at room temperature that is soluble in organic solvents. Oil aerosols are not soluble in water. (2) Regardless of the series of

respirator, filters must be changed when they become dirty or damaged, lose their shape, or become difficult to breathe through.

Filters. For the filters in each category of respirator, there is a percentage efficiency rating that indicates the percentage of particles removed from the air. The ratings are 95%, 99%, and 99.7%. For purposes of filter efficiency, the 99.7% is referred to as 100%. The filter efficiency used will depend upon the size of the particle that has to be filtered out and the permissible exposure limit (PEL) of the contaminant.

Powered air purifying respirators (PAPR) are equipped with battery operated blowers that force outside air through filters into the face piece. The air in the face piece is positive compared to air outside the face piece (they are not negative pressure respirators). This prevents entry of contaminant into the face piece if there is a leak in the face piece because of a poor fit or other reason. (See Figure 16-2.)

Gas masks are negative pressure air purifying respirators and are rated to protect against specific gases. Air is inhaled through a canister filter that contains an absorbing media that purifies the air before it reaches the face piece. Air in the face piece is negative in relation to outside air. Canisters have limited protection periods that can vary from fif-

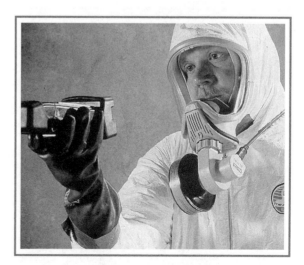

FIGURE 16-2 *OptimAir MM PAPR with Ultra Elite face piece* (*Courtesy of* MSA [Mine Safety Appliances Company])

teen to thirty minutes, depending upon the contaminant. (See Figure 16-3.)

> *Note:* Air purifying respirators are not approved for **oxygen deficient** or immediately dangerous to life or health (IDLH) atmospheres. Oxygen deficient atmospheres are atmospheres where the oxygen content is less than 19.5% by volume.

Atmosphere Supplying. **Atmosphere supplying respirators** provide air from a compressed air tank, gas cylinder, or compressor. They do not rely on outside air for the air supply (except for the type B supplied air). They consist of supplied air respirators, self-contained breathing apparatuses (SCBAs), and combination SCBA and supplied air.

Supplied air respirators get their air from compressed air tanks or compressors and are classed as Type A, Type B, and Type C.

Type A has air blown into the face piece through a hose by a blower. The air is supplied by a hand or power driven pump.

Type B has air brought into the face piece by inhalation through a long hose (up to 75 feet long). The hose inlet has a screen to keep particulates that might be in the air from getting into the hose. The hose must be placed in an area where the air is clean.

Type C is called an airline respirator and consists of continuous flow, demand, and pressure demand.

- Continuous flow delivers air to the face piece at a minimum of 4 cubic feet per minute (cfm). (See Figure 16-4.)
- Demand delivers air on the demand of the wearer when inhalation creates a negative pressure in the face piece.
- Pressure demand provides positive pressure in the face piece when face-piece pressure is reduced by inhalation. This provides a constant positive pressure in the face piece. Pressure demand prevents leakage into the face piece if there is a poor face-piece seal. Air is delivered at a minimum of 4 cfm. (See Figure 16-5.)

> *Note:* Types A, B, and C supplied air respirators can be used in oxygen deficient atmospheres but not IDLH atmospheres. They must be equipped with full face pieces.

Self-contained breathing apparatuses (SCBAs) consist of oxygen cylinder rebreathing, self-generating, demand, pressure demand, and combination SCBA and Type C supplied air respirator.

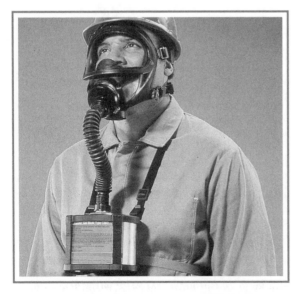

FIGURE 16-3 *Industrial size gas mask* (*Courtesy of* MSA [Mine Safety Appliances Company])

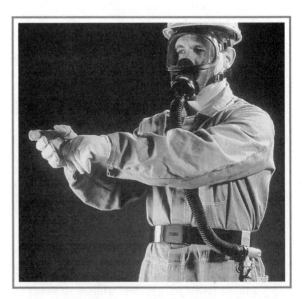

FIGURE 16-4 *Continuous flow airline respirator* (*Courtesy of* MSA [Mine Safety Appliances Company])

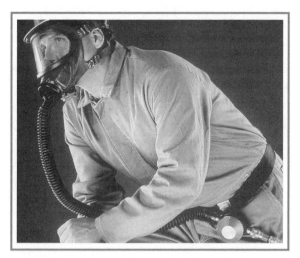

FIGURE 16-5 *Pressure demand airline respirator*
(*Courtesy of* MSA [Mine Safety Appliances Company])

Oxygen cylinder rebreathing consists of an oxygen cylinder that is carried on the back of the wearer. The oxygen is removed from the carbon dioxide in the exhaled breath in a chemical container that is worn on the front and then sent to a breathing bag where it mixes with the oxygen coming from the cylinder. It is this mixture that the wearer breathes. The supply of oxygen for breathing determines how long the respirator can be used. It can vary from one to four hours. (See Figure 16-6.)

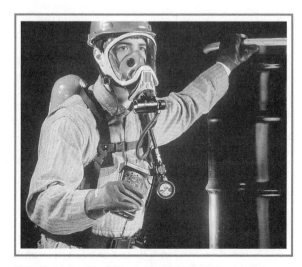

FIGURE 16-6 *WorkMask MMR SCBA* (*Courtesy of*
MSA [Mine Safety Appliances Company])

Self-generating consists of a chemical container worn on the front of the wearer (there is no back-worn cylinder). The oxygen supply comes solely from the oxygen separated from the exhaled carbon dioxide in the container. This is the oxygen the wearer breathes.

Demand consists of a high pressure cylinder and demand regulator connected to the cylinder. Air to the face piece is regulated when a negative pressure is created in the face piece by inhalation.

Pressure demand consists of air supplied by a cylinder that is sent to the face piece when positive pressure in the face piece is reduced by inhalation. This provides a constant pressure in the face piece, which protects against leakage into the face piece if there is a poor seal.

Combination SCBA and type C supplied air respirator consists of a type C (airline) and auxiliary SCBA. If the supply is cut off, the wearer can switch over to the SCBA to escape the contaminated atmosphere. The capacity of the SCBA determines how long the air supply will last. It can vary from three to fifteen minutes.

> **Note:** The oxygen cylinder rebreathing, self-generating, and demand SCBAs can be used in oxygen deficient atmospheres but not IDLH atmospheres. They must be equipped with full face pieces. The pressure demand SCBA and combination Type C airline and SCBA can be used in both oxygen deficient and IDLH atmospheres. They must be equipped with full face pieces.

Combination Air Purifying and Supplied Air Respirator. The combination air purifying and supplied air respirator consists of an airline and an air purifying respirator that is used as an auxiliary or escape respirator. The airline can be of the continuous flow or pressure demand type. If the air supply to the airline fails, the air purifying respirator takes over so there can be a safe escape from the contaminated atmosphere.

> **Note:** The combination air purifying and supplied air respirator cannot be used in either oxygen deficient or IDLH atmospheres.

CHAPTER REVIEW

Multiple Choice

Select the best answer from the choices provided.

1. One of the modes of operation for a Type C supplied air respirator is
   a. self-generating   c. demand
   b. rebreathing   d. negative pressure

2. Quantitative fit testing involves
   a. smelling or tasting the test material
   b. feeling the test material
   c. measuring the amount of leakage in the face piece
   d. placing the hands over the inhalation valve

3. A Type B supplied air respirator can have a hose length up to
   a. 25 feet long   c. 75 feet long
   b. 50 feet long   d. 100 feet long

4. Oxygen cylinders must be tested and maintained in accordance with
   a. OSHA   c. ANSI
   b. NIOSH   d. DOT

5. Respirators used for emergency purposes must be inspected at least
   a. weekly
   b. monthly
   c. every three months
   d. yearly

True/False

Indicate whether the statement is true or false by circling T or F.

6. T F Negative pressure air purifying respirators can be used in oxygen deficient atmospheres.

7. T F Pressure demand is one type of air supplying respirator.

8. T F Engineering and work practice controls are not needed if a respirator protects adequately.

9. T F N series particulate respirators can be used only in clean environments.

10. T F Fit testing is the responsibility of the employee.

11. T F Any employee can repair a respirator.

12. T F Facial hair prevents the proper wearing of a tight fitting air purifying respirator.

13. T F The employee must do the worksite analysis when updating respirator use.

14. T F A gas mask is an air purifying respirator.

15. T F Respirator training must be conducted every three months.

Matching

Match the terms in column 1 with the definitions in column 2.

Column 1	Column 2
16. SCBA respirator	a. Can be used in both IDLH and oxygen deficient atmospheres
17. Air purifying respirator	b. Can be used in oxygen deficient but not IDLH atmospheres
18. Type C airline and SCBA	c. Atmosphere supplied respirator
19. Type A, B, and C supplied air	d. Cannot be used in IDLH or oxygen deficient deficient atmospheres
20. P series particulate respirator	e. Can be used for oil-containing particulates

Short Answer

Briefly but thoroughly answer each statement.

21. Discuss why it is important that the employee undergo another fit test if he/she changes respirators.

22. Why is it important to determine the level of airborne contaminant in the workplace?

23. Discuss why engineering and work practice controls must be used whenever feasible instead of using respirators.

24. Describe some of the physical conditions that might prevent an employee from wearing a respirator.

25. Explain the major differences between air purifying and air supplying respirators.

CHAPTER 17

Infectious Diseases

OBJECTIVES

After studying this chapter, you should be able to

➤ List the various infectious diseases.

➤ Identify their symptoms.

➤ Identify their causes.

➤ Identify who may be exposed.

➤ Discuss protection of pregnant women who may be exposed.

➤ Explain the use of personal protective equipment.

INTRODUCTION

Allied health professionals, by the nature of their responsibilities, should already have extensive knowledge of infectious diseases. This chapter serves as a reminder on the precautions to be taken to prevent spread of these diseases. Not only can these diseases be transmitted from patient to provider, but they can also be brought into the health care setting from outside. The information in this chapter is geared to the health care provider and does not cover patient protection. It is designed to serve as a reminder in order for the allied health professional to adequately protect himself/herself when administering to patients.

Where not specifically indicated, it is always prudent for a pregnant woman to seek medical advice if she thinks she has been exposed to an infectious disease.

ACQUIRED IMMUNE DEFICIENCY SYNDROME

Acquired immune deficiency syndrome (AIDS) is caused by the human immunodeficiency virus (HIV) and is found in blood; semen; vaginal secretions; and cerebrospinal, lung, pericardial, and amniotic fluid.

HIV is spread when there is unprotected sexual activity (vaginal and anal sex) and when infected drug needles are shared. In extremely rare cases, hospital workers may become infected when they inadvertently stick themselves with an infected needle or when persons receive infected blood during a transfusion.

Persons with AIDS may develop fevers, weight loss, a feeling of tiredness, diarrhea, and swollen lymph glands. There is also a susceptibility to Karposi's sarcoma, which is a form of skin cancer, and to a form of pneumonia called PCP.

Anyone exposed to bodily fluids is at risk.

It is the responsibility of the employer to implement an exposure control plan that meets the requirements of OSHA 29 CFR 1910.1030 bloodborne pathogens standard (see Chapter 15). The exposure control plan must be in writing and include the source of exposure, methods used to comply, training, and recordkeeping.

Recent drugs that have been developed (protease inhibitors, ZDV, and AZT) control the severity of the disease in some afflicted persons. This has increased survival rates.

A vaccine for AIDS called AIDS-VAX is being tested. It is made from genetically engineered proteins that comprise the outer shell of HIV.

Infected pregnant women can spread the disease to the fetus before birth and when breast feeding.

AMEBIASIS (AMEBIC DYSENTERY)

Amebiasis is caused by a parasite. The cyst stage of the parasite enters the body when contaminated food or water is ingested. It is also spread from the fecal to oral route when an infected person does not wash his/her hands after toileting and touches food or drink.

Symptoms include nausea, diarrhea, weight loss, and abdominal tenderness. The disease is diagnosed by examination of stool samples.

Health care employees should wear gowns and impervious gloves and wash hands with soap and water, particularly after each toilet visit.

Recovery does not make a person immune. Subsequent exposure could result in getting the disease again.

The disease can weaken the mother, which in turn can affect the fetus. Pregnant women should avoid contact with persons suspected or known to have the disease.

ANTHRAX

Anthrax is caused by **bacteria** that are inhaled from contaminated soil or from handling the wool and hair of infected animals. Undercooked meat from infected animals can also cause the disease in the person eating the meat. The disease cannot be spread from person to person.

Symptoms include boils and lesions on the skin (from skin contact), swollen underarm lymph glands, and cold-like symptoms.

Health care workers should wear gowns and impervious gloves when treating patients.

After recovery from the disease, immunity is usually obtained.

A vaccine is available for workers who are at risk. Penicillin or tetracycline is used in treating anthrax.

BABESIOSIS

Babesiosis is a tickborne disease. When an infected tick bites a person, it injects a red blood parasite into the blood. The tick is usually found on deer, meadow voles, mice, rats, and chipmunks. The disease can also be transmitted by blood transfusion from infected blood.

It is diagnosed by examining the blood under microscope.

Malaise, fatigue, anorexia, headache, nausea, vomiting, abdominal pain, depression, and dark urine are symptoms. These symptoms can last from a few days to several months and may take one to twelve months to appear. People may also be infected without evidence of any symptoms.

Impervious gloves should be worn by health care employees when in contact with infected persons.

Infected persons can be treated with clindamycin and quinine.

BOTULISM

Botulism is caused by a bacteria-produced toxin. Persons get it when they eat contaminated food that is undercooked or when food is not prepared properly.

When canned food is bulging, there is a good probability the bacteria are present.

It is not spread from person to person.

Blurred vision, weakness, poor reflexes, and swallowing difficulties are symptoms. They can appear in twelve to thirty-six hours after ingestion of contaminated food.

Immunity is not obtained after recovery.

If a pregnant woman suspects she has the disease, she should consult a physician as soon as possible. The unborn child is at risk and can die if the disease is not treated.

BRUCELLOSIS

Brucellosis is caused by bacteria present in unpasteurized milk from diseased cows and in discharges from diseased cattle and goats that abort their fetuses.

It is not spread from person to person.

Fever, headache, weakness, sweating, chills, weight loss, and body aches are symptoms. The symptoms can appear in five to thirty days.

Health care workers who treat infected patients should wear gowns and impervious gloves.

Persons who recover from the disease acquire immunity. Brucellosis is treated with **antibiotics**. Antibiotics are a variety of natural and synthetic substances that retard or destroy the growth of microorganisms.

CHICKEN POX *(VARICELLA ZOSTER)*

Chicken pox is caused by a virus that is extremely communicable. It is transmitted when an infected person coughs or sneezes and the droplets carrying the virus are inhaled and by airborne spread of discharges from an infected person's nose and throat. It can also be spread when articles are soiled with the discharges from an infected person's skin lesions.

Fever and a feeling of weakness and tiredness are symptoms. Blisters appear that dry and form crusty scabs. The scabs may appear on the scalp, armpits, trunk, eyelids, and mouth. These scabs may appear from eleven to twenty-one days after infection.

The disease can be transmitted from five days before the rash appears to about six days after appearance of the first lesion.

The disease may be hidden and appear a number of years later as herpes zoster (shingles) in adults.

Chicken pox in adults can cause pneumonia.

Health care workers who are not sure if they are immune should wear masks, impervious gloves, and gowns when treating patients.

Health care workers who are considered unvaccinated or who cannot document immunity should receive the recently developed live, attenuated varicella virus vaccine.

Pregnant women and persons with suppressed immune systems should not be vaccinated with the varicella vaccine.

Those at risk, such as newborns, exposed pregnant women, and those with suppressed immune systems should be given the varicella-zoster (VZIG) vaccine.

Persons who recover from chicken pox usually develop lifetime immunity.

A pregnant woman who has chicken pox can harm the fetus.

An exposed pregnant woman should ask parents or relatives if she ever had chicken pox, check the medical records of her family physician or pediatrician, or have a lab test that would tell if she was ever infected and is now immune.

If she is not sure of her immunity, she should consult with her physician immediately regarding the risk to herself and the fetus.

CHOLERA

Cholera is caused by bacteria that infect the intestinal tract. It is transmitted by eating or drinking the food and water that is contaminated from an infected person's fecal waste.

Diarrhea, vomiting, and dehydration that appear six hours to five days after being exposed are symptoms.

Health care employees should wear gowns and impervious gloves when treating patients.

Immunity is not acquired after recovery from the disease.

The vaccine gives immunity for only two to six months and is administered to persons going to countries where cholera has occurred.

The disease is treated with fluids to prevent dehydration and with antibiotics.

DIPHTHERIA

Diphtheria is caused by bacteria. It may cause a membrane to form in the throat that can suffocate the person. The disease also results in an infection of the nose, throat, tonsils, and larynx. Diphtheria of the skin produces a skin rash or ulcer.

It is transmitted when an infected person coughs or sneezes. The skin variety occurs when the open sores or articles that are soiled from lesions of infected persons are touched.

Infected tonsils, sore throat, hoarseness, nasal discharge, and fever are symptoms.

The bacteria can be carried by persons who show no evidence of having the disease. These people can transmit the disease for six months or more, and untreated persons can spread the disease from two to four weeks before the body kills the bacteria.

Health care workers should wear masks, gowns, and impervious gloves when administering to patients.

The vaccine is inactivated diphtheria toxin and is recommended for everyone. It should be given as a combination with tetanus toxoid (Td).

The Td vaccine is not known to have caused problems with pregnant women.

E. COLI (ESCHERICHIA COLI)

E. coli is caused by bacteria that release a toxin in the intestines. It is acquired by eating contaminated food or food that is not adequately cooked. It is also spread when hands are not properly washed after toilet visits.

Diarrhea, abdominal cramps, and bloody stools are symptoms. They appear about one to nine days after exposure.

When treating patients with E. coli, gowns and impervious gloves should be worn by health care workers.

People with E. coli infections must wash their hands with soap and water after toilet visits.

Persons do not become immune after recovery from the disease.

Pregnant women are prone to the disease because the fetus puts pressure on the bladder and ureter. This encourages bacterial growth.

Pregnant women with E. coli infections should consult with their physicians. The infection has caused high blood pressure and premature births.

ENCEPHALITIS

Encephalitis is caused by a virus that causes inflammation of the brain and spinal cord. It results from the bite of an infected tick or mosquito that is carrying the virus. Infections are also known to occur when there is infected feces contaminating food and water.

Convulsions, confusion, stupor, difficulty in speaking, muscle involvement, weakness, rigid eyeball motion, and facial weakness are symptoms. Fever, headache, and stiff neck are symptoms of spinal cord infection.

Health care workers should wear gowns and impervious gloves when treating patients with encephalitis.

People who recover from the disease do not acquire immunity.

The vaccine is restricted to people who will be traveling to areas known to have encephalitis. The vaccine that protects against Japanese encephalitis (JE) consists of three doses.

Pregnant women should not receive the JE vaccine.

FIFTH DISEASE

Fifth disease is caused by a virus that affects the red blood cells. The virus is transmitted via airborne droplets from an infected person who coughs or sneezes.

Low-grade fever and tiredness are symptoms. They appear in one to two weeks after exposure. A rash appears on the face after the third week and by this time, the infected person is no longer contagious.

Health care workers should wear masks when treating patients.

People who recover from the disease acquire lifelong immunity.

Fifth disease infection may cause miscarriage or spontaneous abortion. Pregnant women should consult with their physician if they have been exposed.

GIARDIASIS (BEAVER FEVER)

Giardiasis is caused by a parasite that gets into water. People get the disease when they drink water that has become contaminated by infected feces from people and animals. The parasite has been found in the feces of people, beavers, muskrats, coyotes, deer, elk, cattle, dogs, and cats.

Symptoms include diarrhea with some victims suffering chronic diarrhea that may last several weeks or months. This is usually accompanied by pronounced weight loss. Most times a fever is not present.

Impervious gloves should be worn when changing diapers. When treating patients, health care workers should wear gowns and impervious gloves. Hands must be thoroughly washed after each toilet visit.

Recovery from the disease does not give immunity.

GONORRHEA

Gonorrhea is spread by sexual contact. The germ causing the disease is found in the mucus of the vagina, penis, throat, and rectum. It is spread from penis to vagina, penis to mouth, penis to rectum, and mouth to vagina. Infected persons are capable of spreading the disease until it is treated.

Symptoms include burning during urination and a yellow discharge from the penis in men and from the vagina in women. In men, symptoms appear from two to seven days after infection. Sometimes symptoms do not appear for up to thirty days. If untreated, the disease can cause sterilization, swelling of the penis and testicles, arthritis, and other infections.

The disease can only be spread by sexual contact.

Recovery does not give immunity. In fact, subsequent infections can be more serious.

The disease is treated with penicillin and other antibiotics.

Women with the disease can spread it to their unborn child. Pregnant women who suspect they have the disease should see their physician immediately.

HAEMOPHILUS INFLUENZA TYPE B (Hib)

Haemophilus influenza is caused by bacteria and is prevalent in young children. It can cause meningitis (which is an inflammation of the covering of the spinal cord and brain), blood infections, pneumonia, and arthritis.

Fever, vomiting, lethargy, and stiff neck are symptoms. They usually appear within ten days from exposure. Contagion lasts as long as the nose and throat are infected and can continue after symptoms are no longer evident.

When treating patients with the disease, a mask and impervious gloves should be worn.

Recovery does not give immunity.

The vaccination should not be given after exposure to the disease; it takes too long to develop an immune response.

The Hib vaccine can be given with the DPT (diphtheria, pertussis, and tetanus), MMR (measles, mumps, and rubella), and polio vaccines.

Antibiotics are used to treat the more serious infections of Hib.

The antibiotic rifampin used to treat the disease is not recommended for pregnant women. They should consult with their physician for treatment.

HEPATITIS B (HBV)

Hepatitis B is caused by a virus that infects the liver. It is spread when people come in contact with infected blood. It is also spread through needle sticks and sharing of body fluids such as lung, synovial, and cerebrospinal fluid and vaginal secretions. It has an incubation period of 30–180 days.

Fatigue, loss of appetite, fever, vomiting, joint pain, hives, or rash are symptoms. The urine changes to a dark color and yellowing of the skin and whites of the eyes occurs (jaundice).

The symptoms appear within two to six months after exposure, and the virus can be in the blood and other body fluids for several weeks before symptoms appear.

The employer must follow OSHA 29 CFR 1910. 1030 bloodborne pathogens standard for workers who are exposed to HBV. An exposure and infection control program must be implemented as described in Chapter 15 covering the OSHA bloodborne pathogens standard.

Without proper immunization, persons can get the disease again after recovery.

HBV vaccine is a series of three shots given in the upper arm. The second shot is given one month after the first shot and the third shot is given six months after the first.

There is an HBV immune globulin vaccine that can be given to persons who have been exposed. It is given with the HBV vaccine.

HBV immune globulin and HBV vaccine can safely be administered to pregnant women. The shots can be given during pregnancy and during lactation.

Pregnant women should be tested for HBV infection because the disease can affect the fetus.

HISTOPLASMOSIS

Histoplasmosis is a fungus infection that gets into the lungs and other parts of the body. The fungal spores can be found in bird droppings (mostly pigeons, blackbirds, and chickens), bats, dogs, cats, rats, skunks, opossum, and fox feces.

It is spread when the fungal spores are inhaled.

Headache, fever, malaise, muscle aches, and chest pain are symptoms. They appear from five to eighteen days after exposure.

Health care workers should wear gowns, masks, and impervious gloves when treating patients.

People who recover from the disease usually get partial immunity because they develop a stronger resistance to the disease.

The disease is treated with an antibiotic.

LEGIONELLOSIS (LEGIONNAIRES DISEASE)

Legionellosis is caused by bacteria that infect the lungs, which results in pneumonia. The bacteria can be present in creeks, ponds, hot and cold sink water, in the water in cooling towers, evaporative condensers, water systems, and in excavated soil. It has been implicated in wound infections, pericarditis, and endocarditis without the presence of pneumonia. The disease is acquired by inhalation of water aerosols containing the organism. It is not transmitted from person to person.

Common sources of this disease are

- Cooling towers, evaporative condensers, fluid coolers that use evaporation to reject heat
- Domestic hot water systems that operate below 140°F and deliver hot tap water below 122°F
- Humidifiers and fountains that spray water at favorable growth temperatures
- Spas and whirlpools
- Dental rinse water kept at 68°F or above
- Stagnant water in fire sprinkler systems and warm water used in eye wash stations and safety showers

Fever, chills, diarrhea, muscle aches, headaches, tiredness, and a dry cough are symptoms. Severity ranges from a mild cough and low fever to progressive pneumonia and coma. Symptoms appear within two to ten days after exposure. A blood test is required to confirm a diagnosis. A detection of the antigen in urine is also an indicator of the presence of the disease.

Health care employees should wear masks when treating people with this disease.

A knowledge of the building water system is important. This includes plumbing, HVAC, water reservoirs, fountains, misters, whirlpools, spas, eye washes, and safety showers. Know where stagnant water accumulates.

Conduct a walk through investigation that includes the following:

- Measuring and recording water temperatures
- Evaluating cooling towers, evaporative condensers, and fluid coolers for biofilm growth, scale buildup, and turbidity
- Recording the condition of the cooling tower; evaluating cooling tower sumps
- Checking maintenance on the water system
- Assessing the results of the investigation

Additional controls include

- Disinfecting by heat treatment or by the use of chlorination
- Eliminating dead legs (where hot water stagnates) in plumbing systems; installing devices that maintain proper water temperatures; insulating plumbing lines
- Using biocides (chlorine and bromine have proven effective)
- Cleaning the cooling tower at least twice a year.
- Running domestic hot water pumps continuously
- Maintaining domestic cold water below 20°C
- Insulating cold water lines that are close to hot water lines
- Maintaining HVAC systems
- Minimizing use of water reservoirs, sumps, and pans
- Draining water pumps when not in use
- "Bleeding" water pumps so that dissolved solids do not form sediments in the sump
- Locating HVAC fresh air intakes so that they do not draw mist from cooling towers, evaporative condensers, or fluid coolers into the system

- Using steam or atomizing humidifiers instead of units that use recirculated water (do not use steam from the central heating boiler because it contain corrosives and other contaminants)
- Using contaminant-free water in atomizing humidifiers

Recovery from the disease does not give immunity. The disease is treated with an antibiotic (erythromycin and rifampin).

LEPTOSPIROSIS (WEIL'S DISEASE)

Weil's disease is a bacterium that is harbored in animals. Infected animal urine causes its transmission.

Rash, jaundice, fever, vomiting, headache, and chills are symptoms. They appear from four to ten days after exposure. If the disease is not treated, there is risk of kidney damage and death.

It is diagnosed by specific blood tests.

Health care workers should wear impervious gloves when treating patients with the disease.

Weil's disease is caused by several strains of bacteria. After recovery from one strain, the person is immune to that strain of bacteria but can get the disease again from a different strain.

The disease is treated with antibiotics.

LYME DISEASE

Lyme disease is caused by a deer tick bite from a tick that is infected with the spirochete borrelia burgdorferi. The tick is found on deer, mice, dogs, and oppossums.

The tick, when biting the skin, releases the spirochete into the bloodstream.

Skin rash that appears circular, chills, fever, fatigue, headache, pains in the muscles and joints, and swollen lymph nodes are symptoms.

A blood test is required to confirm the diagnosis.

A vaccine has been developed that may prove 80 percent effective in preventing the disease and 100 percent effective in preventing cases where symptoms of infection are not manifested. The vaccine creates antibodies that recognize the outer protein of the lyme bacterium in the tick's saliva (Osp-A) and neutralizes it. The vaccine blocks the transmission of the bacterium where it occurs on the skin. Present studies have indicated that it takes at least three doses of the vaccine for maximum protection. The last dose is given one year after the first. Studies are also being done to determine how often booster shots will have to be given and the effects the vaccine may have on persons with arthritis. The vaccine is designed for persons from fifteen to seventy years old.

Currently, persons who recover from the disease can get it again, if exposed.

Pregnant women who get the disease can, in rare cases, infect the fetus and cause stillbirth. If a pregnant woman believes she has been exposed, she should see her physician immediately.

MALARIA

Malaria is caused by a bite from the female Anopheles mosquito. After sucking the blood of an infected person, the mosquito spreads the disease by biting into another person and injecting the blood parasite. Untreated or poorly treated malaria victims can transmit the disease anywhere from one to three years.

Chills, fever, headache, sweats, jaundice, shock, central nervous system disorders, kidney and liver failure, and coma are symptoms. They usually appear from twelve to thirty days after being exposed.

When treating patients with malaria, impervious gloves should be worn by health care workers.

Repeated infection can cause a partial immunity. Persons who have a sickle cell trait are immune to certain forms of malaria.

There is presently no vaccine for malaria. It is treated with antibiotics.

Pregnant women are at increased risk of getting the disease because pregnancy lowers the resistance to infection. Malaria can cause spontaneous abortion, stillbirth, and low birth weight.

Pregnant women who get malaria should be immediately treated with chloroquine or quinine. Sulfadoxine, tetracycline, and primaquinine should not be administered because of their detrimental effects on the fetus.

MEASLES

Measles is a very contagious disease that is caused by a virus. Transmission is by airborne droplets that are spread into the air and inhaled when an infected person coughs, sneezes, or talks. It can also be transmitted when an infected person touches someone else or touches an item that is touched by a person who is not infected.

More severe forms can cause diarrhea, ear infections, and pneumonia.

Rash, fever, runny nose, cough, and watery eyes are symptoms that can last one to two weeks. They appear from ten to twelve days after being infected and usually are accompanied by a facial rash that spreads to other parts of the body. Diarrhea, ear infections, and pneumonia are the more serious effects of the disease.

A person is contagious when the fever develops until four to nine days after the rash appears.

Health care workers should wear masks, gowns, and impervious gloves when treating patients.

At risk people such as health care workers should be vaccinated if they are not sure of their immunity.

The vaccine is a weakened live virus and is given as a measles only, MR, or MMR vaccine. When given within seventy-two hours of exposure, it can provide immunity. MR is measles and rubella and MMR is measles, mumps, and rubella vaccine.

Persons with severe allergies to eggs should not be vaccinated, nor should persons who have a severe allergy to neomycin.

Pregnant women infected with measles run the risk of miscarriage or premature delivery. Measles is also suspected of causing birth defects, although not proven.

Neither the live measles vaccine nor the MR and MMR vaccines should be given to pregnant women or to women who want to become pregnant within the next three months. Women who receive the measles only vaccine should not become pregnant for at least thirty days after the vaccination.

Pregnant women who are exposed to measles should get the immune globulin (IG) as soon as possible.

MENINGOCOCCAL MENINGITIS (SPINAL MENINGITIS, CEREBROSPINAL FEVER, MENINGOCOCCEMIA)

Meningitis is caused by bacteria that infect the blood and meninges, which is the lining of the brain and spinal cord.

It is spread by the nose and throat discharges of an infected person.

Rash, stiff neck, fever, headache, and vomiting are symptoms. They appear from two to ten days after infection, and the disease can be transmitted until the fever stage is over.

Health care workers should wear gowns and impervious gloves when treating patients. When close contact is required, workers should take a sulfa drug prescribed by a physician.

Casual contact will not cause transmission of the disease.

Recovery does not make a person immune.

A vaccine is available that protects against two strains of meningitis. It is usually administered only in high-risk cases or when traveling to an area where outbreaks have occurred.

MUMPS

Mumps is caused by a virus and is transmitted when an infected person coughs, sneezes, or talks. It can also be transmitted when there is contact with the saliva of an infected person or when an infected person touches something which in turn is touched by a non-infected person.

The virus is also found in urine, body tissue, and breast milk.

Swollen glands under the jaw, headache, fever, neck or ear pain, tiredness, and a mild form of meningitis are symptoms. They can appear within fourteen to twenty days after exposure.

Some males will get a painful swelling of the testicles. This does not make the man sterile.

The disease can be transmitted from three days before the disease is active to the fourth day of the disease.

Health care workers who are not sure of their immunity should wear masks when treating patients.

Persons not sure of their immune status should get vaccinated.

The vaccine is a live mumps vaccine and can be given as mumps only, MR, or MMR vaccine.

Side effects of the vaccine include a low-grade fever and swollen salivary glands.

Persons with allergies that have caused hives, mouth and throat swelling, breathing difficulties, hypotension, or shock after eating eggs, as well as persons allergic to the antibiotic neomycin, should consult with a physician before being vaccinated.

Mumps infection during the first trimester has been associated with an increased chance of miscarriage (not premature delivery or birth defects).

Because there is a question concerning the vaccine's effects on the fetus, pregnant women or those considering pregnancy within three months, should not receive the vaccine.

If a pregnant woman becomes infected, she should see her physician immediately.

PERTUSSIS (WHOOPING COUGH)

Pertussis is caused by bacteria that get into the lungs, which can cause pneumonia.

It is transmitted when an infected person coughs, sneezes, or talks or when the mucous discharge is touched.

A low-grade fever, coughing, a runny nose, and sneezing are symptoms. The cough can last as long as ten weeks. Complications of the disease include ear infection, loss of appetite, and dehydration.

The symptoms appear within five to ten days after infection and can last as long as ten weeks.

Health care workers who are not immune should wear masks when treating patients.

Health care workers who have not been immunized and who have infected children at home, should receive antibiotics to minimize transmission.

Persons who recover from the disease develop immunity.

The vaccine is a killed whole cell pertussis and is given with diphtheria and tetanus toxoid (DTP). The side effects of the vaccine include fever and soreness and swelling at the vaccination site.

Vaccination for pertussis is not recommended for adults. Adults should be given antibiotics to reduce risk.

PLAGUE

Plague is caused by bacteria that are found in fleas that live on rodents. It can also be transmitted by handling the tissue of infected animals, from droplets coughed or sneezed into the air from infected persons (pneumonic plague), from pets that have pneumonic plague, and by exposure in the laboratory.

Fever and swollen lymph glands near the flea bite are symptoms. Blood infection and pneumonia are the result as the disease progresses. Symptoms appear from one to six days after exposure, and if the disease goes untreated, it can result in death.

Gowns and impervious gloves should be worn by health care workers when treating patients with bubonic plague. Masks, gowns, and impervious gloves should be worn by health care personnel when treating patients with pneumonic plague.

Immunity varies after recovery. In some cases complete protection against getting the plague again is not achieved.

The vaccine is killed bacteria and is used only for people going to areas where plague has occurred. Antibiotics are used to treat the disease.

Pregnant women who suspect they have been exposed should consult with their physician immediately for treatment. The vaccination treatment should be determined by a physician.

POLIO

Polio is caused by a virus that is transmitted from the fecal to oral route. It can cause paralysis severe enough so that infected people are unable to move their arms or legs. If the respiratory system is affected, breathing becomes difficult and the patient may require a respirator to breathe.

The incubation period is six to twenty days after onset of infection and for paralytic cases, three to thirty-five days. Persons are most contagious seven to ten days before and after the symptoms appear, but infected persons are contagious as long as the virus remains in the throat and feces.

Fever, malaise, vomiting, nausea, headache, sore throat, stomach ache, severe muscle pain, and breathing difficulties are symptoms.

Day-care workers who have suppressed immune systems can become infected when diapering children who have been recently vaccinated with the live polio vaccine (OPV).

When treating polio patients, health care employees should wear gowns and impervious gloves.

The polio virus vaccine gives immunity to those who receive the series. People who recover from polio are immune to the strain of virus that caused their polio but can get the disease caused by a different strain.

There are two types of vaccines. One is the live oral vaccine (OPV), and the other is the inactive vaccine (IPV).

The IPV is a killed virus and is given as a shot. The OPV is a live weakened virus vaccine and is given as a series of oral drops.

For full protection, it is necessary to take four doses of either OPV or IPV.

There is no evidence that the polio vaccine causes problems with the fetus. Physicians generally do not recommend giving drugs or vaccines to pregnant women unless it is necessary. If a pregnant woman needs protection, she should receive the OPV.

PSITTACOSIS (PARROT FEVER)

Psittacosis is transmitted from birds such as parrots, pigeons, and turkeys when the dried droppings are inhaled and from handling infected birds.

Chills, fever, headache, and pneumonia are symptoms and appear from four to fifteen days after being infected. The disease can result in death if left untreated.

Health care workers should wear masks, gowns, and impervious gloves when treating patients.

Recovery from the disease does not give immunity.

The disease is treated with antibiotics.

RABIES

Rabies is caused by a virus that attacks the central nervous system. Transmission is from the bite of an infected animal such as a bat, raccoon, fox, skunk, and similar animals.

Transmission can also occur if the saliva or nervous tissue from a rabid animal gets into an open wound or mucous membranes. Animals can transmit the disease for as long as five days without showing any signs of the disease, and the disease can incubate in an animal or person from two weeks to three months before showing any symptoms.

Animals with rabies usually exhibit paralysis of the hind legs and throat, aggressiveness, and friendliness. Irritability, fever, headache, and an itching or pain at the bite site are symptoms in people. As the disease spreads, paralysis sets in. There are spasms of the throat muscles, delirium, convulsions, and death.

Health care employees are susceptible if bitten when they treat patients with rabies. They should wear gowns and impervious gloves.

Employers should train health care workers. Information should include the following:

- How rabies is transmitted
- How to avoid saliva and what should be done if exposed
- Why preexposure rabies vaccine for high-risk employees is recommended
- The use of personal protective equipment

If a person is bitten, the wound site should be cleaned with soap and water. The series of rabies shots must be given immediately.

High-risk employees should receive the preexposure series, which is a series of three injections in the arm.

The rabies vaccination does not pose a hazard to the mother or fetus. If a pregnant woman is bitten by a rabid animal, she should immediately get the rabies series of shots if she has not had the preexposure series.

REYE'S SYNDROME

The suspected cause of Reye's Syndrome is a virus, but this is not confirmed. It is not known whether it is hereditary or caused by exposure to toxic materials. The disease affects the liver and the brain and follows infections such as chicken pox, influenza, upper respiratory infection, coxsackie virus, herpes simplex virus, and adenovirus.

Diagnosis is made from blood tests, biopsies, and tissue examination.

Unconsciousness, hypoglycemia, swelling of the brain, and fatty liver and kidney tubules are symptoms. They appear from one to three days after infection, and death may occur if the disease goes untreated.

Employees that handle toxic materials must be properly protected against exposure. Protection may consist of engineering or work practice controls or the wearing of personal protective equipment. Immunization against chicken pox and influenza also controls the disease.

It is not known if recovery gives immunity to the disease.

It is prudent for pregnant women to be immunized against chicken pox and influenza.

ROCKY MOUNTAIN SPOTTED FEVER (TICKBORNE TYPHUS FEVER)

Rocky Mountain spotted fever is caused by a rickettsial organism. People get it from the bite of an infected American dog tick and other ticks. The tick injects the organism into the blood causing the infection. The disease is not spread from one person to another.

High fever, headache, chills, rash, fatigue, and muscle pain are symptoms. The rash, which spreads to all parts of the body, can last two to three weeks. The rash first appears on the arms and legs and then progresses to the feet, palms, and body. Symptoms usually appear in about two weeks after the tick bite.

Recovery gives immunity to the disease.

RUBELLA (GERMAN MEASLES)

Rubella is transmitted by a virus when an infected person coughs, sneezes, or talks. It is also transmitted when an infected person or item is touched by a noninfected person.

Fever, a rash that starts on the face and spreads to the feet, swollen lymph nodes that remain for several weeks, and joint pain are symptoms.

The disease is highly contagious when the rash appears and can be transmitted from one week before to seven days after the appearance of the rash. The virus incubates from twelve to twenty-three days before onset of infection.

Health care workers should wear masks when treating patients and thoroughly wash hands after patient contact.

After recovery from rubella, there is usually lifelong immunity.

The vaccine is a live rubella virus and can be given as a rubella only, MR, or MMR.

Workplace programs should include the vaccination of health care workers who have not been vaccinated.

Side effects of the vaccination may include rash, joint pain, fever, and swollen lymph nodes. Persons with a high fever because of an illness should not be vaccinated until they recover.

Rubella can harm the fetus. The disease can cause hearing loss, mental retardation, heart defects, loss of weight, and death of the fetus. All women of childbearing age should be vaccinated. Once a woman becomes pregnant, she should not be immunized.

Women who want to become pregnant and are not immunized should receive the vaccine at least three months before they become pregnant. The vaccine is not recommended too close to pregnancy.

SALMONELLOSIS

Salmonellosis is transmitted by bacteria that get into the intestine and bloodstream. People get the disease by eating or drinking contaminated food and water and by person-to-person or person-to-animal contact through the fecal to oral route.

The bacteria are found in raw meat and eggs, unpasteurized milk and cheese products, pet turtles, chicks, dogs, and cats.

Vomiting, fever, and diarrhea are symptoms. They appear one to three days after becoming infected. The bacteria can be carried by a person from several days to several months.

Health care workers should wear gowns and impervious gloves when treating patients. To prevent spread of the disease, workers should wash hands with soap and water after bathroom visits and before and after handling food.

After recovery from the disease, a person does not become immune.

SCABIES

Scabies is a disease that affects the skin when scabies mites burrow into it. This produces an irritation that looks like a pimple. It is transmitted from skin-to-skin contact. It is also contracted when infected people spread the mite to bedclothes and other garments. Sexual contact can also spread the disease.

The disease is spread until the mites are destroyed by treatment.

Itching around the webs and sides of the fingers, wrists, elbows, armpits, breasts, nipples, genitalia, waist, thighs, and lower buttocks are symptoms.

When treating patients with scabies, health care workers should wear impervious gloves and gowns.

Treatment consists of skin lotion applications to the entire body except head and neck.

The fetus is not endangered if the mother has scabies. She should be treated by a physician for the condition.

SHIGELLOSIS (SHIGELLA DYSENTERY)

Shigellosis is caused by bacteria that get into the intestines. It is transmitted when food and water are contaminated by infected people. Direct contact can also spread the disease.

The disease can be passed in the stool for up to two weeks, and if hands are not washed after bathroom visits, it can be spread through the fecal to oral route.

Blood and mucus in the stool, fever, and diarrhea are symptoms. They can appear from one to seven days after being exposed.

Persons who have diarrhea should not return to work until they are cured. It is very important that all workers wash their hands with soap and water after each bathroom visit and before and after handling food.

Fluids should be taken to prevent dehydration. Antibiotics are administered for severe cases.

Immunity is not obtained after recovery.

Pregnant women should see their physician if they have the disease. The disease should not affect the fetus, but diarrhea and dehydration can weaken the mother, which in turn can affect the unborn child.

SHINGLES *(HERPES ZOSTER)*

The identical virus that causes chicken pox causes shingles. The disease results when the dormant chicken pox virus is reactivated in the system.

It occurs more frequently in persons with suppressed immune systems and persons who have suffered trauma and from sun exposure.

People who have shingles can spread chicken pox when contact is made with the fluid in blisters. Shingles on the upper half of the face can damage the eyes and cause blindness. In some cases it can cause facial paralysis, damage to the ear, and encephalitis.

Itching, sharp pain, and a tingling feeling are symptoms. In several days, a rash appears around the side of the trunk or face. This rash becomes blisters that dry out and crust over and then disappear in about three to five weeks.

Health care workers who are not immune to chicken pox can get shingles.

Impervious gloves and gowns should be worn when treating patients.

Immunity is obtained after recovery, but persons with suppressed immune systems may get the disease again.

Like chicken pox, the disease can affect the unborn child. Pregnant women exposed to the disease should follow the same precautions described for chicken pox. If the woman is not sure of her immunity, the degree of exposure should be ascertained and a physician consulted to determine the risk to herself and the fetus.

SYPHILIS

Syphilis is a sexually transmitted disease that is spread by bacteria. It is usually spread through sexual contact when there is contact with the moist lesions caused by the disease or mucous membranes of the infected person. Syphilis can be spread from up to two years, and the sores may not be visible. As the disease progresses, it could infect the skin, central nervous system, bones, and heart and could shorten life.

Symptoms appear ten to ninety days after infection and consist of sores at the site of contact. Glands become swollen about one week after the sores appear. The sores usually disappear within five weeks.

The second phase of symptoms appears about six weeks after the appearance of the sores. The symptoms during this phase include rash, tiredness, sore throat, fever, headache, swollen glands, loss of appetite, and hoarseness. These symptoms last from two to six weeks and eventually disappear.

Impervious gloves should be worn when there is possible contact with lesion secretions and blood.

Immunity to the disease is not obtained after recovery.

The disease is treated with antibiotics.

The disease can be passed to the unborn child from an infected mother. This can cause deformity or death. Pregnant women and infants should be tested for syphilis at time of delivery.

TETANUS (LOCKJAW)

Tetanus is the result of bacteria that invade the body through punctures, cuts, lacerations, and burns in the skin. If the wound is contaminated with tetanus bacteria that are in soil, dust, animal feces, or injected street drugs, this will infect the person with the wound. The bacteria can be present anywhere. The disease is generally not spread from person to person.

Weakness, cramping, stiffness, and difficulty in chewing or swallowing food are symptoms. The jaw,

face, and neck muscles, and eventually the muscles of the arms and legs become stiff.

Health care workers should wear impervious puncture-resistant gloves when treating patients. Immunity is not obtained after recovery. Immunity is only achieved by getting the tetanus toxoid vaccination and required boosters.

The vaccine is an inactivated tetanus toxin. It is usually given with a diphtheria toxoid (Td). If there is difficulty in breathing after having received a dose of tetanus toxoid, the person should not get additional doses.

Reactions to the vaccine are not serious. There is usually a redness, swelling, and tenderness at the injection site. A fever may also result.

The tetanus toxoid vaccination poses no danger to pregnant women.

TOXIC SHOCK SYNDROME

Toxic shock syndrome is a bacterial infection caused by bacteria that release a toxin. It is predominantly caused by the use of tampons and barrier contraceptives but can also be caused by infected surgical wounds and lesions.

Shock, low blood pressure, high fever, vomiting, diarrhea, and rash are symptoms.

Health care workers should wear impervious gloves and gowns when treating patients.

Treatment consists of administering antibiotics and controlling blood pressure.

TRICHINOSIS

Trichinosis is caused by a roundworm that is mainly found in improperly cooked pork and pork products. Pigs are mostly infected, but other animals such as dogs, cats, rats, foxes, wolves, and bears can also harbor the parasite.

Swelling around the eyes, fever, muscle soreness, pain, thirst, sweating, chills, and tiredness are symptoms. They can appear anywhere from five to forty days after infection.

Partial immunity may be obtained after recovery.

TUBERCULOSIS

(Tuberculosis is described under infectious diseases as a reference. A more detailed description concerning OSHA and CDC requirements is described in the TB guidelines [Chapter 14].)

Tuberculosis is a bacterial infection that invades the lungs. It can also infect the lymph nodes, kidneys, joints, and bones (extrapulmonary TB).

There are two stages of the disease: People who are infected but do not have active bacteria and cannot spread the disease; and people who have active TB who can spread the disease when they cough, sneeze, or talk. When this happens, airborne droplets get into the air that can be inhaled.

TB infection could last throughout the person's life and never develop into TB. The active TB stage can occur in two to three weeks after infection, or it could develop many years later. The more time that passes, the less the risk.

If TB is not treated, persons can become severely ill and die.

Fever, sweats, cough, weight loss, and fatigue are symptoms. Most infected people never develop TB.

See Chapter 14 for employer responsibilities involving high-risk employees.

Employers must use engineering and work practice controls to control exposure and have employees wear HEPA or N100 or P100 filter respirators. N100 is to be used in non-oil aerosol environments and P100 used in oil aerosol environments.

After recovery from active TB, reinfection can occur.

TULAREMIA

Tularemia is a disease caused by bacteria that can occur in both people and animals. Rabbits are frequently infected.

It is spread when the blood and tissue of infected animals come in contact with the skin or mucous membranes. It can also be transmitted by fluids from infected deer flies or ticks or by eating improperly cooked rabbit meat. Lesser modes of transmission include drinking contaminated water, inhaling contaminated dust, and handling contaminated animal pelts and paws.

Swollen glands, lesions, intestinal pain, vomiting, and diarrhea are symptoms. They appear in two to ten days after infection.

Health care workers should wear gowns and impervious gloves when treating patients.

Long-term immunity is obtained after recovery.

TYPHOID FEVER

Typhoid fever is a disease that infects the intestinal tract and, infrequently, the bloodstream. It is passed in the urine and feces of infected persons and is spread by eating food or drinking water that has become infected. It is a variety of bacteria that is the cause of salmonella.

People can be infectious for several days or up to several years.

Diarrhea, constipation, fever, headache, enlarged liver or spleen, and the appearance of rose colored spots on the body are symptoms.

Health care workers should wear impervious gloves and gowns when treating patients.

Immunity is not obtained after recovery.

The vaccination is usually only given to people who will be traveling to areas where there have been outbreaks of typhoid fever. There is a live bacteria vaccine called Ty21a, which is an oral vaccine. The other vaccine is a parenteral inactivated bacterial vaccine.

The Ty21a vaccine may cause abdominal discomfort, rash, nausea, and vomiting. The parenteral vaccine may cause discomfort at the injection site, malaise, fever, and headache.

Vaccinating pregnant women with either vaccine is not recommended because there is no information concerning the effects of the vaccine on the mother or unborn child. Pregnant women who believe they have been exposed should consult their physician promptly.

TYPHUS

Typhus is contracted from the bite of an infected flea from a rat host or from a person who has body lice.

The organism is called rickettsiae, and the incubation period is from ten to fourteen days.

The various types of typhus include epidemic typhus (spread person to person from body lice); murine typhus (spread by fleas from rat hosts); Brill-Zinsser disease (contracted by persons who have had epidemic typhus); scrub or miteborne typhus (contracted from the bite of an infected mite); and tick typhus (contracted from the bite of an infected tick).

Symptoms include severe headache; back, arm, and leg pain; weakness; rapid rise in fever within two to three days; weak and rapid pulse; trembling tongue; tongue coated with white fur; pupil contraction; muscle contraction; and delirium. In severe cases, the tongue becomes black and rolls up like a ball in the back of the mouth.

Health care workers should wear impervious gloves when treating patients. Fluids must be considered contaminated, and universal precautions as dictated by the OSHA bloodborne pathogen standard must be followed. This standard is described in Chapter 15 covering bloodborne pathogens.

Immunity is not obtained after recovery.

Typhus is treated with antibiotics.

Pregnant women traveling to areas known to have typhus should consult with their physician.

YELLOW FEVER

Yellow fever is caused by a virus that is carried by a mosquito. The mosquito bite injects the virus into the bloodstream.

Backache, headache, and vomiting are symptoms. Progression of the disease causes slow and weak pulse, bleeding gums, bloody urine, and jaundice. They occur three to six days after exposure.

Recovery from the disease gives the person permanent immunity.

The vaccine is a one-dose live vaccine and may be given with the vaccination for measles, smallpox, and hepatitis B.

Reactions to the vaccine include rash, headache, and fever.

The vaccine can infect the fetus. It is not recommended that pregnant women travel to yellow fever-infected areas.

YERSINIOSIS

Yersiniosis is caused by a bacterial infection of the intestinal tract. It is spread by the fecal to oral route when a person drinks water or eats food that is contaminated.

The bacteria is found in raw milk, lakes, streams, ice cream, improperly pasteurized chocolate milk, tofu, shellfish, and animals. Animals are the main cause of the disease because their feces may contaminate food and water.

The bacteria can be passed in the feces for a few weeks to a few months.

Symptoms include cramps, fever, and diarrhea.

Gowns and impervious gloves should be worn when treating patients.

Immunity is not obtained after recovery.

The disease is treated with antibiotics.

CHAPTER REVIEW

Multiple Choice

Select the best answer from the choices provided.

1. AIDS is caused by
   a. bacteria
   b. using utensils of an infected person
   c. a virus
   d. touch

2. Chicken pox can be hidden and appear later as
   a. meningitis
   b. herpes zoster
   c. hepatitis B
   d. E. coli

3. Legionnaires disease
   a. is caused by transmission from person to person
   b. is caused by a virus
   c. is caused by inhalation of water aerosols containing the organism
   d. cannot be confirmed by a blood test

4. Hepatitis B
   a. is spread by infected blood
   b. vaccine cannot safely be given to pregnant women
   c. cannot be contracted by persons who have recovered from the disease
   d. symptoms appear right after infection

5. Syphilis
   a. is a sexually transmitted disease
   b. is spread by a virus
   c. symptoms never disappear
   d. cannot be passed from the mother to the fetus

True/False

Indicate whether the statement is true or false by circling T or F.

6. T F There are diseases where it is not necessary for pregnant women to consult a physician.

7. T F Many diseases manifest identical symptoms.

8. T F Susceptibility to disease depends upon various circumstances.

9. T F There is a vaccination for just about every disease.

10. T F Every disease will have symptoms to indicate infection.

Matching

Match the terms in column 1 with the definitions in column 2.

Column 1
11. Rabies
12. Haemophilus influenza type B
13. Toxic shock
14. Lyme disease
15. AIDS

Column 2
a. Caused by infected blood
b. Caused by a deer tick bite
c. Caused by a bite from an infected animal
d. Can cause meningitis
e. Caused sometimes by infected surgical wounds

Short Answer

Briefly but thoroughly answer each statement.

16. What are some of the personal protective equipment that should be worn to protect against infectious diseases?

17. Describe some of the body fluids that can cause AIDS.

18. Describe your facility's training concerning infectious diseases.

19. Explain why tuberculosis is making a comeback.

20. Explain how the OSHA bloodborne pathogens standard fits into infectious disease control.

Infection Control

After studying this chapter, you should be able to

➤ Identify proper infection control procedures.
➤ Describe proper handwashing.
➤ Discuss the components of an infection control program.
➤ Identify the procedures for disinfecting equipment.
➤ Explain proper disposal of infectious materials.

An effective infection control program is essential in any health care facility if the spread of microbes is to be minimized. This requires the cooperation of housekeeping, maintenance, health care staff, and patients.

It is important that the employees in health care facilities know how infectious diseases are spread so that they can take the appropriate safeguards. This chapter describes the general guidelines for infection control that detail recommended procedures to follow to protect employees and patients. Many of the procedures described in this chapter, when followed, will assist the health care professional to be in compliance with the OSHA bloodborne pathogens standard.

GUIDELINES FOR HANDWASHING AND HOSPITAL ENVIRONMENTAL CONTROL

Handwashing is the single most important procedure for preventing nosocomial infections (infections acquired in the hospital). Environmental control is also essential to prevent the spread of infection.

Handwashing

Handwashing is defined as a vigorous, brief rubbing together of all surfaces of lathered hands, followed by rinsing under a stream of water. Although various products are available, handwashing can be classified simply by whether plain soap or detergents or antimicrobial-containing products are used. Handwashing with plain soaps or detergents (in bar, granule, leaflet, or liquid form) suspends microorganisms and allows them to be rinsed off; this process is often referred to as mechanical removal of microorganisms. In addition, handwashing with antimicrobial-containing products kills or inhibits the growth of microorganisms; this process is often referred to as chemical removal of microorganisms. Routine handwashing is discussed in this Guideline.

Epidemiology. The microbial flora of the skin consist of resident and transient microorganisms; the resident microorganisms survive and multiply on the skin and can be repeatedly cultured, while the transient microbial flora represent recent contaminants that can survive only a limited period of time. Most resident microorganisms are found in superficial skin layers, but about 10–20 percent can inhabit deep epidermal layers. Handwashing with plain soaps and detergents is effective in removing many transient microbial flora. Resident microorganisms in the deep layers may not be removed by handwashing with plain soaps and detergents, but usually can be killed or inhibited by handwashing with products that contain antimicrobial ingredients.

Many resident skin microorganisms are not highly virulent and are not implicated in infections other than skin infections. However, some of these microorganisms can cause infections in patients when surgery or other invasive procedures allow them to enter deep tissues or when a patient is severely immunocompromised or has an implanted device, such as a heart valve. In contrast, the transient microorganisms often found on the hands of hospital personnel can be pathogens acquired from colonized or infected patients and may cause nosocomial infections. Several recent studies have shown that transient and resident hand carriage of aerobic gram-negative microorganisms by hospital personnel may be more frequent than previously thought. More study on the bacteriology of hands is needed to fully understand the factors that contribute to persistent hand carriage of such microorganisms.

Control Measures. The absolute indications for, and the ideal frequency of, handwashing are generally not known because of the lack of well-controlled studies. Listing all circumstances that may require handwashing would be a lengthy and arbitrary task. The indications for handwashing depend on the type, intensity, duration, and sequence of activity. Prolonged and intense contact with any patient should probably be followed by handwashing. In addition, handwashing is indicated before performing invasive procedures, before taking care of particularly susceptible patients, such as those who are severely immunocompromised or newborn infants, and before and after touching wounds. Moreover, handwashing is indicated, even when gloves are used, after situations during which microbial contamination of the hands is likely to occur, especially those involving contact with mucous membranes, blood and body fluids, and secretions or excretions, and after touching inanimate sources that are likely to be contaminated, such as urine-measuring devices. In addition, handwashing is an important component of the personal hygiene of all hospital personnel, and handwashing should be encouraged when personnel are in doubt about the necessity for doing so.

The circumstances that require handwashing are frequently found in high-risk units, because patients in these units are often infected or colonized with virulent or multiply-resistant microorganisms,

and are highly susceptible to infection because of wounds, invasive procedures, or diminished immune function. Handwashing in these units is indicated between direct contact with different patients and often is indicated more than once in the care of one patient—for example, after touching excretions or secretions, before going on to another care activity for the same patient.

The recommended handwashing technique depends on the purpose of the handwashing. The ideal duration of handwashing is not known, but washing times of fifteen seconds or less have been reported as effective in removing most transient contaminants from the skin. Therefore, for most activities, a vigorous, brief (at least ten seconds) rubbing together of all surfaces of lathered hands followed by rinsing under a stream of water is recommended. If hands are visibly soiled, more time may be required for handwashing.

The absolute indications for handwashing with plain soaps and detergents versus handwashing with antimicrobial-containing products are not known because of the lack of well-controlled studies comparing infection rates when such products are used. For most routine activities, handwashing with plain soap appears to be sufficient, because soap will allow most transient microorganisms to be washed off.

Handwashing products for use in hospitals are available in several forms. It is important, however, that the product selected for use be acceptable to the personnel who will use it. When plain soap is selected for handwashing, the bar, liquid, granule, or soap-impregnated tissue form may be used. It is preferable that bar soaps be placed on racks that allow water to drain. Because liquid-soap containers can become contaminated and might serve as reservoirs of microorganisms, reusable liquid containers need to be cleaned when empty and refilled with fresh soap. Completely disposable containers obviate the need to empty and clean dispensers but may be more expensive. Most antimicrobial-containing handwashing products are available as liquids. Antimicrobial-containing foams and rinses are also available for use in areas without easy access to sinks.

In addition to handwashing, personnel may often wear gloves as an extra margin of safety. As with handwashing, the absolute indications for wearing gloves are not known. There is general agreement that wearing sterile gloves is indicated when certain invasive procedures are performed or when open wounds are touched. Nonsterile gloves can be worn when hands are likely to become contaminated with potentially infective material such as blood, body fluids, or secretions, since it is often not known which patients' blood, body fluids, or secretions contain hepatitis B virus or other pathogens. Further, gloves can be worn to prevent gross microbial contamination of hands, such as when objects soiled with feces are handled. When gloves are worn, handwashing is also recommended because gloves may become perforated during use and because bacteria can multiply rapidly on gloved hands.

The convenient placement of sinks, handwashing products, and paper towels is often suggested as a means of encouraging frequent and appropriate handwashing. Sinks with faucets that can be turned off by means other than the hands (e.g., foot pedals) and sinks that minimize splash can help personnel avoid immediate recontamination of washed hands.

Although handwashing is considered the most important single procedure for preventing nosocomial infections, two reports showed poor compliance with handwashing protocols by personnel in medical intensive care units, especially by physicians and personnel taking care of patients on isolation precautions. Failure to wash hands is a complex problem that may be caused by lack of motivation or lack of knowledge about the importance of handwashing. It may also be caused by obstacles such as understaffing, inconveniently located sinks, absence of paper towels, an unacceptable handwashing product, or the presence of dermatitis caused by previous handwashing. More study is needed to identify which of these factors, alone or in combination, contribute significantly to the problem of poor compliance with handwashing recommendations.

Recommendations.

1. *Handwashing Indications.* In the absence of a true emergency, personnel should always wash their hands before performing invasive procedures; before taking care of particularly susceptible patients, such as those who are severely immunocompromised and newborns; before and after touching wounds, whether surgical, traumatic, or associated with an invasive device; after situations during which microbial contamination of hands is likely to occur, especially those involving contact with mucous membranes, blood or body fluids, secretions, or excretions; after touching inanimate sources that are likely to be contaminated with virulent or epidemiologically important microorganisms (these sources include urine-measuring devices or secretion collection apparatuses); after taking care of an infected patient or one who is likely to be colonized with microorganisms of special clinical or epidemiologic significance (for example, multiply-resistant bacteria); and between contacts with different patients in high-risk units. Most routine hospital activities involving indirect patient contact, e.g., handing patients medications, food, or other objects—do not require handwashing).

2. *Handwashing Technique.* For routine handwashing, a vigorous rubbing together of all surfaces of lathered hands for at least ten seconds, followed by thorough rinsing under a stream of water is recommended.

3. *Handwashing with Plain Soap.* Plain soap should be used for handwashing unless otherwise indicated. If bar soap is used, it should be kept on racks that allow drainage of water. If liquid soap is used, the dispenser should be replaced or cleaned and filled with fresh product when empty; liquids should not be added to a partially full dispenser.

4. *Handwashing with Antimicrobial-Containing Products (Health Care Personnel Handwashes).* Antimicrobial handwashing products should be used for handwashing before personnel care for newborns and when otherwise indicated during their care, between patients in high-risk units, and before personnel take care of severely immunocompromised patients. Hospitals may choose from products in the product category defined by the FDA as health care personnel handwashes. Persons responsible for selecting commercially marketed an-

timicrobial health care personnel handwashes can obtain information about categorization of products from the Center for Drugs and Biologics, Division of OTC Drug Evaluation, FDA, 5600 Fishers Lane, Rockville, MD 20857. In addition, information published in the scientific literature, presented at scientific meetings, documented by manufacturers, and obtained from other sources deemed important may be considered. Antimicrobial-containing products that do not require water for use, such as foams or rinses, can be used in areas where no sinks are available.

5. *Handwashing Facilities.* Handwashing facilities should be conveniently located throughout the hospital. A sink should be located in or just outside every patient room. More than one sink per room may be necessary if a large room is used for several patients. Handwashing facilities should be located in or adjacent to rooms where diagnostic or invasive procedures that require handwashing are performed (e.g., cardiac catheterization, bronchoscopy, sigmoidoscopy, etc.).

Cleaning, Disinfecting, and Sterilizing Patient-Care Equipment

Cleaning, the physical removal of organic material or soil from objects, is usually done by using water with or without detergents. Generally, cleaning is designed to remove rather than to kill microorganisms. Sterilization, on the other hand, is the destruction of all forms of microbial life; it is carried out in the hospital with steam under pressure, liquid or gaseous chemicals, or dry heat. Disinfection, defined as the intermediate measures between physical cleaning and sterilization, is carried out with pasteurization or chemical germicides.

Chemical germicides can be classified by several systems. We have used the system originally proposed by Spaulding in which three levels of disinfection are defined: high, intermediate, and low. In contrast, EPA uses a system that classifies chemical germicides as sporicides, general disinfectants, hospital disinfectants, sanitizers, and others. Formulations registered by the EPA as sporicides are considered sterilants if the contact time is long enough to destroy all forms of microbial life, or high-level disinfectants if contact times are shorter. Chemical germicides registered by the EPA as sanitizers probably fall into the category of low-level disinfectants. Numerous formulations of chemical germicides can be classified as either low- or intermediate-level disinfectants, depending on the specific label claims. For example, some chemical germicide formulations are claimed to be efficacious against *Mycobacterium tuberculosis;* by Spaulding's system, these formulations would be classified at least as intermediate-level disinfectants. However, chemical germicide formulations with specific label claims for effectiveness against *Salmonella choleraesuis, Staphylococcus aureus,* and *Pseudomonas aeruginosa* (the challenge microorganisms required for EPA classification as a "hospital disinfectant") could fall into intermediate- or low-level disinfectant categories.

The rationale for cleaning, disinfecting, or sterilizing patient-care equipment can be understood more readily if medical devices, equipment, and surgical materials are divided into three general categories (critical items, semicritical items, and noncritical items) based on the potential risk of infection involved in their use. This categorization of medical devices also is based on the original suggestions by Spaulding.

Critical items are instruments or objects that are introduced directly into the bloodstream or into other normally sterile areas of the body. Examples of critical items are surgical instruments, cardiac catheters, implants, pertinent components of the heart-lung oxygenator, and the blood compartment of a hemodialyzer. Sterility at the time of use is required for these items; consequently, one of several accepted sterilization procedures is generally recommended. Items in the second category are classified as semicritical in terms of the degree of risk of infection. Examples are noninvasive flexible and rigid fiber-optic endoscopes, endotracheal tubes, anesthesia breathing circuits, and cystoscopes. Although these items come in contact with intact mucous membranes, they do not ordinarily penetrate body surfaces. If steam sterilization can be used, it is often cheaper to sterilize many of these items, but sterilization is not absolutely essential; at a minimum, a high-level disinfection procedure that can be expected to destroy vegetative microorganisms, most fungal spores, tubercle bacilli, and small nonlipid viruses is recommended. In most cases, meticulous physical cleaning followed by an appropriate high-level disinfection treatment gives the user a reasonable degree of assurance that the items are free of pathogens.

Noncritical items are those that either do not ordinarily touch the patient or touch only intact skin. Such items include crutches, bed boards, blood pressure cuffs, and a variety of other medical accessories. These items rarely, if ever, transmit disease. Consequently, depending on the particular piece of equipment or item, washing with a detergent may be sufficient.

The level of disinfection achieved depends on several factors, principally contact time, temperature, type and concentration of the active ingredients of the chemical germicide, and the nature of the microbial contamination. Some disinfection procedures are capable of producing sterility if the contact times used are sufficiently long; when these procedures are continued long enough to kill all but resistant bacterial spores, the result is high-level disinfection. Other disinfection procedures that can kill many types of viruses and most vegetative microorganisms (but cannot be relied upon to kill resistant microorganisms such as tubercle bacilli, bacterial spores, or certain viruses) are considered to be intermediate or low-level disinfection.

The tubercle bacillus, lipid and nonlipid viruses, and other groups of microorganisms are used in the context of indicator microorganisms that have varying degrees of resistance to chemical germicides and not necessarily because of their importance in causing nosocomial infections. For example, cells of *M. tuberculosis* or *M. bovis,* which are used in routine efficacy tests, are among the most resistant vegetative microorganisms known and, after bacterial endospores, constitute the most severe challenge to a chemical germicide. Thus, a tuberculocidal chemical germicide may be used as a high- or intermediate-level disinfectant targeted to many types of nosocomial pathogens but not specifically to control respiratory tuberculosis.

Control Measures. Because it is neither necessary nor possible to sterilize all patient-care items, hospital policies can identify whether cleaning, disinfecting, or sterilizing of an item is indicated to decrease the risk of infection. The process indicated for an item will depend on its intended use. Any microorganism, including bacterial spores that come in contact with normally sterile tissue can cause infection. Thus, it is important that all items that will touch normally sterile tissues be sterilized. It is less important that objects touching mucous membranes be sterile. Intact mucous membranes are generally resistant to infection by common bacterial spores but are not resistant to many other microorganisms, such as viruses and tubercle bacilli; therefore, items that touch mucous membranes require a disinfection process that kills all but resistant bacterial spores. In general, intact skin acts as an effective barrier to most microorganisms; thus, items that touch only intact skin need only be clean.

Items must be thoroughly cleaned before processing, because organic material (e.g., blood and proteins) may contain high concentrations of microorganisms. Also, such organic material may inactivate chemical germicides and protect microorganisms from the disinfection or sterilization process. For many noncritical items, such as blood pressure cuffs or crutches, cleaning can consist only of washing with a detergent or a disinfectant-detergent, rinsing, and thorough drying.

Steam sterilization is the most inexpensive and effective method for sterilization. Steam sterilization is unsuitable, however, for processing plastics with low melting points, powders, or anhydrous oils. Items that are to be sterilized but not used immediately need to be wrapped for storage. Sterility can be maintained in storage for various lengths of time, depending on the type of wrapping material, the conditions of storage, and the integrity of the package.

Several methods have been developed to monitor steam sterilization processes. One method is to check the highest temperature that is reached during sterilization and the length of time that this temperature is maintained. In addition, heat- and steam-sensitive chemical indicators can be used on the outside of each pack. These indicators do not reliably document sterility, but they do show that an item has not accidentally bypassed a sterilization process. As an additional precaution, a large pack might have a chemical indicator both on the outside and the inside to verify that steam has penetrated the pack.

Microbiological monitoring of steam sterilizers is recommended at least once a week with commercial preparations of spores of *Bacillus stearothermophilus* (a microorganism having spores that are particularly resistant to moist heat, thus assuring a wide margin of safety). If a sterilizer is working properly and used appropriately, the spores are usually killed. One positive spore test (spores not killed) does not necessarily indicate that items processed in the sterilizer are not sterile, but it does suggest that the sterilizer should be rechecked for proper temperature, length of cycle, loading, and use and that the test be repeated. Spore testing of steam sterilization is just one of several methods for assuring adequate processing of patient-care items.

Implantable items, such as orthopedic devices, require special handling before and during sterilization; thus, packs containing implantable objects need to be clearly labeled so that they will be appropriately processed. To guarantee a wide margin of safety, it is recommended that each load of such items be tested with a spore test and that the sterilized item not be released for use until the spore test is negative at forty-eight hours. If it is not possible to process an implantable object with a confirmed forty-eight-hour spore test before use, it is recommended that the unwrapped object receive the equivalent of full-cycle steam sterilization and not flash sterilization. Flash sterilization (270°F [132°C] for three minutes in a gravity displacement steam sterilizer) is not recommended for implantable items because spore tests cannot be used reliably and the margin of safety is lower.

Because ethylene oxide gas sterilization is a more complex and expensive process than steam sterilization, it is usually restricted to objects that might be damaged by heat or excessive moisture. Before sterilization, objects also need to be cleaned thoroughly and wrapped in a material that allows the gas to penetrate. Chemical indicators need to be used with each package to show that it has been exposed to the gas sterilization process. Moreover, it is recommended that gas sterilizers be checked at least once a week with commercial preparations of spores, usually *Bacillus subtilis var. niger*. Because ethylene oxide gas is toxic, precautions (e.g., local exhaust ventilation) should be taken to protect personnel. All objects processed by gas sterilization also need special aeration according to manufacturer's recommendations before use to remove toxic residues of ethylene oxide.

Powders and anhydrous oils can be sterilized by dry heat. Microbiological monitoring of dry heat sterilizers and following manufacturers' recommendations for their use and maintenance usually provides a wide margin of safety for dry heat sterilization.

Liquid chemicals can be used for sterilization and disinfection when steam, gas, or dry heat sterilization is not indicated or available. With some formulations, high-level disinfection can be accomplished in ten to thirty minutes, and sterilization can be achieved if exposure is for significantly longer times. Nevertheless, not all formulations are equally applicable to all items that need to be sterilized or disinfected. No formulation can be considered as an "all purpose" chemical germicide. In each case, more detailed information can be obtained from the EPA, descriptive brochures from the manufacturers, peer-review journal articles, and books. The most appropriate chemical germicide for a particular situation can be selected by responsible personnel in each hospital based on the object to be disinfected, the level of disinfection needed, and the scope of services, physical facilities, and personnel available in the hospital. It is also important that the manufacturer's instructions for use be consulted.

Gloves may be indicated to prevent skin reactions when some chemical disinfectants are used. Items subjected to high-level disinfection with liquid chemicals need to be rinsed in sterile water to remove toxic or irritating residues and then thoroughly dried. Subsequently, the objects need to be handled aseptically with sterile gloves and towels and stored in protective wrappers to prevent recontamination.

Hot-water disinfection (pasteurization) is a high-level, nontoxic disinfection process that can be used for certain items (e.g., respiratory therapy breathing circuits).

In recent years, some hospitals have considered reusing medical devices labeled disposable or single use only. In general, the primary, if not the sole, motivation for such reuse is to save money. For example, the disposable hollow-fiber hemodialyzer has been reprocessed and reused on the same patient in hemodialysis centers since the early 1970s. By 1984, 51 percent of the 1,200 U.S. dialysis centers were using dialyzer reprocessing programs. It has been estimated that this practice saves more than $100 million per year. When standard protocols for cleaning and disinfecting hemodialyzers are used, there does not appear to be any significant infection risk to dialysis patients. Moreover, the safety and efficacy of dialyzer reuse programs are supported by several major studies. Few, if any, other medical devices that might be considered candidates for reprocessing have been evaluated in this manner.

Arguments for and against reprocessing and reusing single-use items have been summarized. Because there is lack of evidence indicating increased risk of nosocomial infections associated with reusing all single-use items, a categorical recommendation against all types of reuse is not considered justifiable. Rather than recommending for or against reprocessing and reuse of all single-use items, it appears more prudent to recommend that hospitals consider the safety and efficacy of the reprocessing procedure of each item or device separately and the likelihood that the device will function as intended after reprocessing. In many instances it may be difficult if not impossible to document that the device can be reprocessed without residual toxicity and still function safely and effectively. Few, if any, manufacturers of disposable or single-use medical devices provide reprocessing information on the product label.

Hydrotherapy pools and immersion tanks present unique disinfection problems in hospitals. It is generally not economically feasible to drain large hydrotherapy pools that contain thousands of gallons of water after each patient use. Typically, these pools are used by a large number of patients and are drained and cleaned every one to two weeks. The water temperature is typically maintained near 37°C (98.6°F). Between cleanings, water can be contaminated by organic material from patients, and high levels of microbial contamination are possible. One method to maintain safe pool water is to install a water filter of sufficient size to filter all the water at least three times per day and to chlorinate the water so that a free chlorine residual of approximately 0.5 mg/l is maintained at a pH of 7.2 to 7.6. Local public health authorities can provide consultation regarding chlorination, alternate halogen disinfectants, and hydrotherapy pool sanitation.

Hubbard and immersion tanks present entirely different problems than large pools, since they are drained after each patient use. All inside surfaces need to be cleaned with a disinfectant-detergent, then rinsed with tap water. After the last patient each day, an additional disinfection step is performed. One general procedure is to circulate a chlorine solution (200–300 mg/l) through the agitator of the tank for fifteen minutes and then rinse it out. It is also recommended that the tank be thoroughly cleaned with a disinfectant-detergent, rinsed, wiped dry with clean cloths, and not filled until ready for use.

An alternative approach to control of contamination in hydrotherapy tanks is to use plastic liners and create the "whirlpool effect" without agitators. Such liners make it possible to minimize contact of contaminated water with the interior surface of the tank and also obviate the need for agitators that may be very difficult to clean and decontaminate.

Recommendations.

1. *Cleaning.* All objects to be disinfected or sterilized should first be thoroughly cleaned to remove all organic matter (blood and tissue) and other residue.

2. *Indications for sterilization and high-level disinfection.* Critical medical devices or patient-care equipment that enter normally sterile tissue or the vascular system or through which blood flows should be subjected to a sterilization procedure before each use. Laparoscopes, arthroscopes, and other scopes that enter normally sterile tissue should be subjected to a sterilization procedure before each use; if this is not feasible, they should receive at least high-level disinfection. Equipment that touches mucous membranes—e.g., endoscopes, endotracheal tubes,

anesthesia breathing circuits, and respiratory therapy equipment—should receive high-level disinfection.

3. *Methods of Sterilization.* Whenever sterilization is indicated, a steam sterilizer should be used unless the object to be sterilized will be damaged by heat, pressure, or moisture or is otherwise inappropriate for steam sterilization. In this case, another acceptable method of sterilization should be used. Flash sterilization (270°F [132°C] for three minutes in a gravity displacement steam sterilizer) is not recommended for implantable items.

4. *Biological Monitoring of Sterilizers.* All sterilizers should be monitored at least once a week with commercial preparations of spores intended specifically for that type of sterilizer (i.e., *Bacillus stearothermophilus* for steam sterilizers and *Bacillus subtilis* for ethylene oxide and dry heat sterilizers). Every load that contains implantable objects should be monitored. These implantable objects should not be used until the spore test is found to be negative at forty-eight hours. If spores are not killed in routine spore tests, the sterilizer should immediately be checked for proper use and function and the spore test repeated. Objects, other than implantable objects, do not need to be recalled because of a single positive spore test unless the sterilizer or the sterilization procedure is defective. If spore tests remain positive, use of the sterilizer should be discontinued until it is serviced.

5. *Use and Preventive Maintenance.* Manufacturers' instructions should be followed for use and maintenance of sterilizers.

6. *Chemical Indicators.* Chemical indicators that will show a package has been through a sterilization cycle should be visible on the outside of each package sterilized.

7. *Use of Sterile Items.* An item should not be used if its sterility is questionable—e.g., its package is punctured, torn, or wet.

8. *Reprocessing Single-Use or Disposable Items.* Items or devices that cannot be cleaned and sterilized or disinfected without altering their physical integrity and function should not be reprocessed. Reprocessing procedures that re-

sult in residual toxicity or compromise the overall safety or effectiveness of the items or devices should be avoided.

Microbiologic Sampling

Before 1970, regularly scheduled culturing of the air and environmental surfaces such as floors, walls, and table tops was widely practiced in U.S. hospitals. By 1970, CDC and the American Hospital Association were advocating that hospitals discontinue routine environmental culturing, because rates of nosocomial infection had not been related to levels of general microbial contamination of air or environmental surfaces, and meaningful standards for permissible levels of microbial contamination of environmental surfaces did not exist. Between 1970 and 1975, 25 percent of U.S. hospitals reduced the extent of such routine environmental culturing, and this trend has continued.

In the last several years, there has also been a trend toward reducing routine microbiologic sampling for quality control purposes. In 1982, CDC recommended that the disinfection process for respiratory therapy equipment should not be monitored by routine microbiologic sampling. Moreover, the recommendation for microbiologic sampling of infant formulas prepared in the hospital has been removed from this Guideline, because there is no epidemiologic evidence to show that such quality control testing influences the infection rate in hospitals.

Control Measures. The only routine or periodic microbiologic sampling that is recommended is of the water and dialysis fluids used with artificial kidney machines in hospital-based or freestanding chronic hemodialysis centers. Microbiologic sampling of dialysis fluids and water used to prepare dialysis fluids is recommended because gram-negative bacteria are able to grow rapidly in water and other fluids associated with the hemodialysis system; high levels of these microorganisms place dialysis patients at risk of pyrogenic reactions, bacteremia, or both. It is suggested that the water that is used to prepare dialysis fluid also be sampled periodically, because high levels of bacteria in water often become amplified downstream in a hemodialysis system and are sometimes predictive of bacterial contamination in dialysis fluids. Although it is difficult to determine the exact frequency of such a sampling program in the absence of pyrogenic reactions and bacteremia, sampling water and dialysis fluid monthly appears to be reasonable.

Routine microbiologic sampling of patient-care items purchased as sterile is not recommended because of the difficulty and expense of performing adequate sterility testing with low-frequency contamination.

Microbiologic sampling is indicated during investigation of infection problems if environmental reservoirs are implicated epidemiologically in disease transmission. It is important, however, that such culturing be based on epidemiologic data and follow a written plan that specifies the objects to be sampled and the actions to be taken based on culture results.

Recommendations.

1. *Routine Environmental Culturing of Air and Environmental Surfaces.* Routine microbiologic sampling of the air and environmental surfaces should not be done.
2. *Microbiologic Sampling of Dialysis Fluids.* Water used to prepare dialysis fluid should be sampled once a month; it should not contain a total viable microbial count greater than 200 colony-forming units (CFU)/ml. The dialysis fluid should be sampled once a month at the end of a dialysis treatment and should contain less than 2,000 CFU/ml.
3. *Microbiologic Sampling for Specific Problems.* Microbiologic sampling, when indicated, should be an integral part of an epidemiologic investigation.
4. *Sampling for Manufacturer-Associated Contamination.* Routine microbiologic sampling of patient-care objects purchased as sterile is not recommended. If contamination of a commercial product sold as sterile is suspected, infection control personnel should be notified, suspect lot numbers should be recorded, and items from suspected lots should be segre-

gated and quarantined. Appropriate microbiologic assays may be considered; however, the nearest district office of the FDA, local and state health departments, and CDC should be notified promptly.

Infective Waste

Because a precise definition of infective waste that is based on the quantity and type of etiologic agents present is virtually impossible, the most practical approach to infective waste management is to identify those wastes that represent a sufficient potential risk of causing infection during handling and disposal and for which some special precautions appear prudent. Hospital wastes for which special precautions appear prudent include microbiology laboratory waste, pathology waste, and blood specimens or blood products. Moreover, the risk of either injury or infection from certain sharp items (e.g., needles and scalpel blades) contaminated with blood also needs to be considered when such items are disposed of. Although any item that has had contact with blood, exudates, or secretions may be potentially infective, it is not normally considered practical or necessary to treat all such waste as infective. CDC has published general recommendations for handling infective waste from patients on isolation precautions.

Additional special precautions may be necessary for certain rare diseases or conditions such as Lassa fever. The EPA has published a draft manual (Environmental Protection Agency, Office of Solid Waste and Emergency Response, Draft Manual for Infectious Waste Management, SW-957, 1982, Washington, 1982) that identifies and categorizes other specific types of waste that may be generated in some research-oriented hospitals. In addition to the above guidelines, local and state environmental regulations may also exist.

Control Measures. Solid waste from the microbiology laboratory can be placed in steam-sterilizable bags or pans and steam-sterilized in the laboratory. Alternatively, it can be transported in sealed, impervious plastic bags to be burned in a hospital incinerator. A single bag is probably adequate if the bag is sturdy (not easily penetrated) and if the waste can be put in the bag without contaminating the outside of the bag; otherwise, double-bagging is indicated. All slides or tubes with small amounts of blood can be packed in sealed, impervious containers and sent for incineration or steam sterilization in the hospital. Exposure for up to ninety minutes at 250°F (121°C) in a steam sterilizer, depending on the size of the load and type container, may be necessary to assure an adequate sterilization cycle. After steam sterilization, the residue can be safely handled and discarded with all other nonhazardous hospital solid waste. All containers with more than a few milliliters of blood remaining after laboratory procedures and/or bulk blood may be steam sterilized, or the contents may be carefully poured down a utility sink drain or toilet.

Waste from the pathology laboratory is customarily incinerated at the hospital. Although no national data are available, in one state 96 percent of the hospitals surveyed reported that they incinerate pathology waste. Any hospital incinerator should be capable of burning, within applicable air pollution regulations, the actual waste materials to be destroyed. Improper incineration of waste with high moisture and low energy content, such as pathology waste, can lead to emission problems.

Disposables that can cause injury, such as scalpel blades and syringes with needles, should be placed in puncture-resistant containers. Ideally, such containers are located where these items are used. Syringes and needles can be placed intact directly into the rigid containers for safe storage until terminal treatment. To prevent needle-stick injuries, needles should not be recapped, purposely bent, or broken by hand. When some needle-cutting devices are used, blood may be aerosolized or spattered onto environmental surfaces; however, currently no data are available from controlled studies examining the effect, if any, of the use of these devices on the incidence of needle-transmissible infections.

It is often necessary to transport or store infective waste within the hospital prior to terminal treatment. This can be done safely if proper and common-sense procedures are used. The EPA draft manual mentioned earlier contains guidelines for the storage and transport, both on-site and off-site, of infective waste. For unique and specialized problems, this manual can be consulted.

Recommendations.

1. *Identification of Infective Waste.* Microbiology laboratory wastes, blood and blood products, pathology waste, and sharp items (especially needles) should be considered as potentially infective and handled and disposed of with special precautions. Infective waste from patients on isolation precautions should be handled and disposed of according to the current edition of the Guideline for Isolation Precautions in Hospitals. (This recommendation is not categorized because the recommendations for isolation precautions are not categorized.)

2. *Handling, Transport, and Storage of Infective Waste.* Personnel involved in the handling and disposal of infective waste should be informed of the potential health and safety hazards and trained in the appropriate handling and disposal methods. If processing and/or disposal facilities are not available at the site of infective waste generation (i.e., laboratory, etc.) the waste may be safely transported in sealed impervious containers to another hospital area for appropriate treatment. To minimize the potential risk for accidental transmission of disease or injury, infective waste awaiting terminal processing should be stored in an area accessible only to personnel involved in the disposal process.

3. *Processing and Disposal of Infective Waste.* Infective waste, in general, should either be incinerated or should be autoclaved prior to disposal in a sanitary landfill. Disposable syringes with needles, scalpel blades, and other sharp items capable of causing injury should be placed intact into puncture-resistant containers located as close to the area in which they were used as is practical. To prevent needle-stick injuries, needles should not be recapped, purposely bent, broken, or otherwise manipulated by hand. Bulk blood, suctioned fluids, excretions, and secretions may be carefully poured down a drain connected to a sanitary sewer. Sanitary sewers may also be used

for the disposal of other infectious wastes capable of being ground and flushed into the sewer. (Special precautions may be necessary for certain rare diseases or conditions such as Lassa fever.)

Housekeeping

Although microorganisms are a normal contaminant of walls, floors, and other surfaces, these environmental surfaces rarely are associated with transmission of infections to patients or personnel. Therefore, extraordinary attempts to disinfect or sterilize these environmental surfaces are rarely indicated. However, routine cleaning and removal of soil are recommended.

Control Measures. Cleaning schedules and methods vary according to the area of the hospital, type of surface to be cleaned, and the amount and type of soil present. Horizontal surfaces (for example, bedside tables and hard-surfaced flooring) in patient-care areas are usually cleaned on a regular basis, when soiling or spills occur, and when a patient is discharged. Cleaning of walls, blinds, and curtains is recommended only if they are visibly soiled. Disinfectant fogging is an unsatisfactory method of decontaminating air and surfaces and is not recommended.

Recommendations against use of carpets in patient-care areas have been removed from this Guideline, because there is no epidemiologic evidence to show that carpets influence the nosocomial infection rate in hospitals. Carpets, however, may contain much higher levels of microbial contamination than hard-surfaced flooring and can be difficult to keep clean in areas of heavy soiling or spillage; therefore, appropriate cleaning and maintenance procedures are indicated.

Disinfectant-detergent formulations registered by the EPA can be used for enviromental surface cleaning, but the actual physical removal of microorganisms by scrubbing is probably as important, if not more so, than any antimicrobial effect of the cleaning agent used. Therefore, cost, safety, and acceptability by housekeepers can be the main criteria for selecting any such registered agent. The manufacturers' instructions for appropriate use should be followed.

Special precautions for cleaning incubators, mattresses, and other nursery surfaces with which neonates have contact have been recommended, because inadequately diluted solutions of phenolics used for such cleaning and poor ventilation have been associated with hyperbilirubinemia in newborns.

Recommendations.
1. *Choice of Cleaning Agent for Environmental Surfaces in Patient-Care Areas.* Any hospital-grade disinfectant-detergent registered by the EPA may be used for cleaning environmental surfaces. Manufacturers' instructions for use of such products should be followed.
2. *Cleaning of Horizontal Surfaces in Patient-Care Areas.* Uncarpeted floors and other horizontal surfaces, for example, bedside tables, should be cleaned regularly and if spills occur. Carpeting should be vacuumed regularly with units designed to efficiently filter discharged air, cleaned if spills occur, and shampooed whenever a thorough cleaning is indicated.
3. *Cleaning Walls, Blinds, and Curtains.* Terminal cleaning of walls, blinds, and curtains is not recommended unless they are visibly soiled.
4. *Disinfectant Fogging.* Disinfectant fogging should not be done.

Laundry

Although soiled linen has been identified as a source of large numbers of pathogenic microorganisms, the risk of actual disease transmission appears negligible. Rather than rigid rules and regulations, hygienic and common sense storage and processing of clean and soiled linen are recommended.

Control Measures. Soiled linen can be transported in the hospital by cart or chute. Bagging linen is indicated if chutes are used, because improperly designed chutes can be a means of spreading microorganisms throughout the hospital.

Soiled linen may or may not be sorted in the laundry before being loaded into washer/extractor units. Sorting before washing protects both machinery and linen from the effects of objects in the linen and reduces the potential for recontamination of clean linen that sorting after washing requires. Sorting after washing minimizes the direct exposure of laundry personnel to infective material in the soiled linen and reduces airborne microbial contamination in the laundry. Protective apparel and appropriate ventilation can minimize these exposures.

The microbicidal action of the normal laundering process is affected by several physical and chemical factors. Although dilution is not a microbicidal mechanism, it is responsible for the removal of significant quantities of microorganisms. Soaps or detergents loosen soil and also have some microbicidal properties. Hot water provides an effective means of destroying microorganisms, and a temperature of at least 71°C (160°F) for a minimum of twenty-five minutes is commonly recommended for hot-water washing. Chlorine bleach provides an extra margin of safety. A total available chlorine residual of 50-150 ppm is usually achieved during the bleach cycle. The last action performed during the washing process is the addition of a mild acid to neutralize any alkalinity in the water supply, soap, or detergent. The rapid shift in pH from approximately 12 to 5 also may tend to inactivate some microorganisms.

Recent studies have shown that a satisfactory reduction of microbial contamination can be achieved at lower water temperatures of 22°-50°C (71.6°-122°F) when the cycling of the washer, the wash formula, and the amount of chlorine bleach are carefully monitored and controlled. Instead of the microbicidal action of hot water, low temperature laundry cycles rely heavily on the presence of bleach to reduce levels of microbial contamination. Regardless of whether hot or cold water is used for washing, the temperatures reached in drying and especially during ironing provide additional significant microbicidal action.

Recommendations.

1. *Routine Handling of Soiled Linen.* Soiled linen should be handled as little as possible and with minimum agitation to prevent gross microbial contamination of the air and of persons handling the linen. All soiled linen should be bagged or put into carts at the location where it was used; it should not be sorted or prerinsed in patient-care areas. Linen soiled with blood or body fluids should be deposited and transported in bags that prevent leakage. If laundry chutes are used, linen should be bagged, and chutes should be properly designed.
2. *Hot-Water Washing.* If hot water is used, linen should be washed with a detergent in water at least 71°C (160°F) for twenty-five minutes.
3. *Low-Temperature Water Washing.* If low temperature (less than or equal to 70°C [158°F]) laundry cycles are used, chemicals suitable for low-temperature washing at proper use concentration should be used.
4. *Transportation of Clean Linen.* Clean linen should be transported and stored by methods that will ensure its cleanliness.

GUIDELINES FOR INFECTION CONTROL IN HOSPITAL PERSONNEL

The organization of a health service for hospital personnel will depend on many factors—for example, the size of the institution, the number of personnel, and the services offered. These factors will determine the size, location, and staffing of the service. Regardless of how the service is provided, certain elements will assist in effectively attaining infection control goals:

1. Placement evaluations
2. Personnel health and safety education
3. Immunization programs
4. Protocols for surveillance and management of job-related illnesses and exposures to infectious diseases
5. Counseling services for personnel regarding infection risks related to employment or special conditions
6. Guidelines for work restriction because of infectious disease
7. Maintenance of health records

Placement Evaluations

When personnel are initially appointed or are reassigned to different jobs or areas, a placement evaluation can be used to ensure that persons are not placed in jobs that would pose undue risk of infection to them, other personnel, patients, or visitors. A health inventory is an important part of this evaluation. This inventory can include determining a health worker's immunization status and obtaining a history of any conditions that may predispose the health worker to acquiring or transmitting infectious diseases—for example, a history of such childhood diseases as chickenpox and measles; history of exposure to or treatment for tuberculosis; history of hepatitis, dermatologic conditions, chronic draining infections or open wounds, and immunodeficient conditions. Physical examinations may be useful to detect conditions that may increase the likelihood of transmitting disease to patients, or unusual susceptibility to infection, and to serve as a baseline for determining whether any future problems are work-related. There are no data, however, to suggest that routine complete physical examinations are needed for infection control purposes. Neither are there data to suggest that routine laboratory testing (such as complete blood counts, serologic tests for syphilis, urinalysis, chest roentgenograms) or pre-employment screening for enteric or other pathogens are cost-beneficial. The health inventory can be used to determine whether physical examinations or laboratory tests are needed. In some areas, however, local public health ordinances may still mandate that certain screening procedures be used.

It is important that initial placement evaluations be done when personnel are hired or as soon after as possible. After the placement evaluation, later appraisals may be done as needed for ongoing programs or evaluation of work-related problems.

Personnel Health and Safety Education

Personnel are more likely to comply with an infection control program if they understand its rationale. Thus, staff education should be a central focus of the infection control program. Clearly written policies, guidelines, and procedures are needed in many instances for uniformity, efficiency, and effective coordination of activities. Because job categories vary, not all personnel need the same degree of instruc-

tion in infection control. Educational programs should be matched to the needs of each group.

Immunization Programs

Because hospital personnel are at risk of exposure to and possible transmission of vaccine-preventable diseases because of their contact with patients or material from patients with infections, maintenance of immunity is an essential part of a hospital's personnel health and infection control program. Optimal use of immunizing agents will not only safeguard the health of personnel but also protect patients from becoming infected by personnel. Following a consistent program of immunizations could eliminate the problem of susceptible personnel and avoid unnecessary work restrictions.

Protocols

Immunization recommendations are made by the U.S. Public Health Service Immunization Practices Advisory Committee (ACIP) and are published periodically in the Morbidity and Mortality Weekly Report (MMWR). Indications for use of licensed vaccines are generally the same for hospital personnel as for the general population; however, immunity to some diseases, such as rubella, may be more important for persons who work in hospitals. Decisions about which vaccines to include in immunization programs can be made by considering 1) the risk of exposure to an agent in a given area, 2) the nature of employment, and 3) the size and kind of institution. The suggestions included in this guideline summarize ACIP recommendations as they apply to hospital personnel. The categories reflect the views of the Working Group for this guideline. The ACIP guidelines should be consulted for a detailed discussion of the rationale for active or passive immunization of hospital personnel and the general population. The ACIP guidelines can be requested from Public Inquiries, Building 1, Room B63, Centers for Disease Control, Atlanta, Georgia 30333.

Screening for Susceptibility to Hepatitis B or Rubella. The decision to screen potential vaccine recipients for susceptibility to hepatitis B virus (HBV) is an economic one, because vaccinating HBV carriers or persons already immune does not appear to present a hazard. In the United States the prevalence of previous infection in any targeted group, the cost of screening, and the cost of immunizing personnel determine whether screening would be cost-effective.

Routinely performing serologic tests to determine susceptibility to rubella to be sure that vaccine is given only to proven susceptibles may be very expensive. The ACIP believes that rubella immunization of men and women not known to be pregnant is justifiable without serologic testing.

Vaccine Administration. The most efficient use of vaccines with high-risk groups is to immunize personnel before they enter high-risk situations. It is crucial that persons administering immunizing agents be well-informed about indications, storage, dosage, preparation, and contraindications for each of the vaccines, toxoids, and immune globulins they may use. Product information should be available at all times, and pertinent health history should be obtained from each health worker before an agent is given.

How immunizations are provided to personnel and who pays for vaccines are topics not addressed in this guideline.

Work Restrictions and Management of Job-Related Illnesses and Exposures

The major functions of health counseling by the health service for personnel include arranging for prompt diagnosis and management of job-related illnesses and providing prophylaxis for certain preventable diseases to which personnel may be exposed. If susceptible personnel contract a serious infection that is potentially transmissible or are exposed to an illness that leads to a period during which infection may be spread, the hospital's responsibility to prevent the spread of infection to patients and other personnel may sometimes re-

quire that these persons be excluded from direct patient contact. For any exclusion policy to be enforceable and effective, all personnel—especially department heads, area supervisors, and head nurses —must know when an illness must be reported. Any policy for work restriction should be designed to encourage personnel to report their illnesses or exposures and not penalize them with loss of wages, benefits, or job status.

Health Counseling

Access to health counseling about illnesses they may acquire from or transmit to patients is especially important for all hospital personnel, but particularly for women of childbearing age and persons with special clinical conditions. All personnel should know about infection risks related to employment. Female personnel who may be pregnant or who might become pregnant should know about potential risks to the fetus due to work assignments and preventive measures that will reduce those risks. Among the diseases with potential for risk to a fetus if contracted by the mother are cytomegalovirus infection, hepatitis B, and rubella.

Coordinated Planning with Other Departments

For infection control objectives to be achieved, the activities of the personnel health service must be coordinated with the infection control program and with various hospital departments. This coordination will help assure adequate surveillance of infections in personnel and maintenance of effective infection control programs. During case investigations, outbreaks, and other epidemiologic studies that involve hospital personnel, coordinating activities will help to assure that investigations can be conducted efficiently and control measures implemented promptly.

CHAPTER REVIEW

Multiple Choice

Select the best answer from the choices provided.

1. The most important procedure for preventing infection is
   a. ventilating
   b. mopping
   c. handwashing
   d. spraying

2. Handwashing facilities should be located
   a. outside the hospital
   b. near the bathrooms
   c. throughout the hospital
   d. in the maintenance department

3. Infectious waste can be made noninfectious by
   a. rinsing in hot water
   b. sterilization and autoclaving
   c. rinsing in cold water
   d. putting it in an oven

4. Soiled linen can be transported by
   a. cart or chute
   b. rolling it along the floor
   c. tossing to one another
   d. putting it into paper bags

5. Infective waste should be
   a. incinerated
   b. buried
   c. burned in a bonfire
   d. dumped into the nearest waterway

True/False

Indicate whether the statement is true or false by circling T or F.

6. T   F   Hot water at a temperature of 50°F (10°C) can destroy microorganisms.

7. T   F   Rubbing of the hands with lather for ten seconds is effective handwashing.

8. T   F   Health counseling is not a part of an infection control program.

9. T   F   Protocols must be established for vaccinating personnel.

10. T   F   Cleaning agents should be approved by OSHA.

Matching

Match the terms in column 1 with the definitions in column 2.

Column 1
11. Ethylene oxide
12. Fogging
13. Vaccinations
14. Chlorine bleach
15. Incinerator requirements

Column 2
a. Part of an infection control program
b. Air pollution regulations
c. Air pollution regulations
d. Sterilizing agent
e. Extra margin of safety in sterilization

Short Answer

Briefly but thoroughly answer each statement.

16. Explain the infection control measures used at your health care facility.

17. Describe some of the elements you would include in an infection control program.

18. Identify how you would handle infectious waste.

19. Describe how the soiled linens are handled at your facility.

20. Explain the vaccination protocols in effect at your facility.

CHAPTER 19

Hazardous Medications

After studying this chapter, you should be able to

➤ State the categories of drugs that can be hazardous in their preparation.

➤ Define the procedures to use in storage and preparation areas.

➤ Identify those drugs covered under the OSHA hazard communication standard.

➤ Explain the categories and uses of biological safety cabinets.

➤ Discuss the use of personal protective equipment in drug preparation and disposal.

DRUGS INVOLVED

There are thousands of workers in the health care industry who are exposed to the growing health hazard of dangerous medications. These drugs can cause cancer and reproductive abnormalities.

The employer should control the exposure of his/her employees through engineering controls, work practice controls, and hygiene practices. If these controls are not feasible, then personal protective equipment should be furnished to employees at risk.

Drugs administered to patients by health care workers, such as anticancer agents and anesthetic gases, can cause side effects to both patients and employees. Hospital workers who are exposed can develop serious health problems. Some of these health effects are

- Genetic damage
- Cancer
- Birth defects
- Fertility problems (both men and women)
- Toxic effects to organs

Antineoplastic drugs are drugs that fight cancers by preventing the growth of cancerous cells. They not only fight cancer but can also cause cancerous growths in humans. These drugs have caused leukemia and related cancers, spontaneous abortions, birth of malformed infants, and ectopic pregnancies in hospital workers.

Anesthetics (drugs that cause partial or complete loss of sensation) used in hospital operating rooms are known to cause nerve and brain damage, as well as reproductive damage to animals and exposed workers.

Low doses of **antiviral drugs** (drugs that inhibit viruses) given to animals have caused damage to the reproductive system of the person giving the drug. These doses are generally lower than doses absorbed by nurses administering the same drugs to humans. The American Society of Health-System Pharmacists (ASHP) recommends that pharmaceutical agents that are animal carcinogens be considered as human carcinogens.

Some drugs have several health effects—such as aerosolized pentamidine, which is used to prevent *Pneumo-cystis carinii* in HIV patients and to control TB in patients with active TB. The administration of aerosolized drugs has caused harmful concentrations in the breathing zone of workers. Zidovudine, used in the treatment of AIDS patients, is known to cause health effects in health care workers. **Cytotoxic drugs** (cell destroying), when not used in biological safety cabinets (BSCs), were found to accumulate in the breathing zone of workers. Various health effects have been noted among pharmaceutical workers in the manufacturing of estrogens and opiates.

Liver damage has been reported in nurses working in cancer wards. This was related to the concentrations in the air and the length of exposure to antineoplastic drugs. Light-headedness, dizziness, nausea, and allergic reactions have occurred in workers after the administration of these drugs in areas that were not ventilated.

OSHA considers drugs or pills that are crushed or in the aerosolized form to be a hazardous substance. Employees exposed to this form of drug or medication must be included in any hazard communication program. Drugs and medication in the solid form are not considered to have the potential for exposure and are not defined as hazardous substances by OSHA. Solid-form drugs and medications do not have to be included in the hazardous communication program.

RECOMMENDED EXPOSURE LIMITS

A **recommended exposure limit (REL)** is a recommended exposure limit for a toxic substance that is recommended based on studies of the substance.

The National Institute for Occupational Safety and Health (NIOSH), which is the federal agency responsible for conducting research and making recommendations for the prevention of work-related illnesses and injuries, has recommended exposure limits (RELs) for some anesthetic gases such as **halothane** and **nitrous oxide**. There are no established OSHA permissible exposure limits (PELs) indicating exposure levels for most hazardous medications. It is difficult to establish safe levels of exposure based on current information, but there is strong evidence of the toxicity of these drugs if controls are not put into effect.

WORK AND PREPARATION AREAS

The following activities can cause exposure to hazardous drugs:

- Needle withdrawal from drug vials
- Transferring drugs when using syringes, needles, or filter straws
- Breaking open ampules
- Expelling air from drug-filled syringes

Drug preparation should be done in a controlled, centralized area. Unauthorized personnel should be kept out of the area and appropriate signs posted. Spill and emergency procedures should be posted that indicate what to do in the event of skin or eye contact.

Smoking, eating, drinking, and applying cosmetics should not be done in these areas because they increase the chance of exposure.

WASTE DRUG DISPOSAL

Properly labeled, covered, and sealed containers should be used for the disposal of contaminated gloves, gowns, syringes, and vials. If these items are contaminated with blood or other infectious or potentially infectious materials, the OSHA bloodborne pathogens standard must be followed (see Chapter 15).

Unused commercial chemical product drugs considered by the **Environmental Protection Agency (EPA)** to be toxic wastes must be disposed of as hazardous wastes in accordance with the Resource Conservation and Recovery Act (RCRA).

Waste bags should be kept in covered waste containers and labeled **"HD Waste Only."** Waste should remain in the area where the drug is prepared or administered and not moved to other areas. After the bag is full, it should be sealed and the container taped.

The employer must make sure that all employees involved in drug preparation and disposal are trained in the handling of spills.

Workers disposing of the waste should wear gowns and gloves. If the outside of the container becomes contaminated, it should be placed in another container. Care should be taken to ensure that the outer container does not become contaminated. Workers disposing of hazardous drug waste, should receive training as specified in OSHA 29 CFR 1910.1200 Hazard Communication. (Chapter 26 describes the required training content.)

Drug and related waste should be kept separate from regular hospital waste. Disposal must be in accordance with federal, state, and local laws. Before the waste is picked up, it must be kept in a secure area and stored in covered, labeled drums equipped with plastic liners.

HAZARDOUS DRUG SAFETY AND HEALTH PLAN

The American Society of Health-System Pharmacists recommends that a written Hazardous Drug and Health Plan be developed that mandates the following:

- Standard operating procedures that protect health care workers who are exposed to hazardous drugs.
- The employer's use of engineering controls, personal protective equipment, and hygiene practices to reduce exposure.
- That ventilation systems be kept in proper operating condition.
- That employees exposed to hazardous drugs be given information and training concerning safe handling of the drugs.
- How the criteria are formulated for specific drug use that requires prior approval by the employer.
- Medical examinations of exposed and potentially exposed workers.
- Designation of employees responsible for the operation of the Hazardous Drug Safety and Health Plan. This includes the designation of a Hazardous Drug Officer (person who has the required drug expertise) and the forming of a Hazardous Drug and Chemical Committee.
- Establishing a Hazardous Drug Management Area.
- Using biological safety cabinets (BSCs).
- Proper procedures for removal of contaminated waste.
- Decontamination procedures.

The ASHP recommends that the plan be reviewed and reevaluated at least annually and updated whenever necessary.

BIOLOGICAL SAFETY CABINETS (BSC)

Biological safety cabinets enable drug preparation to be done in enclosed areas that keep the contaminated air from the breathing zone of the worker. The cabinets will vary as follows:

- By the volume of air recirculated within the cabinet.
- If the air is exhausted into the room or to the exterior of the building.
- If the ducts are under positive or negative pressure. This will relate to the fan operation.

Class II or III cabinets that meet the National Sanitation Foundation (NSF) standard should be used in the preparation of hazardous drugs.

BSC Types

The employer should determine which cabinet will best meet the requirements for the activities that will be performed. Room size, material being processed, cabinet location, and the room ventilation system are factors to be considered.

Class II Cabinets. *Type A* cabinets recirculate 70 percent of the air in the cabinet through HEPA (high-efficiency particulate air) filters. The remaining air is discharged into the room through a HEPA filter. The ducts are under positive pressure.

Type B1 cabinets have higher air volumes and flow, and recirculate 30 percent of the air in the cabinet. The remaining air is exhausted to the exterior through HEPA filters. The ducts and plenums are under negative pressure.

Type B2 cabinets are similar to Type B1 except that cabinet air is not recirculated.

Type B3 cabinets are similar to Type A except that the remaining 30 percent of air is exhausted to the exterior and the ducts are under negative pressure.

Class III Cabinets. These cabinets are totally enclosed and have a gas-tight construction. The cabinet is under negative pressure, and the preparation is done by using gloves that are attached to the cabinet. The entire air goes through HEPA filters.

Cabinet Vented Air. Air that is exhausted to the outside must be kept away from air intakes to avoid reentrainment and away from pedestrian walks. Reentrainment is the process whereby exhausted airborne contaminants get back into the building.

Cabinet Operation. The fan or blower should operate constantly, except when the hood is being repaired or moved. Whenever the fan is turned off, the cabinet should be decontaminated before it is used.

The cabinet should have a monitoring device to indicate if there is adequate airflow and whether it is operating properly.

It should be placed in a location that minimizes the effects of air turbulence. This excludes proximity to doors or where there is heavy pedestrian traffic.

The manufacturer's instructions should be reviewed to ensure proper operation of the cabinet.

Cabinet Decontamination. Cabinets should be cleaned in accordance with manufacturer's instructions. This could be weekly, when spills occur, when it is moved, or when it is serviced.

Fumigation with a germicidal agent is not approved because it does not remove or inactivate the drug.

The worker should wear the appropriate PPE. The cabinet sash should remain in the down position during cleaning. If the sash is lifted, the worker should wear a respirator approved by the National Institute for Occupational Safety and Health (NIOSH) for that particular hazard. The exhaust fan or blower should remain on during the cleaning operation.

Cleaning should be from the least to most contaminated area. The drain trough should be cleaned at least twice. All collected materials from the cleaning should be considered hazardous drugs and disposed of in accordance with federal, state, and local laws.

Cabinet Servicing. A qualified technician should service the cabinet every six months or whenever it is moved or repaired. The technician must be made aware of the hazards and be trained in accordance with the OSHA hazard communication standard. He/she should also wear the appropriate PPE.

HEPA filters should be replaced when they restrict airflow or if they become contaminated. Filters that are removed should be placed in plastic bags and disposed of as a hazardous drug.

Whenever the cabinet is moved or turned off, it should be sealed in a plastic cover.

BSC Work Practices. Handling of drugs in the BSC should not be done close to the surface. Unsterilized items should be kept downstream from working areas. Entry and exit should be perpendicular to the front of the cabinet, and there should be no rapid hand movements.

PERSONAL PROTECTIVE EQUIPMENT (PPE)

The National Study Commission on Cytotoxic Exposure recommends that gowns, latex gloves, and chemical splash goggles be worn when administering hazardous drugs.

Gowns

Disposable gowns should have

- Resistance to permeability.
- Closed fronts, long sleeves, and elastic or closed cuffs.
- Outer glove worn over the cuff and inner glove under.
- Inner glove removed last when gown is removed.

Gowns and gloves should not be worn outside of the preparation area.

Gloves

Thick latex gloves are considered most effective when handling hazardous drugs, unless it is stipulated by the drug manufacturer that another glove gives better protection. Gloves that do not have powder are preferred because the powder can absorb the drug.

Double gloving is recommended because of drug permeability. Gloves should be changed hourly, or immediately if torn, punctured, or contaminated by a spill. Hands should be washed before gloves are put on and after they are removed. Employees should be trained in the proper way to remove gloves.

Respirators

When biological safety cabinets are not available in the preparation of hazardous drugs, a NIOSH-approved respirator must be worn appropriate for the hazard. The respirator use must comply with OSHA 29 CFR 1910.134 respirator protection standard. (Chapter 16 describes respiratory protection.) Surgical masks cannot be used in drug preparation because they do not prevent the penetration of aerosols upon inhalation.

Respirators *should not* be considered substitutes for engineering controls (BSC).

Face and Eye Protection

When hazardous drug splashes, sprays, or aerosols can impact the eyes or face, face and eye protection is required. This protection must conform to OSHA 29 CFR 1910.133 Subpart I. (Chapter 20 describes PPE.) Eye protection with temporary side shields is not appropriate protection.

Goggles should be cleaned with a detergent and rinsed thoroughly.

If eye protection is to be worn with a respirator, the following combinations should be used: a respirator with full face piece, or a plastic face shield or splash goggles when using a respirator with less than a full face piece. (*Note:* Eyewash stations should be available.)

Administration Kit

Protective and administration kits can be prepared that contain PPE and cleanup materials. These kits should include

- Personal protective equipment.
- 4" × 4" gauze for cleaning up.
- Alcohol wipes.
- Disposable plastic backed absorbent liners.
- Puncture-resistant container for needles and syringes.
- A thick plastic bag (sealable) with warning label.
- Supplemental warning labels.

  Note: The complete kit should be disposed of after use. Waste bag disposal should be in accordance with hazardous drug disposal requirements and unused drugs returned to the pharmacy.

PPE Disposal and Decontamination

Gowns, gloves, and other disposable materials should be disposed of in accordance with the facility's drug waste procedures and in accordance with federal, state, and local laws. Goggles, face shields, and respirators can be cleaned for reuse with approved mild detergents and water.

EQUIPMENT

The National Institutes of Health (NIH) recommend that the preparation of hazardous drugs be done in BSCs on disposable plastic backed paper liners. The liner should be replaced after preparation is completed for the day or shift, and after a spill.

Syringes and IV sets with Luer-lock fittings should be used for hazardous drugs.

A covered disposable container should be available to take excess solution. A covered sharps container should be kept in the BSC.

Hazardous drug labeled plastic bags should be available for contaminated materials and disposed of in accordance with American Society of Hospital Pharmacists' recommendations.

PPE should be put on prior to working in the BSC and all necessary items placed in the BSC before work is done.

Labeling

Syringes and IV bags containing hazardous drugs should have labels on them that state "Special Handling/Disposal Precautions." Those hazardous drugs that are included under OSHA 29 CFR 1910.1200 Hazard Communication must also have the label required by the standard.

Specific Guidelines for Handling Drugs

Drug administration sets, needles, ampules, and vials should have specific guidelines when handled. These guidelines should be followed.

Needles. The American Society of Health-System Pharmacists (ASHP) recommends that syringes and needles used to prepare drugs be placed in "sharps" containers for disposal and not clipped or capped.

Priming. Drug administration sets should be primed within the BSC before the drug is added. **Priming** prepares the drug administration set for use. If priming is done at the site where the drug is administered, the intravenous line should be primed with a fluid that does not contain a drug, or a backflow system should be used.

Vials. Both negative and positive pressure extremes should be avoided in vials. Venting devices (filter needles and dispensing pins) can be used to let outside air replace the withdrawn fluid. Another technique that can be used is to add small amounts of **diluent** slowly to the vial and letting the displaced air go into the syringe. Additional air can be withdrawn after all the diluent has been added to create a slight negative pressure in the vial. This air should then be injected into a vacuum vial or left in the syringe to be discarded.

Ampules. Dry material in ampules should be tapped down before breaking. Before breaking the top, a sterile gauze pad should be wrapped around the neck.

Any diluent that is added to an ampule should be slowly injected down the side.

A needle withdrawn from the ampule should be cleaned by holding it vertically with the point turned up. Tap the syringe to remove any air bubbles and expel the bubbles into a closed container.

Transportation of Hazardous Drugs. Bags and bottles containing hazardous drugs should be wiped with moist gauze on the outside and the opening wiped with moist alcohol pads and then capped. Containers used in transport should not be breakable and should be sealed in plastic bags.

Workers performing transport duties should be trained in spill procedures, which includes sealing off the contaminated area and calling for assistance if a spill occurs.

Receipt of Damaged Hazardous Drug Packages. Damaged packages should be opened in isolated areas or in a BSC by workers wearing appropriate protective equipment. These workers should be trained in this procedure.

The ASHP recommends that broken containers and contaminated packaging mats be put in sharps containers and then into hazardous drug disposal bags. The bags should be closed and then placed in covered receptacles as described under waste disposal.

Hazardous drugs that are also included under Environmental Protection Agency regulations as hazardous waste must be packaged and transported to meet the requirements of the Department of Transportation (DOT).

Hazardous Drugs in Solid Form. A BSC should be used when counting tablets that may produce dust upon handling. The BSC used should be reserved for only hazardous drugs. If an enclosed process isolates the hazard, only then can automatic counting machines can be used.

Compounding should be done in the BSC, and gown and gloves should be worn. A NIOSH-approved respirator should be worn if the work cannot be done in a BSC.

Aerosolized Drugs. These drugs, particularly pentamidine and ribavirin, should be administered in booths with local exhaust systems designed for this purpose or in isolation rooms with HEPA filtration. This protection is also needed when performing endotracheal tube administration.

Anesthetic gases also require the use of engineering controls to limit employee exposure.

Spills. The material safety data sheet (MSDS) for the drug should be consulted concerning the recommended method and procedure for cleanup and disposal of the spill. Emergency procedures to be followed for spills should be incorporated in the health care safety and health program.

Small spills. The ASHP defines a small spill as one involving less than 5 ml or 5 gm. If it occurs outside a BSC, it should be cleaned up immediately. Workers doing the cleanup must wear gowns, double latex gloves, and proper eye protection. If the drug can become airborne, an appropriate respirator must be worn.

Liquids are to be wiped up with absorbent gauze pads and solids with wet absorbent gauze. The spill area should then be wiped clean at least three times with a detergent solution followed by a clean water rinse.

Broken glass should be picked up with a scoop and placed in a "sharps" container. The container is then placed in a hazardous drug disposal bag with the absorbent pads and any other contaminated waste. The scoop should be cleaned as indicated for reusable items.

Large spills. Large spills are defined as those involving more than 5 ml or 5 gm.

The area should be isolated and airborne contamination controlled. Carefully cover the spill area with absorbent sheets or spill control pads or pillows. A damp cloth or towel can be used for powders. Workers cleaning up large spills must be trained.

The same protective equipment that is worn for small spills should be worn for large spills.

The area should be cleaned the same way as for small spills and contaminated absorbent materials placed in hazardous drug bags and disposed of properly.

BSC spills. All interior surfaces of the BSC must be decontaminated after cleanup of a spill. The ASHP recommends this procedure for spills larger than 150 ml or if a vial is spilled. If the HEPA filter becomes contaminated, the BSC should be sealed in plastic until the filter is changed and disposed of properly. Workers doing the filter change must wear proper protective equipment.

Patient Care for Those on Hazardous Drugs

Health care workers must follow proper procedures and take the necessary precautions to avoid being exposed to toxic drugs. Even low-level exposure over long periods of time can be harmful.

Universal Precautions. Universal precautions assume that all blood and other potentially infectious materials are contaminated. Workers must take the necessary precautions as specified in OSHA 29 CFR 1910.1030 Bloodborne Pathogens.

PPE. When handling excreta, particularly urine of patients who have received hazardous drugs within the last forty-eight hours, workers should wear latex or other approved gloves and disposable gowns. These items should be disposed of after use or when contaminated.

Eye and face protection should be worn if there is a splash hazard. Hands should be washed after gloves are removed or after contacting contaminated substances.

Linens. Linen soiled with blood or other potentially infectious materials from patients who have received hazardous drugs within the past forty-eight hours must be handled in accordance with the OSHA bloodborne pathogens standard.

MEDICAL SURVEILLANCE

Workers who are exposed or potentially exposed to hazardous drugs should be monitored to prevent occupational injury and disease.

Surveillance should be performed on workers

- Before they are placed in the job where there is exposure or potential exposure (initial examinations).
- Periodically during the course of their employment.
- After there has been an acute exposure.
- When the job is terminated or there is a transfer.

Preplacement Medical Examinations

The initial examination should include a patient history; physical examination that emphasizes the skin, mucous membranes, cardiopulmonary and lymphatic systems and liver; and lab studies. The employer should give the examining physician the following information:

- A description of the employee's duties as these relate to the exposure.
- The employee's exposure levels or expected levels.
- The personal protective equipment that is used or will be used.
- Information from previous exams not available to the examining physician.

Periodic Medical Examinations

Periodic examinations are recommended in order to update the employee's medical, reproductive, and exposure histories. They should be conducted yearly or every two to three years, depending upon the advice of the examining physician.

Post-Exposure Examinations

The post-exposure examination is designed for the type of exposure, whether it be after a spill, a needle stick, or some other incident. The examination should evaluate the affected area as well as skin, mucous membranes, and pulmonary system. The occurrence causing the exposure should be included on an incident report.

Exit Examinations

The exit examination concludes the information on the employee's medical, reproductive, and exposure histories. The worker's exposure history and the procedures for the periodic examination should be used as a guide for the exit examination and laboratory evaluation.

A database should be kept that includes information concerning the worker's medical and reproductive history as well as information involving epidemiologic evaluation.

CONSIDERATIONS OF THE EXAMINING PHYSICIAN AND FACILITY

The hazardous nature of these drugs on the reproductive system should be explained by the examining physician to workers who will be exposed. The health care facility should have a policy that describes the reproductive toxicity of hazardous drugs for both males and females. Workers should understand the reproductive and carcinogenic hazards of these drugs. The avoidance of exposure should be emphasized, particularly in early pregnancy. Updated information should be supplied to employees on a regular basis and when their duties involve new hazards. Medical personnel and other staff who are not hospital employees must be informed of these policies and be expected to comply.

RECORDKEEPING

The assessment of exposure and maintenance of records for employees exposed to hazardous drugs is crucial. Records have to be kept in accordance with OSHA 29 CFR 1910.1020 Access To Employee Exposure And Medical Records.

Exposure and Medical Records Retention

Retention of these records is as follows:

1. Exposure records are kept for at least thirty years.
2. Medical records are kept for the duration of employment plus thirty years.

Training Records Description and Retention

These records must include

1. Dates of training.
2. What was covered in the training.
3. Names and qualifications of the trainer(s).
4. Names and job titles of trainees.

Training records must be kept for at least three years from the date of the training.

HAZARDOUS DRUGS AND THE HAZARD COMMUNICATION STANDARD

Certain hazardous drugs are included under OSHA 29 CFR 1910.1200 Hazard Communication because the standard includes any substance that is a physical or health hazard.

The standard considers any of the following chemical characteristics hazardous:

- Carcinogen
- Corrosive
- Toxic or highly toxic

- Irritant
- Sensitizer
- **Reproductive toxin** (injurious to tissue of the reproductive system); **hepatotoxin** (attacks liver cells); **nephrotoxin** (attacks kidney cells); **neurotoxin** (attacks nerve cells); or **hematopoietic system toxin** (attacks blood cells)
- Chemicals that affect the lungs, skin, eyes, or mucous membranes.

The Hazard Communication Standard requires that any drug having any of these hazardous characteristics be included. These drugs must be included on employee hazardous chemical exposure lists. The exceptions are drugs in a solid final form (capsules, pills, or tablets) that are directly administered to the patient.

Employee exposure and medical records involving employee exposure to these drugs has to be maintained in accordance with OSHA 29 CFR 1910.1020 Access to Employee Exposure and Medical Records. These records also include any workplace or biological monitoring and material safety data sheets (MSDSs) describing the drugs.

Information and Training

Training under the standard must include any employee exposed, or potentially exposed, to hazardous drugs. This includes

- Health care professionals.
- Physical plant.
- Maintenance.
- Employees involved in drug receiving, transportation, and storage.
- Support personnel.

Training and information must be provided at the time of initial assignment to an area where hazardous drugs are present and before any assignment to areas involving new drug hazards. Refresher training and information must be provided by the employer at least annually.

Information Criteria. Employees must be informed of

1. The requirements of the hazard communication standard.
2. Where hazardous drugs are present at the worksite.
3. Where the written hazard communication program is located.
4. Where other hazardous drugs are located in their areas (other than the ones they are working with).
5. The location of other plans involving hazardous drugs, other than the written hazard communication program.

Training Criteria. Training has to include at least the following:

1. Methods and observations that can be used to detect the presence or release of hazardous drugs in the work area (monitoring, odor, or visual appearance).
2. The physical and health hazards of the hazardous drugs in the work area.
3. The measures employees can take to prevent exposure (identification of the drugs, work practices, and emergency procedures).
4. The use of PPE.
5. Specifics of the employer's hazard communication program.
6. Explanation of the labeling system and MSDSs and how employees can use this information to protect against exposure.
7. An understanding of any carcinogenic and/or reproductive hazards of the drugs. Both males and females should know the importance of avoiding these drugs, particularly women who are pregnant.
8. An explanation of the facility's policy concerning reproductive toxicity.

Employees should receive updated information on hazardous drugs when necessary and when their jobs involve new hazards.

Other health care facility personnel not involved with hazardous drug exposure or potential exposure should be made aware of the facility's policy concerning hazardous drugs and be expected to comply with this policy.

Material Safety Data Sheets (MSDS)

MSDS must accompany initial shipments of all hazardous drugs and pharmaceutical products except drugs in solid form.

All hazardous drugs on site must have the appropriate MSDS available. The MSDS must describe

1. Health hazards.
2. Exposure routes into the body.
3. Carcinogenic evaluations.
4. Treatment for acute exposure.
5. Chemical(s) to use to make the drug inactive.
6. Solubility, volatility, and stability of the drug.
7. PPE required for protection against exposure.
8. Spill and disposal procedures.

The MSDS must be available to employees and OSHA upon request.

Hazard Communication Standard Inclusions

The employer is required to develop a hazard communication program. The requirements are described in Chapter 26. Hazardous drug exposure control is required to be implemented the same way as any other chemical included in the hazard communication standard. The written program must comply with the requirements

1. For labeling and other warnings.
2. That MSDS be available for all hazardous drugs.
3. Describing how employees are being informed of these hazards, including when nonroutine tasks are performed.
4. That describe the methods used to inform personnel from other sites who may become exposed or potentially exposed.

The hazard communication program must be available to employees and OSHA upon request.

HAZARDOUS DRUG LIST

The following is a list of drugs determined to be hazardous after a review by a team of pharmacists and other health care professionals. Various institutions organized these teams for drug evaluation. The hazard involved refers to the preparation of the drugs.

The list is not complete, and drugs should be periodically evaluated and updated as new information is received concerning their hazard status. The chemical or generic name is indicated.

Altretamine	Interferon-A
Aminoglutethimide	Isotretinoin
Azathioprine	Leuprolide
L-Asparaginase	Levamisole
Bleomycin	Lomustine
Busulfan	Mechlorethamine
Carboplatin	Medroxyprogesterone
Carmustine	Megestrol
Chlorambucil	Melphalan
Chloramphenicol	Mercaptopurine
Chlorotrianisene	Methotrexate
Chlorosporin	Mitomycin
Cisplatin	Mitotane
Cyclophosphamide	Mitoxantrone
Cytarabine	Nafarelin
Dacarbazine	Pipobroman
Dactinomycin	Plicamycin
Daunorubicin	Procarbazine
Diethylstilbestrol	Ribavirin
Doxorubicin	Streptozocin
Estramustine	Tamoxifen
Ethinyl Estradiol	Testolactone
Etoposide	Thioguanine
Floxuridine	Thiotepa
Fluorouracil	Uracil Mustard
Flutamide	Vidarabine
Ganciclovir	Vinblastine
Hydroxyurea	Vincristine
Idarubicin	Zidovudine
Ifosfamide	

CHAPTER REVIEW

Multiple Choice

Select the best answer from the choices provided.

1. Hazardous drugs have caused
   a. genetic damage
   b. cancer
   c. difficulty having children
   d. a, b, and c

2. A hazardous drug safety and health plan should be reviewed at least
   a. quarterly   c. annually
   b. semiannually   d. bi-annually

3. Disposable gowns should have
   a. open fronts and open cuffs
   b. resistance to permeability
   c. outer glove worn under the cuff
   d. inner glove worn over the cuff

4. Workers exposed to hazardous drugs should have medical surveillance
   a. after they are put on the job
   b. only once during employment
   c. before there is an acute exposure
   d. before they are placed on the job

5. Universal precautions assume that
   a. all blood and infectious materials are contaminated
   b. most blood and infectious materials are contaminated
   c. only material showing evidence of infectious staining is hazardous
   d. it is not necessary to use PPE if you feel there is no chance of infection

True/False

Indicate whether the statement is true or false by circling T or F.

6. T F OSHA considers drugs that are crushed or in aerosolized form not to be hazardous.

7. T F Needle withdrawal from drug vials can cause a hazardous exposure.

8. T F Type A biological safety cabinets recirculate 30 percent of the air.

9. T F A small spill is less than 5 ml or 5 gm.

10. T F All hazardous drugs are included under OSHA's hazard communication standard.

Matching

Match the terms in column 1 with the definitions in column 2.

Column 1
11. Antineoplastic drug
12. Corrosivity
13. Standard operating procedures
14. Biological safety cabinet
15. Personnel protective equipment

Column 2
a. Enclosed area
b. Gloves
c. Cancer fighter
d. Characteristic of a hazardous waste
e. Part of a hazardous drug safety plan

Short Answer

Briefly but thoroughly answer each statement.

16. Discuss the various types of biological safety cabinets.

17. List the personal protective equipment to be worn when handling hazardous drugs.

18. Discuss why engineering and work practice controls are preferred over personal protective equipment.

19. Discuss some of the points of a hazardous drug safety and health plan.

20. Describe some of the activities that can expose health care employees to hazardous drugs.

SECTION III

Industrial Standards and Guidelines

CHAPTER 20

Personal Protective Equipment

OBJECTIVES

After studying this chapter, you should be able to

➤ Explain the OSHA requirements for personal protective equipment.
➤ Identify the personal protective equipment required for exposures.
➤ Discuss latex allergy.

OSHA 29 CFR 1910 SUBPART I PERSONAL PROTECTIVE EQUIPMENT (PPE)

Personal protective equipment is covered under OSHA 29 CFR Subpart I, General Industry Standards and 29 CFR 1926 Subpart E, Construction Standards.

These standards describe the requirements for eye and face protection; respiratory protection (which is covered in Chapter 16); head protection; foot protection; electrical protective equipment; and hand protection.

The most recent update to this standard adds more responsibility for the employer. There must be an evaluation of worksite hazards before issuing PPE to employees.

General Requirements

Whenever hazards in the workplace expose workers to injuries involving the head, face, body, eye, hands, feet, and respiratory tract, appropriate PPE must be worn.

Employees may provide their own equipment, but it must be inspected and approved by the employer. Respirators, because of their importance as PPE, cannot be supplied by the employee, only by the employer.

The employer is responsible for assessing the workplace to determine the PPE necessary to protect the worker. This assessment should include areas subject to impact, penetration, roll-over, chemical, heat, harmful dust, and light radiation.

Training

The employer is required to train employees in the following regarding PPE:

1. When PPE is required
2. What type is necessary for protection
3. Methods to properly put it on, take it off, and adjust it
4. Its limitations
5. Proper care and maintenance
6. Useful life and disposal

The employer should provide a written policy that clearly defines when PPE must be worn and the consequences for not wearing it. This policy should be made known to all employees who are required to wear PPE, and it should be enforced.

Eye and Face Protection

When employees are exposed to flying particles, molten metal, liquid chemicals, acids, caustic liquids, chemical gases or vapors, or potentially injurious light radiation, they must wear appropriate eye protection.

Side protection is required when there is exposure to flying objects.

If employees wear prescription lenses, the lenses must be part of the eye protection or the eye protection must fit over regular lenses. If protection is worn over the prescription glasses, the prescription glasses or eye protection cannot be altered.

When employees are exposed to welding arcs, they must wear the appropriate lens shade as described in the OSHA welding standard.

Protective eye and face devices purchased after July 5, 1994, must comply with the "American National Standards Institute (ANSI) Standard Practice for Occupational and Educational Eye Protection," Z87.1-1989.

Eye and face protection purchased before July 5, 1994, must comply with "ANSI USA Standard for Occupational and Educational Eye Protection," Z87.1-1968.

The OSHA "Eye and Face Protection Selection Chart" should be consulted to determine the type of protection for the eyes and face that is appropriate for the type of hazard.

For severe face and eye exposure, a face shield worn over eye protection is required. Exposure to chemical splash will require side and top protection and indirect venting for the eyewear.

Foot Protection

When employees' feet are subject to the hazard of falling or rolling objects, objects piercing the sole, or exposure to electrical hazards, appropriate foot protection must be worn.

Foot protection consists of standard steel safety toed shoe or metatarsal protection, depending upon the type of hazard.

Footwear purchased after July 5, 1994, must comply with ANSI standard Z41-1991, "American National Standard for Personal Protection—Protective Footware."

Footwear purchased before July 5, 1994, must comply with ANSI Standard Z41.1-1967, "USA Standard for Men's Safety-Toe Footware."

Hand Protection

When the hands of employees are exposed to skin absorption of harmful substances, severe cuts or lacerations, severe abrasions, punctures, chemical and thermal burns, and harmful temperature extremes, appropriate hand protection must be worn.

Manufacturer's catalogs are extremely helpful when determining the proper hand protection for the hazard.

Recommendations When Using Latex Gloves. Contact and chemical sensitivity dermatitis, as well as latex allergy, have been caused by latex gloves. Health care workers have found that when wearing latex gloves they suffered skin reddening and dryness, hives, and itching. More severe reactions included throat irritation, difficulty breathing, coughing, itchy eyes, and wheezing.

The following are suggested for health care workers to minimize the effects from wearing latex gloves:

- Wear powderless gloves to reduce exposure to the latex protein.
- After removing latex gloves, wash hands with soap and water and dry them thoroughly. Do not use hand creams that contain oil or other lotions with latex gloves.
- If you work with noninfectious materials, wear gloves that do not have latex.
- Vacuum up latex dust that has accumulated on furniture, in ventilation ducts, and other surfaces.
- Health care workers that develop symptoms that indicate sensitivity to latex should see a physician who has a specialty in treating people with this sensitivity. It would be prudent for those that have this sensitivity to wear a medical alert bracelet.

Additional information on latex and the types of problems it can cause can be obtained from: Elastic, P.O. Box 2228, West Chester, PA 19380.

REFERENCE MATERIAL FOR PERSONAL PROTECTIVE EQUIPMENT

A library of catalogs should be kept on file that details the personal protective equipment available from various manufacturers and which hazards they protect against. Selection of the proper PPE is important, and if there are questions concerning this selection, the employer should consult with knowledgeable individuals in the safety profession or with manufacturer's representatives.

CHAPTER REVIEW

True/False

Indicate whether the statement is true or false by circling T or F.

1. T   F   For severe face and eye exposure, a face shield must be worn over eye protection.

2. T   F   Exposure to a welding arc requires a good pair of sunglasses over the eye protection.

3. T   F   A written policy for PPE is not required by the employer as long as he tells employees about the requirements for protective equipment.

4. T   F   Employees may wear their own PPE as long as it is approved by the employer.

5. T   F   Assessment of the workplace is the responsibility of the employee.

Short Answer

Briefly but thoroughly answer each statement.

6.   Describe the activities in your facility and the personal protective equipment you would assign to protect employees.

7.   Discuss some of the ways you would enforce the wearing of PPE.

8.   What are some of the ways you can obtain assistance in selecting PPE?

9.   List the corrective action you can take to avoid latex sensitivity.

10.   Do you think you would require foot protection in a laboratory?

CHAPTER 21

Noise

OBJECTIVES

After studying this chapter, you should be able to

➤ Describe the requirements of the OSHA noise standard.
➤ Define how noise is measured and in what units.
➤ Explain how noise calculations are done to determine exposure.

Noise is covered under OSHA 29 CFR 1910.95 General Industry Standards.

OSHA 29 CFR 1910.95 NOISE

The employer must comply with the noise standard if there is noise above stated OSHA limits.

OSHA Noise Exposure Limits

Noise exposure limits are expressed in **dBA**s. A dBA is the sound level reading in decibels obtained on the A scale of a sound level meter at slow response. The A scale contains the frequency range of the human ear.

Protection against the effects of noise exposure shall be provided when the sound levels exceed those shown in Table G-16 when measured on the A scale of a standard sound level meter at slow response.

When noise levels are determined by octave band analysis, the equivalent A weighted sound level may be determined by using Figure G-9 in the standard (refer to the standard for the table).

Table G-16
90 dBA for more than 8 hours
92 dBA for more than 6 hours
95 dBA for more than 3 hours
100 dBA for more than 2 hours
102 dBA for more than $1\frac{1}{2}$ hours
105 dBA for more than 1 hour
110 dBA for more than $\frac{1}{2}$ hour
115 dBA for $\frac{1}{4}$ hour or less

Continuous noise is noise at intervals less than one second. Impact (impulse) noise is noise at intervals of more than one second. Employees cannot be exposed to impact noise exceeding 140 decibels.

Hearing Conservation Program

The employer shall administer a continuing, effective hearing conservation program whenever employee noise exposures equal or exceed an eight-hour time weighted average (TWA) sound level of 85 decibels measured on the A scale (slow response) or equivalently a dose of 50 percent. This is without any attenuation provided by the use of personal protective equipment.

This eight-hour time weighted average or dose of 50 percent shall also be referred to as the **action level**. This is the level that mandates training, medical surveillance, monitoring, and the use of personal protective equipment (PPE).

The hearing conservation program is described in the following sections.

Monitoring. When information indicates that the employee's exposure may equal or exceed an eight-hour time weighted average of 85 decibels, the employer must implement a monitoring program.

137

The sampling strategy shall be designed to identify employees for inclusion in the hearing conservation program and to enable the proper selection of hearing protectors.

When worker mobility or high variations in sound levels make area monitoring inappropriate, the employer must use representative personal sampling to comply with the monitoring requirements.

All continuous, intermittent, and impulsive sound levels from 80 to 130 decibels shall be integrated into the noise measurements.

Instruments used to measure employee noise exposure shall be calibrated to ensure measurement accuracy.

Monitoring shall be repeated whenever a change in production, process, equipment, or controls increases noise exposures to the extent that additional employees may be exposed above the action level, or the attenuation provided by hearing protectors may be inadequate to meet the requirements of this section.

Employee Notification. The employer shall notify each employee exposed at or above an eight-hour time weighted average of 85 decibels of the results of the monitoring.

Observation of Monitoring. The employer shall allow affected employees or their representatives the opportunity to observe any noise measurements.

Audiometric Testing. The employer shall establish and maintain an audiometric testing program for all employees whose exposures equal or exceed an eight-hour time weighted average of 85 decibels.

The program shall be provided at no cost to employees.

Audiometric tests shall be performed by a licensed or certified audiologist, otolaryngologist, or other physician, or by a technician who is certified by the Council of Accreditation in Occupational Hearing Conservation.

Within six months of an employee's first exposure at or above the action level, the employer shall establish a valid baseline audiogram against which subsequent audiograms can be compared.

Where mobile test vans are used, to meet the audiometric testing requirement, the employer shall obtain a valid baseline audiogram within one year of an employee's first exposure at or above the action level. Where baseline audiograms are obtained more than six months after the employee's first exposure at or above the action level, employees shall wear hearing protectors for any period exceeding six months after first exposure until the baseline audiogram is obtained.

Testing to establish a baseline audiogram shall be preceded by a least fourteen hours without exposure to workplace noise. Hearing protectors may be used as a substitute for the requirement that baseline audiograms be preceded by fourteen hours without exposure to workplace noise.

The employer shall notify employees of the need to avoid high levels of nonoccupational noise exposure during the fourteen-hour period immediately preceding the audiometric examination.

At least annually after obtaining the baseline audiogram, the employer shall obtain a new audiogram for each employee exposed at or above the eight-hour time weighted average of 85 decibels.

Each employee's annual audiogram shall be compared to that employee's baseline audiogram to determine if the audiogram is valid and a **standard threshold shift (STS)** has occurred. An STS is the loss of hearing in either ear of 10 decibels or more at test frequencies of 2,000, 3,000, and 4,000 **hertz (Hz)** (cycles per second) in either ear.

If the annual audiogram shows that the employee has suffered an STS, the employer may obtain a retest within thirty days and consider the results of the retest as the annual audiogram.

The audiologist, otolaryngologist, or physician shall review problem audiograms and shall determine whether there is a need for further evaluation. The employer shall provide to the person performing this evaluation the following information: a copy of the requirements for hearing conservation; the baseline audiogram and most recent audiogram of the employee to be evaluated; measurements of background sound pressure levels in test rooms; and records of audiometer calibrations.

If a comparison of the annual audiogram to the baseline audiogram indicates an STS, the employee must be notified in writing within twenty-one days of the determination.

If an STS occurs, the employer must do the following:

- Employees not wearing hearing protectors must be fitted, trained in their use and care, and required to use them.
- Employees already using protectors shall be re-fitted and retrained in the use of protectors and provided with protectors offering greater attenuation if necessary.
- The employee shall be referred for a clinical audiological evaluation or an otological examination, if additional testing is necessary or if the employer suspects that the protector has aggravated the ear.
- The employee shall be informed of the need for an otological examination if a pathology of the ear unrelated to the use of protectors is suspected.

If subsequent audiometric testing of an employee whose exposure to noise is less than an eight-hour TWA of 90 decibels indicates that an STS is not persistent, the employer shall inform the employee of the new audiometric interpretation and may discontinue the required use of hearing protectors for the employee.

An annual audiogram may be substituted for the baseline audiogram when, in the judgment of the audiologist, otolaryngologist, or physician who is evaluating the audiogram, the STS revealed by the audiogram is persistent or the hearing threshold shown in the annual audiogram indicates significant improvement over the baseline audiogram.

Audiometric Test Requirements. Audiometric examinations shall be pure tone with test frequencies at a minimum of 500, 1,000, 2,000, 3,000, 4,000, and 5,000 Hz. Tests at each frequency shall be taken for each ear.

Examinations shall be conducted in rooms meeting the OSHA requirements for audiometric testing rooms.

The audiometer shall be checked before each day's use and calibrated at least every two years.

Hearing Protectors. Employers shall make hearing protectors available to all employees exposed to an eight-hour time weighted average of 85 decibels or greater at no cost. Protectors shall be replaced as necessary.

Employers shall ensure that hearing protectors are worn:

- By an employee when exposure exceeds that of Table G-16.
- By any employee who is exposed to an eight-hour TWA of 85 decibels or greater.
- By any employee who has not yet had a baseline audiogram.
- By any employee who has experienced an STS.

Employees may select their hearing protection from a variety supplied by the employer.

The employer shall provide training in the use and care of all hearing protectors.

The employer shall ensure proper fitting and supervise the correct use of hearing protectors.

Hearing Protector Attenuation. The employer shall evaluate hearing protector attenuation for the specific noise environment in which the protector will be used.

Hearing protectors must attenuate employee exposure at least to a time weighted average of 90 decibels.

For employees who have experienced an STS, hearing protectors must attenuate employee exposure to an eight-hour TWA of 85 decibels or below.

The adequacy of hearing protector attenuation shall be re-evaluated whenever employee noise exposures increase to the extent that hearing protectors provided may no longer provide adequate attenuation. The employer must provide more-effective hearing protectors where necessary.

Training Program. The employer must institute a training program for all employees who are exposed to noise at or above the eight-hour TWA of 85 decibels and shall ensure employee participation in the program.

The program must be repeated annually for each employee included in the hearing conservation program. Information provided the employee shall be updated when necessary.

The employee must be informed of the following:

- The effects of noise on hearing
- The purpose of hearing protectors; the advantages, disadvantages, and attenuation of various types; and instructions on selection, fitting, use, and care
- The purpose of audiometric testing, and an evaluation of test procedures

Access to Information and Training Materials. The employer must make a copy of the standard available to affected employees and their representatives; make available any material sent by OSHA to the employer; and provide, upon request, all materials related to the employer's training and education program to OSHA.

Recordkeeping. The employer must maintain an accurate record of all employee exposure measurements.

The employer must retain employee audiometric test records. The record must include name and job classification of the employee, date of the audiogram, examiner's name, date of last acoustic or exhaustive calibration of the audiometer, and employee's most recent noise exposure assessment.

The employer shall maintain accurate records of the measurements of background noise in audiometric test rooms.

Noise exposure measurements must be retained for two years.

Audiometric test records must be retained for the duration of employment of the affected employee.

All records shall be provided upon request to employees, former employees, an employee's designated representative, and OSHA.

If an employer ceases to do business, the employer shall transfer to the successor employer all records required to be maintained and the successor shall maintain them for the required periods.

Noise Calculations

If there is more than one period and level of noise in the workplace, the following formula can be used:

$$D(\%) = 100 \, (C_1/T_1 + C_2/T_2 + C_n/T_n)$$

D is the noise level in percentage of dose evaluated from Table A-1 of the OSHA standard.

C_n is total time exposed to a specific noise level.

T_n is the referenced duration for that level from Table G-16a in Appendix A of the OSHA standard.

Example

A worker is exposed to a sound level of 80 dBA for 4 hours and 92 dBA for 4 hours.

Go to Table G-16a.
80 dBA has a T of 32, and 92 dBA has a T of 6.1.

$D = 100(4/32 + 4/6.1)$
$= 100(.79)$
$= 79\%$

Go to Table A-1.
79% converts to an eight-hour time weighted average of 88.4 decibels (TWA closest to 79%). The worker is not overexposed because the TWA is not 90 decibels or above as averaged over eight hours. Because the decibel level is over 85 decibels, the employer must institute a hearing conservation program.

Example

A worker is exposed to a sound level of 92 dBA for 6 hours and 88 dBA for 2 hours.

Go to Table G-16a.
92 dB(A) has a T of 6.1, and 88 dB(A) has a T of 10.6.

$D = 100(6/6.1 + 2/10.6)$
$= 100(1.17)$
$= 117\%$

Go to Table A-1.
117% converts to an eight-hour time weighted average of 91.1 decibels, which exceeds the 90 decibel limit. The employer is required to immediately bring sound levels to below 90 dBA averaged over eight hours.

APPENDIX

This appendix discusses examples of hearing protectors, control, and measuring instruments.

Hearing Protectors

There is a variety of hearing protection available. They can be categorized into ear barriers (muffs), earplugs that can be thrown away after use, molded plugs that fit individual ears, and plugs that are held against the ear by a headband. Protectors are given NRR ratings, which are noise reduction ratings. This is the ability of the protector to reduce (attenuate) the noise level under the protector by the rated amount. An NRR of 10 decibels reduces the noise under the protector by 10 decibels. In the workplace, the NRR rating might not attenuate to its rating because the protectors are usually tested under different conditions by the manufacturer.

Controlling Noise

As with reducing exposure to toxic materials, engineering or work practice controls should always be considered before assigning hearing protection (PPE). If these controls can reduce noise levels below OSHA limits, this would be preferable to having employees wear protectors.

Putting employees in a soundproof booth is an example of an engineering control; reducing the time employees are exposed to noise so that the TWA is less than OSHA limits is an example of a work practice control.

Noise-Measuring Instruments

There are two types of measuring instruments. One is a decibel meter (decimeter). This measures noise levels directly on a scale in decibels. OSHA uses the A scale at slow response because these are the frequencies the human ear hears. The sound level meter is most effective when the employee stays in relatively one spot on the job. When using a sound level meter to get an equivalent sound level when there are different levels in the work area, the calculations at the end of the chapter that determine percent dose that becomes an equivalent dBA level should be used.

The second type of meter is a dosimeter. This meter measures sound levels at different frequencies. It is most effective if the employee has to move to various areas with different sound levels. The readings are at various octave band sound levels and frequencies, which converts to decibels on the A scale by using Table G-9 in the standard.

CHAPTER REVIEW

Multiple Choice

Select the best answer from the choices provided.

1. Continuous noise is noise at intervals of

    a. 2 seconds or less
    b. 5 seconds or less
    c. 1 second or less
    d. no time interval

2. Workers cannot be exposed to impact noise exceeding

    a. 100 decibels   c. 200 decibels
    b. 150 decibels   d. 140 decibels

3. Training of employees is required for those exposed above

    a. 85 dBA   c. 100 dBA
    b. 90 dBA   d. 70 dBA

4. Putting an employee in a soundproof booth is an example of

    a. a work practice control
    b. personal protective equipment
    c. an engineering control
    d. a, b, and c

5. When a standard threshold shift occurs, the employee must be notified within
   a. ten days
   b. twenty-one days
   c. thirty days
   d. fifteen days

True/False

Indicate whether the statement is true or false by circling T or F.

6. T F Employees cannot observe monitoring.

7. T F An exposure of 90 dBA triggers a hearing conservation program.

8. T F Monitoring of employees is required when there is an exposure above 85 dBA.

9. T F A standard threshold shift is an average hearing loss of 50 decibels or more in either ear.

10. T F Reducing the time an employee is exposed to high noise levels is a work practice control.

CHAPTER 22

Ventilation

OBJECTIVES

After studying this chapter, you should be able to

➤ List the various types of ventilation systems.
➤ Explain the requirements for a general exhaust ventilation system.
➤ Describe the types of pressures in exhaust systems.
➤ Discuss the maintenance required for these systems.
➤ Discuss fume hoods and ways they can be used efficiently.

VENTILATION SYSTEMS

A basic understanding of the types of ventilation systems that are used and how they operate is essential for anyone responsible for the safety of workers. Ventilation systems are a very important engineering control and are effective in keeping contaminants below the permissible exposure limits (PELs), as well as maintaining comfort levels. The PELs are the OSHA permissible exposure limits as described in OSHA 29 CFR 1910.1000 Air Contaminants.

A properly designed and installed ventilation system will protect workers and eliminate the need for respirators and respirator programs.

There will be situations where contaminant levels are too high for the ventilation system to bring concentrations to safe levels. Then a ventilation system must be used in conjunction with the proper respirator.

Contaminant levels can also be lowered by opening windows and doors or by using other openings for infiltration. When this method is used it is called **natural ventilation**; when fans are used, it is called **mechanical ventilation**. Natural ventilation is not recommended when contaminant levels are high or when the contaminant is being produced at a consistent rate.

A poorly designed or installed exhaust system can be hazardous. Ventilation systems must be checked periodically to make sure they are exhausting contaminants to safe levels. When a contaminant is being improperly exhausted, high levels of the substance can be inhaled.

This chapter describes general and local exhaust ventilation, which are the basic ventilation systems used to control airborne contaminants.

AIRFLOW PRINCIPLES

Whenever there is a pressure differential, there will be a flow of air from high pressure to low pressure. That is why using a fan to create these pressures to move air is more efficient than depending upon natural ventilation, particularly if contaminant levels are high.

When a fan is on exhaust, the exhaust side of the fan develops low pressure in relation to the room air, which is at higher pressure. This causes the room air to move towards the low pressure created by the fan and be exhausted to the outside. The blower or opposite side of the fan develops positive pressure.

When one fan brings in outside air (OA) (air at positive pressure) while another exhausts the air (air at negative pressure), it is called a "push-pull" effect. Outside air is the air brought in from the exterior.

GENERAL EXHAUST VENTILATION

General exhaust ventilation is a ventilation system designed to dilute contaminated air. It uses outside air to dilute. It is also known as **dilution ventilation**. It is used when sources of contamination generation are spread throughout the room.

General Exhaust Ventilation Criteria

General exhaust ventilation systems have the following limitations:

- The amount of contaminant produced cannot be more than the system can safely exhaust or dilute.
- Workers must be located so their respiratory systems are not exposed to the air being exhausted. They should be away from the point or points where the contaminant is generated.
- For general exhaust to be used safely, the toxicity of the contaminant generated should be below the PEL. Toxicity is also related to the dose rate of the contaminant and the susceptibility of the worker being exposed. The dose rate is the amount of contaminant that can be inhaled during a specified period of time.
- The generation of contaminant should be uniform and not produced at levels that can go up sharply.
- It is not efficient for exhausting fumes and dusts and other particulates because of the high volume of air needed. High exhaust air volumes cause large amounts of heat to be lost from buildings, which is not economical. The system is more efficient when exhausting vapors and gases.

General exhaust ventilation is most effective when:

- The contaminant is being generated at a uniform rate and is below the PEL.
- The contaminant is a gas or vapor and not a particulate.
- The contaminant is dispersed and not near workers.
- The climate conditions are moderate.

- Outside air is used to remove contaminant from the space.
- Concentrations of vapors or gases in enclosures are to be reduced.
- Emissions from portable or mobile sources have to be controlled.

Makeup Air

Makeup air is the air brought into the space to replace the exhausted air. In cold climates it should be heated to prevent heat loss in the building.

When relatively small volumes of air are being exhausted, sufficient makeup air can be introduced into the space naturally by atmospheric pressure through windows, doors, and louvers.

Makeup air can also be supplied mechanically by having fans supply the air into the space. Mechanical makeup air systems can be interlocked with exhaust fans to automatically operate to maintain a constant flow of replacement air.

Whether using natural or mechanical methods, the volume of makeup air should approximately equal the volume of exhausted air. A mechanical system is preferred over a natural system because it prevents:

- A buildup of negative pressure. This can be identified when doors are either difficult to open or slam shut.
- High-velocity air from coming through wall cracks, doors, and windows.
- High heating costs in cold climates because the makeup air can be heated.

Formula to Determine Air Volume Required

To estimate the volume of air required to dilute a specific amount of identified contaminant to the OSHA PEL, the following formula is used:

Volume of air (cfm) =

$$\frac{\text{Volume of vapor} \times 10^6 \times k}{\text{OSHA PEL for contaminant (ppm)}}$$

To determine *volume of vapor:*

Volume of vapor =

$$\frac{\text{Specific gravity} \times 8.31 \times 387}{\text{Molecular weight of contaminant}}$$

1. *Volume of vapor* is determined by obtaining the specific gravity of the contaminant and multiplying it by the weight of a gallon of water (8.31 pounds). The specific gravity of substances can be found in chemistry texts.
2. This product is then multiplied by 387, which is the cubic feet of space occupied by one pound molecular weight of the contaminant. Molecular weights can be found in chemistry texts.
3. The result is divided by the molecular weight of the contaminant.
4. The resulting volume of vapor is expressed in cubic feet per gallon.

To determine *k:*

> *k* is a safety factor that commonly varies from 3 to 6. It is determined by such factors as emission rates, mixing of contaminant, and employee practices. If you feel these factors are good, assign a value of 3; if you think they are poor, assign a value of 5 or 6. In extreme cases when factors are very poor, assign a value of 9 or 10. If this is the case, local exhaust should be considered.

To determine the *OSHA Permissible Exposure Limit (PEL):*

> The OSHA PEL for the contaminant can be obtained from OSHA 29 CFR 1910.1000 Air Contaminants.

The result:

> The resulting volume of air calculated is expressed in cubic feet per minute (cfm) and is the volume of air required to dilute the specified volume of vapor of the contaminant to its PEL.

Formula to Determine Number of Air Changes per Hour

The number of air changes per hour (ACH) is the number of times per hour the entire air in the space is replaced by the ventilation system. The number of ACHs to dilute the contaminant to its PEL is determined by the following formula:

$$\text{ACH} = \frac{\text{Volume of air} \times 60 \text{ minutes/hr.}}{\text{Space volume}}$$

To determine *volume of air:*

> This is the figure obtained from working the preceding formula.

To determine *space volume:*

> Multiply height times width times length of the space. The result is expressed in cubic feet (ft^3).

The resulting ACH:

> The result is expressed in air changes per hour (ACH).

Formula to Determine Flow Rate

The flow rate (V) in feet per minute (fpm) is the air needed to dilute the contaminant to the PEL and is determined by the following formula:

$$\text{V (fpm)} = \frac{\text{Volume of air}}{\text{Width} \times \text{height (area) of wall fan is on}}$$

To determine *volume of air:*

> This is the figure obtained from working the formula given previously.

To determine *area of wall* where the fan(s) are located:

> Multiply the width of the wall by the height. The result is expressed in square feet (ft^2).

Fan Determination

The above three formulas will assist in determining the size of the fan(s) required in order to move the specified volumes of air. Once these three figures are obtained, a fan can be installed that will meet the necessary specifications determined by the calculations. If one fan cannot move the required volume of air, then additional fans may have to be installed, which in combination will do the job.

Remember, general ventilation should be used only when conditions warrant. If there are factors that prohibit this type of system, local exhaust ventilation should be considered.

LOCAL EXHAUST VENTILATION

Local exhaust ventilation is different from general ventilation. This type of system is designed to capture the contaminant at the point where it is generated (source) and to exhaust it outside to another safe location. Under special conditions, the exhausted air may be recirculated. The main components of this system are

- A hood to capture the contaminant.
- Ducts to transport the contaminant to the outside.
- A fan that moves air and exhausts the contaminant.
- A filter or air cleaner that cleans the contaminant before it is exhausted to the outside or other safe location. Exhausted air may be recirculated only under special conditions.
- A stack where the fan is mounted.

Advantages of a Local Exhaust System

This type of system is preferred when the contaminant generated is very toxic, the rate of generation varies, and the points of contaminant generation are stationary.

The design of local exhaust systems should be left to qualified persons. There are many factors used in determining the size and shape of the hood, ductwork, and fan. If the system is not designed or installed properly, it will not exhaust efficiently.

System Design Factors

The following factors must be taken into consideration when designing a local exhaust system:

Static Pressure (SP). Static pressure is the pressure produced by the fan. It is exerted in all directions as it moves through the duct. It is also the algebraic difference between the total pressure and velocity pressure in the duct. It is measured in inches of water. Static pressure is negative upstream from the fan and positive downstream.

$$SP = TP - VP$$

Velocity Pressure (VP). Velocity pressure is the pressure due to the velocity of the air as it travels through the duct. It is exerted in the direction of airflow. It is measured in inches of water. Velocity pressure is positive both upstream and downstream from the fan. It is also the algebraic difference between the total pressure and the static pressure.

$$VP = TP - SP$$

Total Pressure. Total pressure is the algebraic sum of static pressure and velocity pressure. Total pressure is negative upstream from the fan and positive downstream. It is measured in inches of water.

$$TP = SP + VP$$

System Losses. When designing a local exhaust system, qualified personnel determine the losses in pressure due to hood entry, duct friction, duct design, fan, air cleaner, blast gates (vanes in the duct that can be opened and closed), and stack.

Designing a System Using the Velocity Pressure Method

A local exhaust system can be designed by using the **velocity pressure method**. The design is based upon what is to be exhausted, system losses to be considered, location of contaminant generation, and number of generation points. If used correctly, it determines the size and length of duct(s) required, hood size and shape, and size of fan needed.

The procedure can be found in the "Industrial Ventilation Manual" published by the American Conference of Governmental and Industrial Hygienists (ACGIH).

If you are not comfortable using this method to design a system, you should hire a professional engineer.

Hoods. The hood converts duct static pressure into velocity pressure and hood entry losses. In order to minimize these losses, the hood should be enclosed as much as possible. Baffles or curtains can help capture or contain the contaminant and reduce air current effects.

If high velocities are needed to maintain required airflow to capture contaminants, the system should be redesigned. High velocities prevent effective air distribution in the hood.

Locate the hood to prevent the contaminants from passing past the worker's breathing area and interfering with worker activities. Access doors should not be located in the hood because if left open, it affects hood performance.

Hoods must meet the design specifications of the ACGIH Ventilation Manual or OSHA standards.

Hoods will not draw air from considerable distances, so they must be located as close to the source of contamination as possible. The blower side of the fan will move approximately nine times more air than the exhaust side.

Ducts. The duct design should minimize turbulence as the air enters. This transport air can flow at between 2,000 and 6,000 feet per minute (fpm). If the point of contaminate generation is located one-half the duct diameter from the hood, the capture air velocity will be about 30 percent of the air velocity at the hood entrance. This figure tails off dramatically the further the distance from the hood.

Ductwork has to be designed for the contaminant. Where there is duct branching from the main duct, or changes in duct size, or elbows, it adds to friction loss. The system should be designed to minimize these losses as much as possible. Square and rectangular duct will have more friction losses than round duct. Duct branches should never enter at right angles to the main duct. The preferable angle should be between 10 and 60 degrees. The lesser the angle, the less the loss due to friction.

Ducts can be made from galvanized sheetmetal, spiral round sheetmetal, flexible steel, plastic (both flexible and rigid), and other materials. They can be round, square, or rectangular. The type of exhaust determines the duct material. Flammable, toxic, and hot materials should be exhausted through metal duct. If the material exhausted does not pose a fire or toxic threat, other materials can be used.

Fans. The fan is a very important component of the local exhaust system. It supplies the static pressure that helps move air through the duct. A negative pressure is created on the suction or exhaust side of the fan and a positive pressure on the supply or push side of the fan.

There are two types of fans: centrifugal and axial. The centrifugal fan has forward or backward curved blades or radial blades. The axial fan has propeller-type blades.

Fan selection is determined by friction losses that have to be overcome, hood and duct design, required cfm, and static pressure generated.

When determining fan size (particularly after using the velocity pressure method), a manufacturer's fan curve chart should be reviewed. This chart plots fan static pressures against delivered cfm.

Air Cleaners. Different air cleaners will be required to filter out particulates from those filtering out gases and vapors.

High efficiency particulate air (HEPA) filters are used if it is necessary to filter out minute particles 0.3 microns in diameter or larger. The HEPA filter will trap 99.97% of these particles.

Air cleaners that filter out particulates consist of particulate filters, cyclone separators, wet scrubbers, and electrostatic precipitators.

Gas and vapor cleaners consist of wet scrubbers, chemical reaction and catalytic scrubbers, and absorption and adsorption collectors.

Stacks. The stack disperses the exhausted contaminant to the outside air, or safe location. The main hazard is reentrainment (exhaust air getting back into the building) through intake ducts, windows, louvers, or other openings. Reentrainment depends upon location of the stack, the volume exhausted, wind speed and direction, temperature, and location of building openings.

Some helpful hints for stack location include

- Making the stack at least ten feet above adjacent roof lines or air intakes to avoid reentrainment.
- Placing the stack at least fifty feet downwind of air intakes.
- Having a stack velocity at least 1.4 times the wind velocity.
- Keeping rain caps off stacks if they are within fifty feet of air intakes.

Makeup Air. Local ventilation systems that exhaust large volumes of air require makeup air units if air infiltration through doors and windows is insufficient. As with general systems, the makeup air volume should be approximately equal to the exhaust air volume. To reduce building heating costs, heating makeup air should be considered. The criteria for general exhaust makeup air as described under general ventilation can be used for local exhaust systems.

System Maintenance

Local exhaust systems require periodic maintenance if they are to operate properly.

- Local exhaust systems should be checked on a scheduled basis to make sure they are operating in accordance with design specifications.
- A velometer that measures airflow and static pressure at various points in the duct should be used and results compared to system design parameters.
- Any changes should be investigated and corrected.
- Dirty filters must be replaced to avoid static pressure buildup. The duct and hood should be inspected to make sure there is no blockage.
- Fan belts and motors should be checked on a scheduled basis and fan motors lubricated where necessary.
- Ducts should be examined to make sure they are not disconnected. Ascertain that clean-out doors are not left open or leaking, that there are no holes in the ductwork from punctures, and that there is no buildup of exhausted materials.

Recirculation of Air

In some instances it is permissible to recirculate exhausted air back into the ventilation system. This is usually done for economic reasons. In order to maintain employee safety, the following must be considered:

1. Employee protection must be a priority.
2. The contaminant should be removed to below any hazardous levels. This means that recirculation cannot simply ensure that exposure levels are maintained at the PEL.
3. Recirculation cannot increase exposure levels.
4. It cannot be used if there is carcinogenic exposure.
5. The system should have a fail-safe warning feature or backup that notifies when it is not operating.
6. A bypass or auxiliary system should be in place if the main system fails to operate.
7. Continuous and reliable contaminant capture must be maintained by use of cleaning and filtering devices.
8. Devices should be installed to supervise the system and ensure proper operation. This includes monitoring of static pressure, particulates, and amperage.
9. Employees must be trained in system operation.

Laboratory Hoods

Laboratory hoods are local exhaust systems. They are designed specifically to exhaust gases and vapors before they get back into the room and in the breathing zone of the worker.

There are general purpose hoods and auxiliary hoods.

General Purpose Hoods. General purpose hoods exhaust room air through the hood opening. Ideally, the heating, ventilating, and air-conditioning system (HVAC) should automatically compensate for room air loss. When the hoods operate, the HVAC system should automatically supply treated air to the room as needed. This is done on a variable rate through modulating dampers.

Auxiliary Hoods. Auxiliary hoods take air from an outside location and bring it into the room, bypassing the hood opening. This reduces the need for the building HVAC system to increase the supply of treated air to the space.

Hood Performance. For optimal hood performance the following should be considered:

- Hoods should not be located in heavily trafficked paths or by doors and windows. Cross drafts can adversely affect the flow of air into the hood.
- Exhaust fans should be located at the end of the stack outside the building to maintain a negative pressure in the stack. This prevents contaminant leakage from the duct.
- Hood jambs and sills should be designed as an air foil to avoid sharp corners. This helps to prevent turbulence in the hood.
- Laboratories should be provided with conditioned makeup air.
- For best air conservation, horizontal sashes should be used.

Face Velocity of Laboratory Hoods. Face velocity of a hood is the average velocity as measured across the face of the hood in feet per minute (fpm).

A higher face velocity does not mean that the hood will exhaust more efficiently. High face velocities can cause air turbulence in the hood. The contaminant can get back into the room because of this turbulence. The airflow into the hood should be as uniform as possible.

Recommended face velocities for utility hoods (hoods for contaminants with low to average release) should be 100 feet per minute (100 fpm).

Heavy duty hoods (hoods for contaminants with high release) should be 125 fpm. Contaminants requiring velocities greater than 125 fpm should be placed in glove boxes. A glove box totally encloses the generated contaminant. The worker has his/her hands in gloves that are within the box.

Hood Testing and Maintenance. A hand-held velometer can be used across the face of the hood with the sash in the wide open position to determine average face velocity. The readings are totaled and then averaged. If face velocity is not within design specifications, the hood should be examined. The back baffle might need adjustment, there could be blockage in the hood or duct, or the fan may have belt slippage.

Summary

Exhaust systems must be designed and installed properly if they are to do their job. These systems should be on strictly enforced preventative maintenance schedules.

Employee health depends upon the proper functioning of these systems. Workers must be trained to operate them and to make sure they do not inhale contaminant before it gets into the hood or is exhausted outdoors.

CHAPTER REVIEW

Multiple Choice

Select the best answer from the choices provided.

1. Air moves
   a. from low to high pressure
   b. from high to low pressure
   c. downward
   d. upward

2. General exhaust ventilation is most effective when the
   a. contaminant is generated at a uniform rate
   b. climate conditions are moderate
   c. the contaminant is not a gas or vapor
   d. a, b, and c

3. The volume of makeup air should be
   a. equal to the exhaust air
   b. greater than the exhaust air
   c. less than the exhaust air
   d. equal to the exhaust air initially then increased

4. The velocity pressure method determines the specifications for
   a. a general exhaust system
   b. a local exhaust system
   c. reentrainment
   d. makeup air

5. A wet scrubber is an example of
   a. a local exhaust system
   b. a fan
   c. a general exhaust system
   d. an air cleaner

True/False

Indicate whether the statement is true or false by circling T or F.

6. T F Any ventilation system is better than none at all.

7. T F General exhaust ventilation captures the contaminant where it is generated.

8. T F Fans supply the static pressure in ventilation systems that move air.

9. T F Local exhaust is best used when contaminant levels are below the PEL.

10. T F Makeup air must always be considered when installing exhaust systems.

Short Answer

Briefly but thoroughly answer each statement.

11. Discuss the difference between general exhaust and local exhaust ventilation.

12. Describe the procedures you would use to check the performance of a local exhaust system.

13. List the components of a local exhaust system and tell what each does.

14. List the various ways contaminated air can get back into a building and how you could prevent it.

15. Describe where you would place the fume hoods in a laboratory and why.

CHAPTER 23

Control of Hazardous Energy: Lockout/Tagout

OBJECTIVES

After studying this chapter, you should be able to

➤ Describe the OSHA lockout/tagout standard.
➤ Explain the lockout/tagout program where you work.
➤ List the training content for employees in lockout/tagout procedures.

OSHA 29 CFR 1910.147 CONTROL OF HAZARDOUS ENERGY

Lockout/tagout requirements are specified in OSHA 29 CFR 1910.147. These regulations cover employees who service and maintain machines and equipment. The regulations are designed to prevent the unexpected start-up of machines and equipment while employees are working on them.

The standard covers all energy forms. These include electrical, steam, water, vacuum, air, fuel, and atomic.

OSHA included this standard because too many workers were being injured and killed because of the sudden start-up of equipment energy while an employee was working on the machine or equipment.

Definitions

Authorized employee is a person who locks out or tags out machines or equipment in order to perform servicing or maintenance.

Capable of being locked out refers to an energy isolating device capable of being locked out if it has

a hasp or other means of attachment, or through which a lock can be affixed, or it has a locking mechanism built into it.

Energy isolating device is a mechanical device that prevents the transmission or release of energy. It includes circuit breakers, disconnect switches, manually operated switches, line valves, blocks, and push-button selector switches.

Lockout is the placement of a lockout device on an energy isolating device so that the energy isolating device and the equipment to be controlled cannot be operated unless the lockout device is removed.

A *lockout device* is a key or combination type that holds an energy isolating device in a safe position.

Tagout is the placement of a tagout device on an energy isolating device to indicate that the energy isolating device cannot be operated until the tagout device is removed.

Tagout device is a prominent warning device that can be securely fastened to an energy isolating device, and the equipment may not be operated until the tagout device is removed.

Note: The standard does not apply when working on cord and plug connected electrical equipment for which exposure to the hazards of unexpected energization or start-up of the equipment is controlled by the unplugging of the equipment from the energy source and by the plug being under the exclusive control of the employee performing the servicing or maintenance.

Energy Control Program

The energy control program is the program developed for lockout/tagout.

General. The employer shall establish a program consisting of energy control procedures, employee training, and periodic inspections to ensure that before any employee performs any servicing or maintenance on a machine or equipment where the unexpected energizing, start-up, or release of stored energy could occur and cause injury, the machine or equipment shall be isolated from the energy source and rendered inoperative.

Lockout/Tagout. If an energy isolating device is not capable of being locked out, the employer shall utilize a tagout system in accordance with this section.

If an energy isolating device is capable of being locked out, the employer's energy control program shall utilize lockout, unless the employer can demonstrate that tagout will provide full employee protection in accordance with this section.

Since January 20, 1990, whenever new machines or equipment are installed, isolating devices must be capable of being locked out.

Full Employee Protection. When a tagout device is used on an energy isolating device that can be locked out, the tagout device will be attached at the same location where the lockout device would have been attached, and shall provide the same level of protection equivalent to that of the lockout device.

If the employer uses the tagout device, he/she must demonstrate that the tagout program is equivalent to the level of safety as the lockout together with additional elements such as removing an isolating circuit element, blocking of a control switch, opening of an extra disconnect, or the removal of a valve handle.

Energy Control Procedure. Procedures shall be developed, documented, and utilized for the control of potentially hazardous energy when employees are engaged in the activities covered in this section.

The procedures shall clearly outline the scope, purpose, authorization, rules, and techniques to be utilized for the control of hazardous energy, and the means to enforce compliance. The procedures must include specific steps for shutting down, isolating, blocking, and securing machines and equipment; steps for the placement, removal and transfer of lockout devices or tagout devices and the responsibility for them; and requirements for testing a machine or equipment to determine and verify the effectiveness of the lockout or tagout device.

Protective Materials and Hardware. Locks, chains, wedges, key blocks, adapter pins, self-locking fasteners, or other hardware for securing machines and equipment must be supplied by the employer.

Lockout and tagout devices must be identified and not used for any other purpose.

Devices must be durable and able to withstand the environment to which they are exposed.

The printing on tagout devices must remain legible and not be affected by the environment to which they are exposed.

Tags shall not deteriorate in corrosive environments.

Standardization. Lockout and tagout devices shall be standardized within the facility.

Devices shall be substantial enough to prevent removal without the use of excessive force.

Tagout devices shall be substantial enough to prevent inadvertent or accidental removal.

Identifiable. Lockout and tagout devices shall identify the employee applying the device(s).

Tagout devices shall warn against hazardous conditions if the machine or equipment is energized and shall include the legend **Do Not Start**, **Do Not Open, Do Not Close, Do Not Energize**, or **Do Not Operate**.

Periodic Inspection. The employer shall conduct a periodic inspection of the energy control procedure at least annually.

The periodic inspection shall be performed by an authorized employee other than the one(s) utilizing the energy control procedure being inspected.

The inspection shall correct any deviations or inadequacies identified.

Where lockout is used, the inspection shall include a review of that employee's responsibility under the energy control program.

Where tagout is used, the inspection shall include a review of that employee's responsibilities under the tagout control program.

The employer must certify that periodic inspections have been performed. The certification shall identify the machine or equipment, the date of inspection, the employees included in the inspection, and the person performing the inspection.

Training and Communication. The employer shall provide training to ensure employee knowledge and skills concerning energy control devices. The training shall include the recognition of hazardous energy sources, type and magnitude of energy available in the workplace, and the methods necessary for energy isolation and control; the purpose and use of energy control procedures; and the instruction of other employees who work in areas where energy control devices may be used that they must not make attempts to re-energize machines and equipment that are locked or tagged out.

When tagout systems are used, employees shall be trained as follows:

- That tags are essentially warning devices and do not provide safe restraint as do locks.
- When a tag is removed from an energy isolating device, it cannot be removed without proper authorization of the person responsible for it, and is never to be bypassed, ignored, or defeated.
- That tags must be legible and understandable.
- That tags and their means of attachment must withstand the conditions in which they are installed.
- That tags evoke a false sense of security.
- That tags must be securely fastened.

Retraining shall be provided as follows:

- Whenever there is a change in job assignments, machines, equipment, or processes that present a new hazard.
- Whenever the employer feels that the employee has inadequacies concerning procedures.
- Whenever new or revised control methods are introduced.

The employer shall certify that training has been done and is being kept up to date. The certification shall contain the employee's name and dates of training.

Energy Isolation. Lockout and tagout shall be performed only by authorized employees who are servicing or maintaining the equipment.

Employee Notification. Affected employees shall be notified by the employer or authorized employee concerning the application and removal of lockout or tagout devices. Notification shall be given before controls are put on and after they are removed.

Lockout or tagout procedures must include the following sequence:

1. The employee must have knowledge about the machine or equipment he/she is turning off.
2. The machine or equipment must be shut down using established procedures.
3. All energy isolating devices that control energy to the machine or equipment must be shut down.
4. Lockout or tagout devices shall be affixed.
5. Lockout devices shall hold energy isolating devices in the "safe" or "off" position.
6. Tagout devices shall be affixed to indicate that the operation or movement of energy isolating devices from the "safe" or "off" position is prohibited.
7. Tagout devices shall be affixed at the same location at which a lock would have been installed.
8. Where a tag cannot be affixed directly to the energy isolating device, it shall be located in a place immediately obvious to anyone attempting to operate the device.

Verification of Isolation. Prior to starting work on machines or equipment that have been secured, the authorized employee shall verify they have been deenergized.

Before lockout or tagout devices are removed and energy restored, the following procedures must be taken:

1. The work area must be inspected to ensure the removal of nonessential items.
2. Employees must be removed from the area.
3. Affected employees must be notified that the lockout or tagout device(s) have been removed.

Each lockout or tagout device shall be removed by the employee who applied the device. When the authorized employee is unavailable to remove the device, it may be removed under the direction of the employer provided that the procedure has been incorporated into the energy control program. The incorporated procedure must include the following: verification that the authorized employee is not at the facility; making all reasonable efforts to contact the authorized employee that his/her lockout or tagout device has been removed; and ensuring that the authorized employee has this knowledge before he/she comes back to work.

Additional Requirements. In situations where lockout and tagout devices must be temporarily removed to test or reposition the machine or equipment, the following sequence must be followed:

1. Clear the machine or equipment of tools and materials.
2. Remove employees from the area.
3. Remove the lockout or tagout device in accordance with proper procedures.

4. Energize and proceed with the testing or positioning.
5. De-energize all systems and reapply energy control measures in accordance with proper procedures.

Whenever outside contractors are to be engaged in activities covered by the lockout/tagout standard, the on-site employer and the outside employer shall inform each other of their respective lockout/tagout procedures.

When servicing or maintenance is performed by a crew, each employee shall affix a personal lockout or tagout device to the group lockout device, group lockbox, or comparable mechanism when he or she begins work and shall remove those devices when he or she stops working on the machine or equipment being serviced or maintained.

Specific procedures shall be utilized during shift or personnel changes to ensure the continuity of protection, including the orderly transfer of lockout or tagout devices protection between off-going and on-coming employees.

APPENDIX

There are various devices available for use as lockout. Circuit breakers can be isolated by specially designed locks. Plugs can be isolated by devices that lock after they enclose the plug. Pipes can be isolated by blanking and blinding, which closes the pipe with a solid plate to prevent the contents from flowing through. Pipes can also be isolated by double block and bleed. This method closes two valves with an open drain or vent in between. Line breaking is another method to isolate pipe flow. This disconnects a section of pipe to prevent flow. There are devices that lock valves. Manufacturer's catalogues are available that describe these devices.

CHAPTER REVIEW

True/False

Indicate whether the statement is true or false by circling T or F.

1. T F Lockout/tagout refers only to electrical energy.

2. T F Tags are to be used only if locks are not feasible.

3. T F Retraining is not required of employees after the initial training.

4. T F Inspections must be done at least annually and certified in writing.

5. T F Any worker can apply the lock to lockout the device.

CHAPTER 24

Confined Spaces

OBJECTIVES

After studying this chapter, you should be able to

➤ Describe the requirements of the permit required confined space standard

➤ State the hazards that may be present in confined spaces.

➤ Identify the difference between a confined space and a permit required confined space.

➤ State the conditions that must be present to reclassify a permit required confined space to a confined space.

➤ Explain the requirements for putting together a permit required confined space program.

OSHA 29 CFR 1910.146 PERMIT REQUIRED CONFINED SPACE

The standard is called a performance standard, which allows the employer some flexibility in methods used to comply.

Definitions

Acceptable entry conditions. Acceptable entry conditions are those conditions that must exist in a permit space to allow entry and to ensure that employees involved with a permit required confined space entry can safely enter into and work within the space.

Attendant. Attendant is an individual stationed outside one or more permit spaces who monitors the authorized entrants and who performs all attendant's duties assigned in the employer's permit space program.

Authorized entrant. Authorized entrant is an employee who is authorized by the employer to enter a permit space.

Blanking or *binding.* Blanking or binding is the absolute closure of a pipe, line, or duct by the fastening of a solid plate (such as a spectacle blind or a skillet blind) that completely covers the bore and that is capable of withstanding the maximum pressure of any pipe, line, or duct with no leakage beyond the plate.

Confined space (CS). A confined space is large enough and so configured that an employee can bodily enter and perform assigned work; has limited or restricted means for entry or exit (e.g., tanks, vessels, silos, storage bins, hoppers, vaults, and pits); and is not designed for continuous employee occupancy.

Double block and bleed. Double block and bleed is the closing of a line, duct, or pipe by closing and locking or tagging two in-line valves and by opening and locking or tagging a drain or vent valve in the line between the two closed valves.

Entry. Entry is the action by which a person passes through an opening into a permit required confined space. Entry includes ensuing work activities in that space and is considered to have occurred as soon as any part of the entrant's body breaks the plane of an opening into the space.

Entry permit. Entry permit is the written or printed document that is provided by the employer to allow and control entry into a permit space and that contains the information specified in this section.

Entry supervisor. Entry supervisor is the person (such as the employer, foreman, or crew chief) responsible for determining if acceptable entry conditions are present at a permit space where entry is planned, for authorizing entry and overseeing entry operations, and for terminating entry as required by this section. An entry supervisor may also serve as an attendant, or as an authorized entrant, as long as that person is trained and equipped as required by this section for each role he or she fills. Also, the duties of entry supervisor may be passed from one individual to another during the course of an entry operation.

Hazardous atmosphere. A hazardous atmosphere is one that may expose employees to the risk of death, incapacitation, impairment of ability to self-rescue (that is, escape unaided from a permit space), injury, or acute illness from one or more of the following causes: flammable gas, vapor, or mist in excess of 10 percent of its lower flammable limit (LFL); airborne combustible dust at a concentration that meets or exceeds its LFL; atmospheric oxygen concentration below 19.5 percent (oxygen deficient) or above 23.5 percent (oxygen enriched); atmospheric concentration of any substance for which a dose or a permissible exposure limit is published in OSHA standards subpart G or Z and that could result in employee exposure in excess of its dose or permissible exposure limit; and any other atmospheric condition that is immediately dangerous to life and health.

Hot work permit. A hot work permit is the employer's written authorization to perform operations (e.g., riveting, welding, cutting, burning, and heating) capable of providing a source of ignition.

Immediately dangerous to life or health (IDLH). IDLH means any condition that poses an immediate threat or delayed threat to life or that would cause irreversible adverse effects or that would interfere with an individual's ability to escape unaided from a permit space.

Non-permit confined space. A non-permit confined space is a confined space that does not contain or, with respect to atmospheric hazards, have the potential to contain any hazard capable of causing death or serious physical injury.

Permit required confined space (PRCS). A PRCS is a confined space that contains or has the potential to contain a hazardous atmosphere; contains a material that has the potential for engulfing the entrant; has an internal configuration such that an entrant could be trapped or asphyxiated by inwardly converging walls or by a floor that slopes downward

and tapers to a smaller cross-section; contains any other recognized serious safety or health hazard.

Permit required confined space program. A permit required confined space program refers to the employer's overall program for controlling, and, where appropriate, for protecting employees from, permit space hazards and for regulating employee entry into permit spaces.

Permit system. A permit system is the employer's written procedure for preparing and issuing permits for entry and for returning the permit space to service following termination of entry.

Prohibited condition. A prohibited condition is any condition in a permit space that is not allowed by the permit during the period when entry is authorized.

Rescue service. Rescue service is the personnel designated to rescue employees from permit spaces.

Retrieval system. Retrieval system means the equipment (including retrieval line, chest or full body harness, wristlets, if appropriate, and a lifting device or anchor) used for non-entry rescue of persons from permit spaces.

Testing. Testing is the process by which the hazards that may confront entrants of a permit space are identified and evaluated. Testing includes specifying the tests that are to be performed in the permit space.

General Requirements

If the workplace contains permit spaces, the employer shall inform exposed employees by posting danger signs (or by any other equally effective means) of the existence and location of and the danger posed by the permit spaces.

A sign reading **Danger—Permit Required Confined Space, Do Not Enter** or using other similar language would satisfy the requirement for a sign.

If the employer decides that its employees will not enter confined spaces, the employer shall take effective measures to prevent employees from entering the permit spaces.

If the employer decides that employees will enter permit spaces, the employer shall develop and implement a written permit-space program that complies with this section. The written program shall be available for inspection by employees and their authorized representatives.

An employer whose employees enter a permit space need not comply with certain sections of the standard (alternate procedures) if certain conditions are met. To do so, the employer must demonstrate that the only hazard posed by the permit space is an actual or potential hazardous atmosphere; must demonstrate that continuous forced air ventilation alone is sufficient to maintain the permit space safe for entry; must maintain employee monitoring and monitoring of the space atmosphere; must make inspection data pertaining to the confined space available to the employee; and must ensure that the permit entry program is implemented when entry is required to reclassify the space from a permit required confined space to a confined space. The employer must understand the conditions that pertain to alternate procedures by referencing the requirements in the standard.

Any conditions making it unsafe to remove an entrance cover shall be eliminated before the cover is removed.

When an entrance cover is removed, the opening shall be promptly guarded by a railing, temporary cover, or other temporary barrier that will prevent an accidental fall through the opening and that will protect each employee working in the space from foreign objects entering the space.

Before an employee enters the space, the internal atmosphere shall be tested with a calibrated direct reading instrument for oxygen content, flammable gases and vapors, and potential toxic air contaminants.

There may be no hazardous atmosphere within the space whenever any employee is inside the space.

Continuous forced air ventilation shall be used as follows:

- An employee may not enter the space until forced air ventilation has eliminated any hazardous atmosphere.
- The forced air ventilation shall be so directed as to ventilate the immediate areas where an employee is or will be present within the space and shall continue until all employees have left the space.

- The air supply for the forced air ventilation shall be from a clean source and may not increase the hazards in the space.
- The atmosphere within the space shall be periodically tested as necessary to ensure that the continuous forced air ventilation is preventing the accumulation of a hazardous atmosphere.
- If a hazardous atmosphere is detected during entry, each employee shall leave the space immediately, the space shall be evaluated to determine how the hazardous atmosphere developed, and measures shall be implemented to protect employees from the hazardous atmosphere before any subsequent entry takes place.

The employer shall verify that the space is safe for entry and that the pre-entry procedures of this section have been taken, through a written certification that contains the date, the location of the space, and the signature of the person providing the certification. The certification shall be made before entry and shall be made available to each employee entering the space.

When there are changes in the use or configuration of a non-permit confined space that might increase the hazards to entrants, the employer shall re-evaluate the space and, if necessary, reclassify it as a permit required confined space.

A permit required confined space may be reclassified as a non-permit confined space under the following procedures: If the permit space poses no actual or potential atmospheric hazards and if all hazards within the space are eliminated without entry into the space, the permit space may be reclassified as a non-permit confined space for as long as the nonatmospheric hazards remain eliminated; and if it is necessary to enter the space to eliminate such hazards, such entry shall be performed in accordance with the proper procedures of this section.

The employer shall document the basis for determining that all hazards in a permit space have been eliminated through a certification that contains the date, the location of the space, and the signature of the person making the determination.

If hazards arise within a permit space that was declassified to a non-permit space, each employee in the space shall exit the space. The employer shall then re-evaluate the space and determine if it should be reclassified.

When an employer (host employer) arranges to have employees of another employer (contractor) perform work that involves space entry, the host employer shall

- Apprise the contractor of the hazards identified and the host's experience with the space that make the space in question a permit space.
- Apprise the contractor of any precautions or procedures that the host employer has implemented.
- Coordinate entry operations with the contractor.
- Debrief the contractor at the conclusion of the entry operations regarding the permit space.

In addition to complying with the permit space requirements that apply to employers, each contractor shall

- Obtain any available information regarding permit space hazards and entry operations from the host employer.
- Coordinate entry operations with the host employer.
- Inform the host employer of the permit space program that the contractor will follow and of any hazards confronted or created.

Permit Required Confined Space Program.
Under the permit required confined space program the employer shall

- Implement the measures necessary to prevent unauthorized entry.
- Identify and evaluate the hazards before employees enter them.
- Develop and implement the means, procedures, and practices necessary for safe permit space entry operations (includes specifying acceptable entry conditions, isolating the permit space, purging, inerting, flushing, or ventilating the permit space, providing pedestrian and vehicular barriers, and verifying that conditions in the permit space are acceptable).
- Provide testing and monitoring equipment.
- Provide ventilation equipment.

- Provide communications equipment.
- Provide personal protective equipment insofar as feasible engineering and work practice controls do not adequately protect employees.
- Provide lighting equipment needed to enable employees to see well enough to do their work and to exit the space quickly in an emergency.
- Provide barriers and shields.
- Provide equipment for safe ingress and egress by authorized entrants.
- Provide rescue equipment, and any other equipment necessary for safe entry and rescue.

Evaluate permit space conditions as follows when entry operations are conducted:

- Test conditions in the permit space to determine if acceptable entry conditions exist before entry is authorized.
- Test or monitor the permit space to determine if acceptable entry conditions are being maintained.
- When testing for atmospheric conditions, test first for oxygen, then for combustible gases and vapors, and then for toxic gases and vapors.

Provide at least one attendant outside the permit space into which entry is authorized for the duration of entry operations.

If multiple spaces are to be monitored by a single attendant, include in the permit program the means and procedures to enable the attendant to respond to an emergency affecting one or more of the permit spaces being monitored without distraction from the attendant's responsibilities.

Designate the persons who are authorized entrants, attendants, entry supervisors, or persons who test or monitor the atmosphere in the permit space. Identify the duties of each employee.

Develop and implement a system for the preparation, issuance, use, and cancellation of entry permits.

Develop and implement procedures to coordinate entry operations when employees of more than one employer are working simultaneously as authorized entrants.

Develop and implement procedures for concluding the entry.

Review entry operations when the employer has reason to believe that the measures taken under the permit space program may not protect employees and revise the program.

Review the permit space program using cancelled permits within one year after each entry, and revise the program to ensure safe entry operations.

Permit System. Before entry is authorized, the employer shall document the completion of measures required by this section by preparing an entry permit.

Before entry begins, the employer shall sign the permit to authorize entry.

The permit shall be posted at the entry portal or by any other equally effective means.

The duration of the permit shall not exceed the time required to complete the task.

The entry supervisor shall terminate entry and cancel the permit when the entry operations covered by the entry permit have been completed or a condition that is not allowed under the entry permit arises in or near the space.

The cancelled permit shall be retained for at least one year.

Entry Permit. The entry permit shall identify the permit space to be entered; the purpose of the entry; the date and the authorized duration of the entry permit; the authorized entrants within the permit space by name; the personnel, by name, currently serving as attendants; the individual, by name, currently serving as entry supervisor; the hazards of the permit space to be entered; the measures used to isolate the permit space; the acceptable entry conditions; the results of initial and periodic tests; the rescue and emergency services that can be summoned; the communication procedures used by authorized entrants and attendants to maintain contact; personal protective equipment, testing equipment, communications equipment, alarm systems, and rescue equipment to be provided; any other information whose inclusion is necessary; and any additional permits, such as hot work, that have been issued.

Training. The employer shall provide training so that all employees whose work is regulated by this section acquire the understanding, knowledge, and skills necessary for the safe performance of the duties assigned under this section.

Training must be provided for each affected employee before the employee is assigned duties under this section; before there is a change in assigned duties; whenever there is a change in permit space operations that presents a hazard about which the employee has not been trained; and whenever there are deviations from the permit space entry procedures.

The training shall establish employee proficiency in all required duties.

The employer shall certify that the training has been accomplished. The certification shall contain each employee's name, the signatures or initials of trainers, and the dates of training.

Duties of Authorized Entrants. The employer shall ensure that all authorized entrants do the following:

- Know the hazards that may be faced during entry, including information on the mode, signs, or symptoms, and consequences of the exposure.
- Properly use equipment.
- Communicate with the attendant.
- Alert the attendant whenever the entrant recognizes any warning signs or symptoms of exposure to a dangerous situation, or the entrant detects a prohibited condition.
- Exit from the space as quickly as possible whenever an order to evacuate is given by the attendant or entry supervisor, the entrant recognizes any warning sign or symptom of exposure to a dangerous situation, the entrant detects a prohibited condition, or an evacuation alarm is activated.

Duties of Attendants. The employer shall ensure that each attendant does the following:

- Knows the hazards that may be faced during entry.
- Is aware of possible behavioral effects of the hazard exposure in authorized entrants.

- Continuously maintains an accurate account of authorized entrants.
- Accurately identifies who is in the space.
- Remains outside the space until relieved by another attendant.
- Communicates with authorized entrants to maintain entrant status.
- Monitors activities inside and outside the space to determine if authorized entrants can remain in the space and orders the authorized entrants to evacuate the permit space immediately if the attendant detects a prohibited condition, if the attendant detects behavioral effects of a hazard in the entrant, if the attendant detects a situation outside the space that could endanger the entrant, or if the attendant cannot effectively communicate with the entrant.
- Summons rescue and emergency services as soon as the attendant determines that entrants may need assistance to escape from the space hazard.
- Takes the following actions when unauthorized persons enter the permit space:
  — Warns unauthorized persons that they must stay away.
  — Advises unauthorized persons that they must exit the space immediately, if they have entered.
  — Informs authorized entrants that unauthorized persons have entered the space.
  — Performs nonentry rescues as specified by the employer's rescue procedures, and performs no duties that might interfere with the attendant's primary duties.

Duties of Entry Supervisor. The employer shall assure that each entry supervisor does the following:

- Knows the hazards that may be faced during entry, including information on the mode, signs or symptoms, and consequences of exposure.
- Verifies by checking that the appropriate entries have been made on the permit, that all tests specified have been conducted, and that all procedures and equipment specified are in place.

- Terminates the entry and cancels the permit as required.
- Verifies that rescue services are available.
- Removes unauthorized individuals who enter or attempt to enter a permit space.
- Determines, whenever responsibility for a permit space operation is transferred and at intervals dictated by the hazards and operations performed within the space, that entry operations remain consistent with the terms of the entry permit and that all acceptable entry conditions are maintained.

Rescue and Emergency Services. An employer who designates rescue and emergency services shall

- Evaluate a prospective rescuer's ability to respond to a rescue summons in a timely manner, considering the hazards identified.
- Evaluate a prospective service's ability, in terms of proficiency with rescue-related tasks and equipment, to function appropriately while rescuing entrants from the particular permit space of types of permit spaces identified.
- Select a rescue team or service from those evaluated that has the capability to reach the victim(s) within a time frame that is appropriate for the permit space hazard(s) identified and is equipped for and proficient in performing the needed rescue services.
- Inform each rescue service or team of the hazards they may confront when called on to perform rescue at the site.
- Provide the rescue team or service selected with access to all permit spaces from which rescue may be necessary so that the rescue service can develop appropriate rescue plans and practice operations.

An employer whose employees have been designated to provide permit space rescue and emergency services shall take the following measures: provide affected employees with the personal protective equipment (PPE) needed to conduct permit space rescues safely and train affected employees so that they are proficient in the use of PPE, at no cost to the employee. The employer must ensure that such employees successfully complete the training required to establish proficiency as an authorized entrant, as provided in the standard; train employees in basic first aid and cardiopulmonary resuscitation (CPR). The employer shall ensure that at least one member of the rescue team or service holding a current certification in first aid and CPR is available; and ensure that affected employees practice making permit space rescue every twelve months, by means of simulated rescue from the actual permit spaces or from representative permit spaces. Representative permit spaces shall, with respect to opening size, configuration, and accessibility, simulate the type of permit spaces from which rescue is to be performed.

To facilitate nonentry rescue, retrieval systems or methods shall be used whenever an authorized entrant enters a permit space, unless the equipment would add to the hazard.

Each authorized entrant shall use a chest or full body harness, with a retrieval line attached at the center of the entrant's back near shoulder level, above the entrant's head, or at another point that the employer can establish presents a profile small enough for the successful removal of the entrant. Wristlets may be used in lieu of the chest or full body harness if the employer can demonstrate that the use of a chest or full body harness is not feasible or creates a greater hazard and the use of wristlets is the safest and most effective alternative.

The other end of the retrieval line shall be attached to a mechanical device (hoist apparatus) or fixed point outside the permit space in such a manner that rescue can begin as soon as the rescuer becomes aware that rescue is necessary. A mechanical device shall be available to retrieve personnel from vertical-type permit spaces more than 5 feet deep.

If an injured entrant is exposed to a substance for which a Material Safety Data Sheet (MSDS) or other similar information is required to be kept at the worksite, the MSDS or written information shall be made available to the medical facility treating the exposed entrant.

APPENDIX

Some of the more common gases and vapors found in confined spaces include carbon monoxide, carbon dioxide, hydrogen sulfide, and methane. Other gases and vapors may be found depending upon the type of space and its location.

CHAPTER REVIEW

Multiple Choice
Select the best answer from the choices provided.

1. A hazard in a PRCS can be
   a. a hazardous atmosphere
   b. a condition that can cause engulfment
   c. a condition that can cause asphyxiation
   d. a, b, and c

2. Training of employees must be done
   a. after entry is permitted
   b. before entry is permitted
   c. during entry
   d. a, b, and c

3. A PRCS permit must include
   a. the names of all employees who work at the facility
   b. the names of only maintenance people
   c. names of employees authorized to enter the PRCS
   d. a cover to keep the permit clean

4. Members of employee rescue services must practice at least every
   a. two months
   b. six months
   c. nine months
   d. twelve months

5. The employer is responsible for training
   a. all employees in PRCS procedures
   b. only PRCS attendants
   c. all employees who enter permit required confined spaces
   d. only rescue personnel

True/False
Indicate whether the statement is true or false by circling T or F.

6. T F A vault is an example of a confined space.

7. T F A space with no hazards is an example of a permit required confined space.

8. T F If the space has only a hazardous atmosphere, only parts of the PRCS standard need be complied with.

9. T F The contractor is not responsible for the host's employees concerning permit required confined spaces.

10. T F A PRCS permit may be used indefinitely.

Matching
Match the terms in column 1 with the definitions in column 2.

Column 1
11. Permit required confined space
12. Confined space
13. Written document
14. Determines if entry is safe
15. Attendant

Column 2
a. Monitors the PRCS
b. Permit
c. Entry supervisor
d. Space with oxygen deficient atmosphere
e. Silo

Short Answer
Briefly but thoroughly answer each statement.

16. Describe the potential hazards of a confined space.

17. Describe the potential hazards of a permit required confined space.

18. List the steps required on a permit for safe entry into a PRCS.

19. List the duties of the entry supervisor.

20. Describe the duties of rescue personnel.

CHAPTER 25

Welding

After studying this chapter, you should be able to

- ➤ Describe the general requirements of the OSHA welding standard.
- ➤ List the various health hazards associated with welding operations.
- ➤ Discuss the personal protective equipment required for welding.
- ➤ Explain why welding in confined spaces must be made safe.
- ➤ State how to ensure that areas are safe for welding.

Welding is covered under the general industry standard 29 CFR 1910.252 Welding, Cutting, and Brazing and under the construction industry standards 29 CFR 1926.350-354 Gas Welding and Cutting; Arc Welding and Cutting; Fire Prevention; Ventilation and Protection in Welding, Cutting, and Heating; Welding, Cutting, and Heating in Way of Preservative Coatings.

This chapter describes the general requirements of the welding and cutting general industry standard. It does not describe the requirements for oxyacetylene or electric arc welding because the scope of this handbook is directed to allied health professionals who may supervise welders. The more detailed coverage is better left for welding manuals directed toward maintenance and custodial supervisors.

OSHA 29 CFR 1910.252 WELDING, CUTTING, AND BRAZING

Health care professionals are often responsible for various maintenance activities. An understanding of the OSHA requirements for these activities is important.

General Requirements

Welding general requirements that pertain to all welding activities are described in this section.

Fire Prevention and Protection. If the object to be welded or cut cannot be readily moved, all movable fire hazards in the vicinity shall be taken to a safe place.

If the object to be welded or cut cannot be moved and if all fire hazards cannot be moved, then guards shall be used to confine the heat, sparks, and slag, and to protect the immovable fire hazards.

Whenever there are floor openings or cracks in the flooring that cannot be closed, precautions shall be taken so that no combustible materials on the floor below will be exposed to sparks that might drop through to the floor. The same precautions shall be observed with regard to cracks or holes in walls, open doorways, and open or broken windows.

Suitable fire extinguishers shall be maintained in a state of readiness for instant use.

An employee on **fire watch** stands guard during welding operations to make sure that no materials are ignited by spark or flame. Fire watchers shall be required whenever welding or cutting is performed in locations where other than a minor fire might develop, or if any of the following conditions exists:

- Appreciable combustible material, in building construction or contents, is more than 35 feet away but is easily ignited.
- Walls or floor openings within a 35-foot radius expose combustible material in adjacent areas including concealed spaces in walls or floors.
- Combustible materials are adjacent to the opposite side of metal partitions, walls, ceilings, or

roofs and are likely to be ignited by conduction or radiation.

Fire watchers shall have extinguishing equipment readily available and be trained in its use. They shall be familiar with procedures for sounding an alarm in the event of fire. They shall watch for fires in exposed areas and try to extinguish them if it is within their capability.

A fire watch shall be maintained for at least one half hour after completion of the welding or cutting operation.

Authorization. Before welding or cutting is permitted, the area shall be inspected by the individual responsible for authorizing welding or cutting. He/she shall designate precautions to be taken in granting authorization.

Floors. Where combustible materials such as clippings, wood shavings, or textile fibers are on the floor, the floor shall be swept clean for a radius of 35 feet. Combustible floors shall be kept wet, covered with damp sand, or protected by fire resistant shields. Where floors have been wet down, personnel operating arc welding or cutting equipment shall be protected from possible shock.

Prohibited Areas. Cutting or welding shall not be permitted in the following situations:

- In areas not authorized by management
- In sprinklered buildings while such protection is impaired
- In the presence of explosive atmospheres (mixtures of flammable gases, vapors, liquids, or dusts in air), or explosive atmospheres that may develop inside uncleaned or improperly prepared tanks or equipment that have previously contained such materials, or that may develop in areas with accumulation of combustible dusts
- In areas near the storage of large quantities of exposed, readily ignitable materials such as bulk sulfur, baled paper, or cotton

Relocation of Combustibles. Where practicable, all combustibles shall be relocated at least 35 feet from the work site. Where relocation is impractica-

ble, combustibles shall be protected with flameproof covers or otherwise shielded with metal or asbestos guards or curtains.

Combustible Walls. Where cutting or welding is done near walls, partitions, ceiling, or roof of combustible construction, fire resistant shields or guards shall be provided to prevent ignition.

Noncombustible Walls. If welding is to be done on a metal wall, partition, ceiling, or roof, precautions shall be taken to prevent ignition of combustibles on the other side, due to conduction or radiation, preferably by relocating combustibles. Where combustibles are not relocated, a fire watch on the opposite side from the work shall be provided.

Combustible Cover. Welding shall not be attempted on a metal partition, wall, ceiling, or roof having a combustible covering nor on walls or partitions of combustible sandwich-type panel construction.

Pipes. Cutting or welding on pipes or other metal in contact with combustible walls, partitions, ceilings, or roofs shall not be done if the work is close enough to cause ignition by conduction.

Management. Management shall recognize its responsibility for the safe use of cutting and welding equipment and, based on fire potentials of plant facilities, establish procedures for cutting and welding in other areas; designate an individual responsible for authorizing cutting and welding operations in areas not specifically designed for such processes; and advise all contractors about flammable materials or hazardous conditions of which they may not be aware.

Supervisor. The supervisor

- Shall be responsible for the safe handling of the cutting and welding equipment and the safe use of the cutting or welding process.
- Shall determine the combustible materials and hazardous areas present or likely to be present in the work location.

- Shall protect combustibles from ignition by having the work moved to a location free from dangerous combustibles, or if the work cannot be moved, having the combustibles moved to a safe distance from the work or having the combustibles properly shielded against ignition.
- Shall see that cutting and welding are so scheduled that plant operations that might expose combustibles to ignition are not started during during cutting or welding.
- Shall secure authorization for cutting or welding operations from the designated management representative.
- Shall determine that the cutter or welder secures his approval that conditions are safe before going ahead.
- Shall determine that fire protection and extinguishing equipment are properly located at the site.

Fire Prevention Precautions. Cutting or welding shall be permitted only in areas that are or have been made fire safe. When work cannot be moved practically, the area shall be made safe by removing combustibles or protecting combustibles from ignition sources.

No welding, cutting, or other hot work shall be performed on used drums, barrels, tanks, or other containers until they have been cleaned so thoroughly as to make absolutely certain that there are no flammable materials present or any substances such as greases, tars, acids, or other materials that, when subjected to heat, might produce flammable or toxic vapors. Any pipelines or connections to the drum or vessel shall be disconnected or blanked.

All hollow spaces, cavities, or containers shall be vented to permit the escape of air or gases before preheating, cutting, or welding. Purging with an inert gas is recommended.

Confined Spaces. When arc welding is to be suspended for any substantial period of time, such as during lunch or overnight, all electrodes shall be removed from holders and the holders carefully located so that accidental contact cannot occur and the machine shall be disconnected from the power source.

In order to eliminate the possibility of gas escaping through leaks or improperly closed valves, torch valves shall be closed and the gas supply to the torch shut off at some point outside the confined space whenever the torch is not to be used for a substantial period of time, such as during lunch or overnight. Where practical, the torch and hose shall be removed from the confined space.

Protection of Personnel. A welder or helper working on platforms, scaffolds, or runways shall be protected from falling. This may be accomplished by the use of railings, lifelines, or some equally effective safeguards.

Welders shall place welding cable and other equipment so that it is clear of passageways, ladders, and stairways.

Eye Protection. Helmets or **hand shields** (shield held over the welder's face to protect the face and eyes from arcs and sparks) shall be used during all arc welding or cutting operations, excluding submerged arc welding. Helpers or attendants shall be provided with proper eye protection.

Goggles or other suitable eye protection shall be used during all gas welding or oxygen cutting operations. Spectacles without side shields, with suitable filter lenses are permitted for use during welding operations on light work, for torch brazing, or for inspection.

All operators and attendants of resistance welding equipment or resistance brazing equipment shall use transparent face shields, or goggles, depending upon the particular job, to protect their faces or eyes, as required.

Helmets and hand shields shall be made of a material that is an insulator for heat and electricity. Helmets, shields, and goggles shall not be readily flammable and shall be capable of withstanding sterilization.

Helmets and hand shields shall be arranged to protect the face, neck, and ears from direct radiant energy from the arc.

Helmets shall be provided with filter plates and cover plates that are easily removed.

Goggles shall be ventilated to prevent fogging of the lenses as much as possible.

Lenses shall bear some permanent distinctive marking by which the source and shade may be readily identified.

The OSHA Shade Number Guide in the welding standard shall be followed to determine the proper lens for the welding operation. Lens shades vary from 2 (for soldering) to 14 (gas shielded arc and carbon arc welding).

Protection from Arc Welding Rays. Where the work permits, the welder should be enclosed in an individual booth painted with a finish of low reflectivity such as zinc oxide (an important factor for absorbing ultraviolet radiations) and lamp black, or shall be enclosed with noncombustible screens similarly painted. Booths and screens shall permit circulation of air at floor level. Workers or other persons adjacent to the welding areas shall be protected from the rays by noncombustible or flameproof screens or shields or shall be required to wear appropriate goggles.

Protective Clothing. Employees exposed to hazards created by welding, cutting, or brazing operations shall be protected by personal protective equipment.

Work in Confined Spaces. A confined space is intended to mean a relatively small or restricted space such as a tank, boiler, or pressure vessel.

Ventilation is a prerequisite to work in confined spaces.

When welding or cutting is being performed in any confined spaces, the gas cylinders and welding machines shall be left on the outside. Before operations are started, heavy portable equipment mounted on wheels shall be securely blocked to prevent accidental movement.

Where a welder must enter a confined space through a manhole or other small opening, means shall be provided for quick removal in case of emergency. An attendant with a preplanned rescue procedure shall be stationed outside to observe the welder at all times and be capable of putting rescue operations into effect.

When arc welding is to be suspended for any substantial period of time, such as during lunch or overnight, all electrodes shall be removed from the holders and the holders carefully located so that accidental contact cannot occur and the machine shall be disconnected from the power source.

In order to eliminate the possibility of gas escaping through leaks of improperly closed valves, when gas welding or cutting, the torch valves shall be closed and the fuel-gas and oxygen supply to the torch positively shut off at some point outside the confined area whenever the torch is not to be used for a substantial period of time, such as during lunch or overnight. Where practical, the torch and hose shall also be removed from the confined space.

After welding operations are completed, the welder shall mark the hot metal or provide some means of warning other workers.

Health Protection and Ventilation. When welding must be performed in a space entirely screened on all sides, the screens shall be so arranged that no serious restriction of ventilation exists. It is desirable to have the screens so mounted that they are about 2 feet above the floor unless the work is performed at so low a level that the screen must be extended nearer to the floor to protect nearby workers from the glare of welding.

Local exhaust or general ventilation systems shall be provided and arranged to keep the amount of toxic fumes and gases below the permissible exposure limits (PELs).

All filler metals and fusible granular materials shall carry the following notice, as a minimum, on tags, boxes, or other containers:

CAUTION
Welding may produce fumes and gases hazardous to your health. Avoid breathing these fumes and gases. Use adequate ventilation. See ANSI Z49.1-1967 Safety in Welding and Cutting published by the American Welding Society.

Brazing (welding) filler metals containing cadmium in significant amounts shall carry the following on tags, boxes, or other containers:

WARNING
CONTAINS CADMIUM—POISONOUS
FUMES MAY BE FORMED ON HEATING
Do not breathe fumes. Use only with adequate ventilation such as fume collectors, exhaust ventilators, or air supplied respirators. See ANSI Z49.1-1967. If chest pain, cough, or fever develops after use, call a physician immediately.

Brazing and gas welding fluxes containing fluorine compounds shall have a cautionary wording to indicate that they contain fluorine compounds. The recommended wording is as follows:

CAUTION
CONTAINS FLUORIDES
This flux when heated gives off fumes that may irritate eyes, nose, and throat.

1. **Avoid fumes—use only in well-ventilated spaces.**
2. **Avoid contact of flux with eyes or skin.**
3. **Do not take internally**

Ventilation for General Welding and Cutting.

Mechanical ventilation shall be provided when welding or cutting is done on metals not covered in this section.

It must be provided as follows:

- In a space of less than 10,000 cubic feet
- In a room having a ceiling height of less than 16 feet
- In confined spaces or where the welding space contains partitions, balconies, or other structural barriers to the extent that they significantly obstruct cross ventilation

Such ventilation shall be at the minimum rate of 2,000 cubic feet per minute per welder, except where local exhaust hoods and booths are used in accordance with this section, or airline respirators approved by the Mine Safety and Health Administration (MSHA) and the National Institute for Occupational Safety and Health (NIOSH).

Mechanical and local exhaust ventilation may be by means of either of the following:

1. Freely movable hoods intended to be placed by the welder as near as practical to the work being welded and provided with a rate of airflow sufficient to maintain a velocity in the direction of the hood of 100 linear feet per minute in the zone of welding when the hood is at its most remote distance from the point of welding. The rates of ventilation required to accomplish this control velocity using a 3-inch-wide flanged suction opening are shown in the following table:

Welding zone	Minimum airflow (cfm)	Duct diameter (inches)
4–6 inches from arc or torch	150	3
6–8 inches from arc or torch	275	3½
8–10 inches from arc or torch	425	4½
10–12 inches from arc or torch	600	5½

When brazing with cadmium-bearing metals or when cutting on such materials, increased rates of ventilation may be required.

Duct diameter is to the nearest half inch based on 4,000 feet per minute velocity in pipe.

2. A fixed enclosure with a top and not less than two sides that surround the welding and cutting operations with a rate of airflow sufficient to maintain a velocity away from the welder of not less than 100 linear feet per minute.

All welding and cutting operations carried out in confined spaces shall be adequately ventilated to prevent accumulation of toxic materials or possible oxygen deficiency. All air replacing that withdrawn shall be clean and respirable.

In such circumstances where it is impossible to provide such ventilation, airline respirators or hose masks approved by MSHA and NIOSH shall be used.

In areas immediately dangerous to life and health (IDLH), self-contained breathing apparatuses (SCBAs) approved for this atmosphere by MSHA and NIOSH shall be used.

Where welding operations are carried out in confined spaces and where welders and helpers are provided with hose masks, hose masks with blowers, or self-contained breathing equipment approved by MSHA and NIOSH, a worker shall be stationed outside of such confined spaces to ensure the safety of those working therein.

Oxygen shall never be used for ventilation.

In confined spaces, welding or cutting involving fluxes, coverings, or other materials that contain fluorine compounds shall be performed in accordance with this section.

In confined spaces, welding or cutting involving zinc-bearing base or filler metals coated with zinc-bearing materials shall be performed in accordance with this section.

In confined spaces, welding involving lead-based metals shall be performed in accordance with this section. When welding involves lead-based metals indoors, it shall be performed in accordance with this section.

In confined spaces or indoors, welding or cutting involving metals containing *lead*, other than as an impurity, or involving metals coated with lead-bearing materials, including paint, shall be performed using local exhaust ventilation or airline respirators. Outdoors, such operations shall be performed using respiratory equipment approved by MSHA and NIOSH. In all cases, workers in the immediate vicinity of the cutting operation shall be protected as necessary by local exhaust ventilation or airline respirators.

Welding or cutting indoors, outdoors, or in confined spaces involving *beryllium*-containing base or filler metals shall be performed using local exhaust ventilation and airline respirators unless atmospheric tests under the most adverse conditions have established that the worker's exposure is below the OSHA permissible exposure limit (PEL). In all cases, workers in the immediate vicinity of the welding or cutting operations shall be protected as necessary by local ventilation or airline respirators.

Welding or cutting indoors or in confined spaces involving *cadmium*-bearing or cadmium-coated base metals shall be performed using local exhaust ventilation or airline respirators unless atmospheric tests under the most adverse condi-

tions have established that the worker's exposure is below OSHA PELs. Outdoors, such operations shall be performed using respiratory protective equipment such as fume respirators approved by MSHA and NIOSH.

Welding or cutting indoors or in confined spaces involving metals coated with *mercury*-bearing materials, including paint, shall be performed using local exhaust ventilation or airline respirators unless atmospheric tests under the most adverse conditions have established that the worker's exposure is below OSHA PELs. Outdoors, such operations shall be performed using respiratory protective equipment approved by MSHA and NIOSH.

In the use of *cleaning materials*, because of their possible toxicity or flammability, appropriate precautions such as manufacturer's instructions shall be followed.

Degreasing and other cleaning operations involving *chlorinated hydrocarbons* shall be so located that no vapors from these operations will reach or be drawn into the atmosphere surrounding any welding operation. In addition, *trichloroethylene* and *perchloroethylene* should be kept out of the atmospheres penetrated by the ultraviolet radiation of gas-shielded welding operations.

Oxygen cutting, using either a chemical flux or iron powder or gas-shielded arc cutting or stainless steel, shall be performed using mechanical ventilation adequate to remove fumes generated.

First aid equipment shall be available at all times. All injuries shall be reported as soon as possible for medical attention. First aid shall be rendered until medical attention can be provided.

Field Shop Operations. When arc welding is performed in wet conditions, or under conditions of high humidity, special protection against electric shock shall be supplied.

APPENDIX

This appendix describes the toxicity of some of the welding gases and fumes.

Beryllium fumes can cause berylliosis, which is granular tumors or growths on the skin or organs.

Fume exposure can also cause chest pain, breathing problems, and general weakness. It is suspected of causing cancer. The eight-hour time weighted average for beryllium is 2 micrograms per cubic meter.

Cadmium fumes affect the lungs, kidneys, and can irritate the nose and throat. Fume exposure can also cause breathing problems, chills, and diarrhea. It is suspected of causing cancer. The eight-hour time weighted average for cadmium is 0.1 milligrams per cubic meter.

Chlorinated hydrocarbons (trichloroethylene and perchloroethylene) can cause irritation to the nose and throat and organ and eye damage. They are suspected of causing cancer. The eight-hour time weighted average for trichloroethylene and for perchloroethylene is 100 parts per million.

Fluorides can cause eye irritation, breathing problems, and skin irritation. The eight-hour time weighted average for fluorides is 2.5 milligrams per cubic meter.

Lead exposure can cause pains in the abdomen, fatigue, aching in joints, and constipation. Lead accumulates in the body. The eight-hour time weighted average for lead is 50 micrograms per cubic meter.

Mercury exposure can cause chills, tremors, breathing problems. It is can also irritate the skin. The eight-hour time weighted average for mercury is 0.05 milligrams per cubic meter.

Zinc exposure can cause metal fume fever, characterized by chills and fever from inhalation of the fumes. The eight-hour time weighted average for zinc is 5 milligrams per cubic meter.

CHAPTER REVIEW

Multiple Choice

Select the best answer from the choices provided.

1. Eye shields and goggles have lens shades ranging from
   a. 1 to 10   c. 2 to 14
   b. 3 to 15   d. 2 to 12

2. When a contractor is welding on the employer's premises, who must tell the contractor where flammable materials are present?
   a. the supervisor
   b. management
   c. the employee
   d. the employee's representative

3. When arc welding in a confined space is stopped, the electrodes must be
   a. placed on a nonconducting surface
   b. placed on the floor of the space
   c. removed and holders kept away from metal surfaces
   d. hung over the welding machine

4. After welding or cutting is stopped, a fire watch must be maintained for at least
   a. thirty minutes
   b. one hour
   c. fifteen minutes
   d. forty-five minutes

5. Welding can only be performed in areas that are
   a. made of metal
   b. wetted wood
   c. fire safe
   d. uncracked surfaces

True/False

Indicate whether the statement is true or false by circling T or F.

6. T   F   Cracks and holes do not have to be covered as long as they are wetted down.

7. T   F   Combustible material on one side of a wall must be moved before welding is performed.

8. T   F   Welders can wear any lens shade to protect the eyes as long as it is polarized.

9. T   F   Ventilation is the most effective means for controlling welding fumes.

10. T   F   Objects that can be moved need not be moved as long as they are covered to prevent sparks from igniting them.

Short Answer

Briefly but thoroughly answer each statement.

11. Describe the personal protective equipment required for welding operations and the part of the body each protects.

12. List some items that cannot be welded and why.

13. Explain the requirements of managers and supervisors for protecting employees who weld.

14. Explain how you would protect a welder in a confined space.

15. Describe some of the toxic fumes you might get from welding operations.

SECTION IV

Chemical and Physical Hazards Standards and Guidelines

CHAPTER 26

Hazard Communication

After studying this chapter, you should be able to

➤ Describe the OSHA hazard communication standard.

➤ Discuss the meaning of a performance standard.

➤ List the information required on a material safety data sheet.

➤ State what is required when training employees.

➤ Describe what constitutes a hazard communication program.

OSHA 29 CFR 1910.1200 HAZARD COMMUNICATION

The OSHA Hazard Communication Standard for General Industry is 29 CFR 1910.1200. It makes it the responsibility of the employer to make sure that all employees exposed to hazardous substances are trained in the handling of these substances and that they have access to information concerning hazardous materials so that they can protect themselves.

This is a **performance standard**, which means that the employer has flexibility in the methods he/she may use to comply as long as the requirements are met.

The hazard communication standard is the standard most often cited by OSHA inspectors because of noncompliance.

Definitions

Chemical element refers to any element, chemical compound, or mixture of elements and/or compounds. Drugs that come in the form of crushed and aerosolized medications are included under the standard. Drugs and pills in solid form have no potential for exposure and are not included under the standard.

Combustible liquid is any liquid having a flash point at or above 100°F but below 200°F.

Compressed gas is a gas or mixture of gases having, in a container, an absolute pressure exceeding 40 psi at 130°F regardless of the pressure at 70°F, or a gas or mixture of gases having, in a container, an absolute pressure exceeding 104 psi at 130°F.

Explosive refers to a chemical that causes a sudden, almost instantaneous release of pressure, gas, and heat when subject to a sudden shock, pressure, or high temperature.

Flammable refers to a chemical that falls into one of the following categories:

• Aerosol—yields a flame projection exceeding 18 inches at full valve opening, or a flashback at any degree of valve opening.

• Gas—at ambient temperature and pressure forms a flammable mixture with air at a concentration of 13 percent by volume or less, at ambient temperature and pressure, forms a range of flammable mixtures with air wider than 12 percent by volume, regardless of the lower limit.

• Liquid—having a flash point below 100°F, except any mixture having components with flash points of 100° or higher, the total of which make up 99 percent or more of the total volume of the mixture.

• Solid—other than a blasting agent or explosive that is liable to cause a fire through friction, absorption of moisture, spontaneous chemical change, or retained heat from manufacturing or processing, or that can be ignited readily.

Flash point is the minimum temperature at which a liquid gives off a vapor in sufficient concentration with air to ignite a material when a source of ignition is present.

Hazardous chemical refers to any chemical that is a physical hazard or a health hazard.

Health hazard refers to a chemical that can cause acute or chronic health effects.

Immediate use means that the hazardous chemical will be under the control of and used only by the person who transfers it from a labeled container and only within the work shift in which it is transferred.

Label is any written, printed, or graphic material displayed on or affixed to containers of hazardous chemicals.

Material safety data sheets (MSDS) are written or printed material concerning a hazardous chemical and containing essential information about the chemical.

Physical hazard refers to a chemical that is a combustible liquid, compressed gas, explosive, flammable, an organic peroxide, an oxidizer, pyrophoric (will ignite spontaneously in air at a temperature of 130°F or below), unstable, or water-reactive.

Unstable refers to a chemical in the pure state that will vigorously polymorize, condense, decompose, or will become self-reactive under conditions of shocks, pressure, or temperature.

Written Hazard Communication Program

The employer shall develop, implement, and maintain at each workplace a written hazard communication program for labels and other forms of warning, material safety data sheets, and employee information and training. The program must also include:

- A list of hazardous materials known to be present. This can be done for the workplace as a whole or for individual work areas.
- The methods the employer will use to inform employees of hazards of nonroutine tasks such

as the hazards associated with chemicals contained in unlabeled pipes.

Employers who use or store hazardous chemicals at a workplace in such a way that other employer(s) of employees may be exposed shall additionally ensure that the hazard communication program will include the following:

- The methods the employer will use to provide these employees access to material safety data sheets for each hazardous chemical to which they may be exposed.
- The methods the employer will use to provide the other employer(s) of employees on-site access to material safety data sheets for each hazardous chemical to which they are exposed.
- The methods the employer will use to inform other employer(s) of any precautionary measures that need to be taken to protect the other employer(s)' employees.
- The methods the employer will use to inform the other employer(s) of the labeling system used in the workplace.

The employer shall make the hazard communication program available, upon request, to employees, their designated representatives, and OSHA.

Where employees must travel between workplaces, the written hazard communication program may be kept at the primary work facility.

Labels and Other Forms of Warning

The chemical manufacturer, importer, or distributor shall ensure that each container of hazardous chemicals leaving the workplace is labeled, tagged, or marked with the following information:

- Identity of the hazardous chemical
- Appropriate hazard warnings
- Name and address of the chemical manufacturer, importer, or other responsible party

If the hazardous chemical is regulated by OSHA in a substance-specific health standard, the chemical manufacturer, importer, distributor, or employer shall ensure that the labels or other forms of warning used are in accordance with that standard.

The employer shall ensure that each container of hazardous chemicals in the workplace is labeled, tagged, or marked with the following identification:

- Identity of the hazardous substance
- Appropriate hazard warnings, or words, pictures, symbols, or combination that provide general information regarding the hazards of the chemicals, and that, in conjunction with other information, will provide specific information regarding physical and health hazards of the hazardous chemical.

The employer is not required to label portable containers into which hazardous chemicals are transferred from labeled containers, and that are intended only for the immediate use of the employee who performs the transfer. Drugs that are dispensed by a pharmacy to a health care provider for direct administration are exempt from labeling.

The employer shall not remove or deface existing labels on incoming containers.

The employer shall ensure that labels or other forms of warning are legible, in English, and prominently displayed on the container. Employers having employees who speak other languages may add the information in that language as long as the information presented is in English as well.

Employers who become aware of any significant information regarding the hazards of a chemical shall revise the label within three months of becoming aware of the new information.

Material Safety Data Sheets (MSDS)

Employers shall have material safety data sheets for each hazardous chemical in the workplace.

Each material safety data sheet shall be in English (the employer may maintain copies in other languages as well) and shall contain at least the following information:

- The identity used on the label.
- If the hazardous chemical is a single substance, its chemical common name.
- If the hazardous chemical is a mixture, the chemical and common name(s) of the ingredients.

- Physical and chemical characteristics of the hazardous chemical (such as vapor pressure and flash point).
- The physical hazards such as potential for fire or explosion, and reactivity.
- The health hazards, including signs and symptoms of exposure, and any medical conditions that are recognized as aggravated by exposure.
- The primary routes of entry.
- The OSHA permissible exposure limit or ACGIH threshold limit value, or any recommended exposure limit.
- Whether the chemical is listed in the National Toxicology Program (NTP) or has been found to be a potential carcinogen.
- Any generally acceptable precautions for safe handling and use.
- Any generally applicable control measures such as appropriate engineering controls, work practices, or personal protective equipment.
- Emergency and first aid procedures.
- The name, address, and telephone number of the chemical manufacturer, importer, employer, or other responsible party preparing or distributing the material safety data sheet.
- If no relevant information is found for any given category, the preparer shall indicate by marking that section to indicate no applicable information available or n/a.

Manufacturers or importers shall ensure that a material safety data sheet accompanies all shipments of hazardous chemicals. If the material safety data sheet is not provided, the employer must obtain one as soon as possible. Manufacturers and importers must also provide material safety data sheets upon request.

When a hazardous chemical has new information, the distributor will provide the updated information on the material safety data sheet with the next shipment to the employer.

Where employees must travel between workplaces, the material safety data sheets may be kept at the primary work location. In this situation, the employer shall ensure that employees can immediately obtain the required information in an emergency.

Material safety data sheets may be kept in any form, but in all cases the employer shall ensure that the required information is provided and readily accessible during each work shift.

Employee Information and Training

Employers shall provide effective information and training on hazardous chemicals in their work areas at the time of initial assignment and whenever a new physical or health hazard is introduced into the workplace. Information and training may be designed to cover categories of hazards (such as flammability, carcinogenicity, or specific chemicals. Chemical specific information shall always be available through labels and material safety data sheets.

Information. Employees shall be informed of

- The requirements of the hazard communication standard.
- The location and availability of the written hazard communication program, including

the list of hazardous chemicals and material safety data sheets.

Training. Employee training shall include

- Methods and observations that may be used to detect the presence or release of hazardous chemicals. This includes monitoring, continuous monitoring devices, visual appearance, odor when released, and so forth.
- The physical and health hazards of the chemicals in the work area.
- The measures the employees can take to protect themselves from these hazards, including specific procedures the employer has implemented to protect employees from exposure such as work practices, emergency procedures, and personal protective equipment to be used.
- The details of the hazard communication program developed by the employer, including explanation of the labeling system and the material safety data sheets and how employees can obtain and use the appropriate information.

CHAPTER REVIEW

True/False

Indicate whether the statement is true or false by circling T or F.

1. T F All employees must be trained in hazard communication.

2. T F Labels are not required on in-house containers.

3. T F A performance standard means that the employer has flexibility in complying with the standard as long as requirements are met.

4. T F The hazard communication program does not have to be written.

5. T F Drugs that are crushed and aerosolized medications are included under the standard.

Matching

Match the terms in column 1 with the definitions in column 2.

Column 1

6. Routes of entry into the body
7. Overexposure prevention
8. Most cited standard by OSHA
9. Description of the training program
10. Identity cross-referenced to the MSDS

Column 2

a. Part of the written hazard communication program
b. Information on container label
c. Part of the training program
d. Part of the MSDS
e. Hazard communication

CHAPTER 27

Hazardous Waste and Regulated Medical Waste

After studying this chapter, you should be able to

➤ Describe the requirements under the OSHA hazardous waste and emergency response standard.

➤ List the requirements for generators and transporters of hazardous waste under the RCRA law.

➤ Describe the requirements for regulated medical waste.

➤ State the associated standards that apply to hazardous waste operations.

➤ List the categories of hazardous waste.

Hazardous waste has become an ever-increasing problem for business and industry, as well as for the health care industry. Every year, more and more of this type of waste has to be disposed of. Fines and criminal penalties from both OSHA and the Environmental Protection Agency (EPA) can be assessed if proper procedures are not used in the disposal process.

Additional federal standards, besides the Hazardous Waste and Emergency Response Standard (HAZWOPER), include the Resource Conservation and Recovery Act (RCRA), which regulates the generation, transportation, treatment, storage, and disposal of hazardous waste incorporated in 40 CFR 262-265 and the requirements for disposal of regulated medical waste (RMW) incorporated in 40 CFR 22 and 259.

OSHA 29 CFR 1910.120 HAZARDOUS WASTE OPERATIONS AND EMERGENCY RESPONSE (HAZWOPER)

This section covers the following cleanup operations:

- Operations required by a governmental body, whether state, federal, local, or other involving hazardous substances that are conducted at uncontrolled hazardous waste sites

- Corrective actions involving cleanup operations covered by the Resource Conservation and Recovery Act (RCRA)

- Voluntary cleanup operations at sites recognized by federal, state, local, or other governmental bodies as uncontrolled hazardous waste sites

- Operations involving hazardous waste that are conducted at treatment, storage, and disposal (TSD) facilities

- Emergency response operations for releases of, or substantial threats of releases of, hazardous substances without regard to the location of the hazard

Definitions

Cleanup operation is an operation by which hazardous substances are removed, contained, incinerated, neutralized, stabilized, cleared-up, or in any manner processed or handled with the ultimate goal of making the site safer for people or the environment.

Decontamination is the removal of hazardous substances from employees and their equipment to the extent necessary to preclude the occurrence of foreseeable adverse health affects.

Emergency response is a response effort by employees from outside the immediate release area or by other designated responders.

Hazardous materials response team (HAZMAT) is an organized group of employees, designated by the employer, who are expected to perform work to handle and control actual or potential leaks or spills of hazardous substances requiring close approach to the substance.

Hazardous substance refers to any substance exposure that results or may result in adverse effects on the health and safety of employees.

Hazardous waste refers to a waste or combination of wastes defined in 49 CFR 171.8 (see the section in this chapter on RCRA).

Hazardous waste operation refers to any operation conducted within the scope of this standard.

Hazardous waste site refers to any facility or location within the scope of this standard at which hazardous waste operations take place.

Health hazard refers to a chemical, mixture of chemicals, or a pathogen for which there is statistical significant evidence that acute or chronic health affects may occur in exposed employees. The term includes carcinogens, toxic or highly toxic agents, reproductive toxins, irritants, corrosives, sensitizers, hepatoxins, nephrotoxins, neurotoxins, agents that act on the hematopoietic system, and agents that damage the lungs, skin, eyes, or mucous membranes.

Immediately dangerous to life or health (IDLH) refers to an atmospheric concentration of any toxic, corrosive, or asphyxiant substance that poses an immediate threat to life or would cause irreversible or delayed adverse health effects or would interfere with an individual's ability to escape from a dangerous atmosphere.

Oxygen deficiency is that concentration of oxygen by volume below which atmosphere supplying respiratory protection must be provided. It exists in atmospheres where the percentage of oxygen by volume is less than 19.5 percent.

Post-emergency response refers to that portion of an emergency response performed after the immediate threat of a release has been stabilized or eliminated and the cleanup of the site has begun.

Site safety and health supervisor is the person located at the hazardous waste site who is responsible to the employer and has the authority and knowledge necessary to implement the site safety and health plan and verify compliance with applicable safety and health requirements.

Uncontrolled hazardous waste sites refers to an area identified as an uncontrolled hazardous waste site by a governmental body—whether federal, state, local, or other—where an accumulation of hazardous substances creates a threat to the safety and health of individuals or the environment. Some sites are found on public lands and private property.

Safety and Health Program

A safety and health plan must be developed by the employer.

General. Employers shall develop a site safety and health plan for their employees involved in hazardous waste operations. The program shall identify, evaluate, and control safety and health hazards, and provide for emergency response. The safety and health plan shall incorporate the following:

- An organizational structure
- A comprehensive work plan
- A site-specific safety and health plan
- The safety and health training program
- The medical surveillance program
- The employer's standard operating procedures for safety and health
- Any necessary interface between general program and site-specific activities.

Employer's contractors and subcontractors who are retained for services for work in hazardous waste operations shall be informed of site emergency response procedures and of any potential fire, explosion, health, safety, or other hazards.

The written safety and health plan must be made available to contractors and subcontractors.

Organizational Structure Part of the Site Program. The organizational structure shall establish the specific chain of command and specify overall responsibilities. It must include the following elements:

- A general supervisor who has the responsibility and authority to direct all hazardous waste operations
- A site safety and health supervisor who has responsibility for the site safety and health plan
- All other personnel needed for hazardous waste site operations and emergency response and their general function and responsibilities
- The lines of authority, responsibility, and communication

The organizational structure shall be reviewed and updated as necessary to reflect the current status of waste site operations.

Comprehensive Workplan Part of the Site Program. This program shall address the tasks and objectives of the site operations and the logistics and resources necessary to reach those tasks and objectives.

It shall:

- Address anticipated cleanup activities as well as normal procedures
- Define work tasks and objectives and identify the methods for accomplishing those tasks and objectives
- Provide for training
- Provide for additional programs
- Provide for medical surveillance.

Site-Specific Safety and Health Plan Part of the Program. This plan must be kept on site, address safety and health hazards, and include requirements for employee protection. The site safety and health plan must address the following:

- A safety or risk hazard analysis
- Employee training assignments
- Personal protective equipment to be used
- Medical surveillance requirements
- Frequency and types of monitoring
- Site control measures
- Decontamination procedures
- An emergency response plan
- Confined space entry procedures
- A spill containment program

Inspections shall be conducted by the site safety supervisor, or other qualified person, to determine the effectiveness of the plan. The site will be evaluated to determine the appropriate safety and health procedures needed to protect employees from hazards.

Preliminary Evaluation. A preliminary evaluation of the site's characteristics must be performed by a qualified person in order to aid in the selection of appropriate protective methods prior to entry.

Hazard Identification. All suspected conditions that may pose an immediately dangerous to life or health (IDLH) hazard shall be identified and evaluated.

Required Information. The following information shall be obtained by the employer prior to allowing employees to enter the site:

- Location and approximate size of the site
- Description of the task to be performed
- Duration of the task
- Site topography and accessibility
- Safety and health hazards
- Pathways for hazardous substance dispersion
- Present status and capabilities of emergency response teams
- Hazardous substances and health hazards involved or expected at the site and their chemical and physical properties

Personal Protective Equipment (PPE). Personal protective equipment shall be provided and used during initial entry in accordance with the following:

- Based upon the results of the preliminary site evaluation, PPE shall be selected and used during initial entry that will adequately protect.
- If positive pressure self-contained breathing apparatus is used, there must be a self-contained breathing apparatus with at least five minutes duration carried by employees during initial entry.

PPE to be selected must be at least from level B PPE if the preliminary site evaluation does not identify the site hazards because of insufficient information.

Level A clothing is to be selected when the greatest level of skin, respiratory, and eye protection is required. This could include National Institute for Occupational Safety and Health (NIOSH) approved self-contained breathing apparatus (SCBA), totally enclosing chemical protective suit, coveralls, long underwear, inner and outer chemical resistant gloves, steel toe boots that are chemical resistant, hard hat, or disposable protective suit, and gloves and boots worn over the totally encapsulating suit.

Level B is the highest level of respiratory protection, but a lesser level of skin protection. This could include SCBA, hooded chemical resistant clothing, coveralls, inner and outer chemical resistant gloves, steel toe boots that are chemical resistant, boot covers, hard hat, and face shield.

Level C is worn when concentrations of hazardous substances are known and the criteria for wearing air purifying respirators are met. This could include full-face or half-mask air purifying respirator, hooded chemical resistant clothing, coveralls, inner and outer chemical resistant gloves, steel toe boots that are chemical resistant, boot covers, hard hat, escape mask, and face shield.

Level D is a work uniform worn when minimal protection is needed, as against nuisance contamination. This could include coveralls, gloves, steel toe boots that are chemical resistant, disposable outer chemical resistant boots, safety or chemical splash goggles, hard hat, escape mask, and face shield.

Monitoring. Monitoring must be conducted during initial entry when site evaluation shows the potential for ionizing radiation or IDLH conditions. Monitoring must be done as follows:

- Use of direct reading instruments
- Visual observation of dangerous conditions
- Implementation of an ongoing air-monitoring program

Risk Identification. Once the presence and concentration of specific hazardous substances has been established, the risks shall be identified.

Employee Notification. Information concerning the chemical, physical, or toxicologic properties of substances known or expected to be present on-site must be conveyed to the employees.

Site Control. Site control procedures, which are part of the employer's site safety and health program, shall be developed during the planning stages of the cleanup. The program must contain a site map, site work zones, the use of a "buddy system," site communications, standard operating procedures, and identification of the nearest medical assistance.

Training. All employees working on-site exposed to hazardous substances, health hazards, or safety hazards, and their supervisors and management responsible for the site must receive training before they engage in hazardous waste operations. Training must include the names of personnel and alternates responsible for safety and health, hazards present at the site, use of PPE, work practices that minimize risks, use of engineering controls and equipment, medical surveillance requirements, and contents of the site safety and health plan.

General site workers (such as equipment operators, general laborers, and supervisory personnel) shall receive a minimum of forty hours of instruction and a minimum of three days of field experience under the supervision of a trained supervisor.

Workers on-site only occasionally for a specific limited task (such as groundwater monitoring, land surveying, or geophysical surveying) and who are unlikely to be exposed over permissible exposure limits must receive a minimum of twenty-four hours of instruction and a minimum of one day field experience under the supervision of a trained supervisor.

Workers regularly on-site who work in areas that have been monitored that show exposures under permissible exposure limits where respirators are not necessary, and there are no other health hazards, shall receive a minimum of twenty-four hours of instruction and a minimum of one day field experience under the supervision of a trained supervisor.

On-site management and supervisors shall receive forty hours initial training and three days of field experience and at least eight additional hours of specialized training to include the employer's safety and health program, employee training program, PPE program, spill containment program, and health hazard monitoring techniques.

Trainers must be qualified.

Employees who respond to hazardous emergency situations must be trained in how to respond to such emergencies.

Employees who are trained must receive refresher training annually.

Medical Surveillance. Medical surveillance must be instituted for the following employees:

- All employees who are or may be exposed above permissible exposure limits for thirty days or more a year
- All employees who wear a respirator for thirty days or more a year
- All employees who are injured or become ill due to overexposure
- Members of HAZMAT teams

    Medical examinations must be given as follows:

- Prior to assignment
- At least every twelve months for each covered employee
- At termination of employment or reassignment where the employee would not be covered if the employee has not had an examination within the last six months
- As soon as possible after the employee has developed signs and symptoms of possible overexposure or that the employee was injured
- At more frequent times if determined by the examining physician

Examinations shall be performed without cost to the employee and at a convenient time and place.

The employer must give the physician a copy of this standard and its appendices, plus the following:

- A description of the employee's duties
- Exposure levels and anticipated levels
- PPE used
- Information from previous examinations
- Information required by the respirator standard 29 CFR 1910.134

The employer shall obtain from the physician and furnish a copy to the employee of the attending physician's opinion. The opinion must contain the physician's recommended limitations on the employee, results of the examination and tests, and a statement that the employee has been informed by the physician of the results.

Records of medical surveillance must be kept by the employer. The record must include the following information:

- The name and social security number of the employee
- Physician's written opinions, limitations, and results of examinations and tests
- Any employee medical complaints related to exposure
- A copy of the information provided to the examining physician by the employer with the exception of the standard and its appendices

Engineering Controls, Work Practices, and Personal Protective Equipment for Employee Protection. Engineering controls, work practices, PPE, or a combination of these shall be used to protect employees.

Engineering controls and work practices shall be used to reduce employee exposure to or below the permissible exposure limits.

When engineering controls and work practices are not feasible or not required, any reasonable combination of engineering controls, work practices, and PPE shall be used. Employee rotation is not permitted to reduce exposure to below permissible exposure limits except when there is no other feasible way of complying with the airborne or dermal dose limits for ionizing radiation.

Published literature and material safety data sheets may be used to determine safe limits of substances.

PPE must be selected based on an evaluation of the performance characteristics of the PPE.

Positive pressure self-contained breathing apparatus, or positive pressure air-line respirators equipped with an escape air supply, shall be used when exposure levels present the possibility of immediate death, serious illness or injury, or impair the ability to escape.

Chemical suits equivalent to level B must be used when skin absorption may result in immediate death, serious illness or injury, or may impair escape.

Monitoring. Monitoring shall be performed when there is a question of employee exposure to hazardous concentrations of substances.

Air monitoring shall be done upon initial entry. Periodic monitoring shall be done when the possibility of an IDLH condition or flammable atmosphere has developed or when it is suspected that exposures have risen over permissible exposure limits.

Information Programs. Employers shall develop a program that is part of the safety and health program to inform employees, contractors, and subcontractors of the level and degree of exposure likely to result from their work.

Handling Drums and Containers. Drums and containers must meet appropriate DOT, OSHA, and EPA regulations.

Drums and containers must be inspected and their integrity assured.

Unlabeled drums shall be assumed to contain hazardous substances until the contents are identified.

Where major spills may occur, a spill containment program, which is part of the safety and health program, must be implemented to control the spill.

Fire extinguishing equipment must be kept on hand in drum areas.

Employees not involved in opening drums must be kept a safe distance away.

If employees must work adjacent to drums, a shield must be erected between the employees and the drums to protect against fire or explosion.

When the possibility of flammable materials could be present, equipment and tools must be of the type that prevents ignition.

Employees cannot stand on drums or work from them.

Material-Handling Equipment. Material-handling equipment used to transfer drums and containers must be selected, positioned, and operated to minimize sources of ignition related to the equipment from igniting vapors released from ruptured drums or containers.

Drums and containers containing radioactive wastes must not be handled until the hazard is assessed.

All nonessential employees must be removed from areas when shock-sensitive waste is handled.

Material-handling equipment must be provided with explosion proof controls or protective shields to protect equipment operators who handle shock-sensitive wastes. An alarm system must be in use when handling shock-sensitive wastes that indicate the beginning and end of handling of this waste.

Continuous communications must be maintained between the employee in charge and both the site safety supervisor and command post until the handling of shock-sensitive waste is completed. The communications equipment must be explosion proof.

Drums and containers containing packaged laboratory wastes must be considered to contain shock-sensitive materials until they have been identified.

Laboratory Waste Packs. Lab packs shall be opened only when necessary.

Crystalline material noted on any container shall be handled as shock-sensitive waste until identified.

Sampling of Drum and Container Contents. Sampling of containers and drums shall be done in accordance with a sampling procedure, which is part of the site safety and health plan.

Shipping and Transport. Drums and containers must be identified before they are packaged for shipment.

Drum staging areas shall be provided with adequate access and egress routes.

Decontamination Procedures. A decontamination procedure shall be developed, communicated to employees, and implemented before any employees or equipment enter the site.

Standard operating procedures shall be developed to minimize employee contact with equipment that has contacted hazardous substances.

All employees leaving a contaminated area shall be appropriately decontaminated.

Decontamination procedures shall be monitored by the site safety and health supervisor.

Decontamination procedures shall minimize exposure of uncontaminated employees.

Personal protective clothing and equipment shall be decontaminated, cleaned, and laundered to maintain its effectiveness.

Employees whose nonimpermeable clothing becomes wetted with hazardous substances must immediately remove the clothing and shower. The clothing must be disposed of or decontaminated.

Unauthorized employees shall not remove protective clothing or equipment from change rooms.

Where the decontamination procedure indicates a need for regular showers and change rooms outside of a contaminated area, they shall be provided in accordance with 29 CFR 1910.141.

Emergency Response by Employees at Uncontrolled Hazardous Waste Sites. An emergency response plan shall be developed and implemented by all employers to handle emergencies prior to the start of hazardous waste operations.

Employers who will evacuate their employees from the danger area when an emergency occurs and who do not permit any of their employees to assist in handling the emergency are exempt from this paragraph if they provide an emergency action plan in complying with 29 CFR 1910.38 (a). This is described in Chapter 6.

The emergency response plan must contain the following:

- Pre-emergency planning
- Personnel roles, lines of authority and communication
- Emergency recognition and prevention
- Safe distances and places of refuge
- Site security and control
- Evacuation routes and procedures
- Decontamination procedures that are not covered by the site safety and health plan
- Emergency medical treatment and first aid
- Emergency alerting and response procedures
- Critique of response and follow-up
- PPE and emergency equipment

The following elements shall also be included in emergency response plans: site topography, layout, and weather conditions; and procedures for reporting incidents to local, state, and federal agencies.

The emergency response plan must be a separate section of the site safety and health plan.

The emergency response plan must be coordinated with the disaster, fire, and/or emergency plans of local, state, and federal agencies.

The plan must be rehearsed regularly and reviewed periodically.

An alarm system must be installed to alert employees of emergency situations.

Sanitation at Temporary Workplaces. Adequate potable water shall be provided at the site.

Portable containers must be tightly closed and equipped with a tap. Water shall not be dipped from containers.

Containers used to distribute water must be clearly marked and not used for any other purpose.

Where single service cups are used, a container must be supplied for their disposal.

Outlets for nonpotable water must be identified.

There cannot be any cross connection between potable and nonpotable water.

At least one toilet facility must be made available.

Hazardous waste sites not provided with a sanitary sewer must be provided with chemical toilets, recirculating toilets, combustion toilets, or flush toilets.

Temporary Sleeping Quarters. When temporary sleeping quarters are provided, they must be heated, lighted, and ventilated.

Washing Facilities. The employer must provide adequate washing facilities. They must be near the worksite and in areas where exposure is below permissible exposure limits.

Showers and Change Rooms. When hazardous waste cleanup commences on-site and the duration of the work will require six months or more to complete, the employer must provide showers and change rooms. The showers and change rooms must be located where exposure is below permissible exposure limits. If this cannot be accomplished, then ventilation must be supplied that will take exposure to below the PELs.

Employers must make sure that employees shower at the end of the work shift and when leaving the hazardous waste site.

Certain Operations Conducted under the Resource Conservation and Recovery Act (RCRA)

Employers conducting operations at treatment, storage, and disposal (TSD) facilities must provide and implement programs for employees working at these facilities who are exposed to hazardous waste.

Safety and Health Plan. The employer shall develop and implement a written safety and health program for employees involved in hazardous waste operations that shall be available for inspection by employees, their representatives, and OSHA. The program shall be designed to identify, evaluate, and control safety and health hazards in their facilities; provide for emergency response; and address site analysis, engineering controls, maximum exposure limits, hazardous waste handling procedures and uses of new technologies.

Hazard Communication Plan. The employer shall implement a hazard communication program meeting the requirements of 29 CFR 1910.1200 (see Chapter 26), a medical surveillance program, decontamination program, a program to introduce new technologies, and a material-handling program.

Training Program. Employees exposed to health hazards at TSD facilities require initial training of twenty-four hours and refresher training for eight hours annually.

Trainers must be qualified.

Emergency Response Program. An emergency response program must be developed and implemented by all employers. The emergency response plan must be a written portion of the safety and health program. Employers who will evacuate their employees from the worksite when an emergency occurs and who do not permit any of their employ-

ees to assist in handling the emergency are exempt if they provide an emergency action plan complying with 29 CFR 1910.38(a). (See Chapter 6.)

The elements of the emergency response plan are as follows:

- Emergency recognition and prevention
- Personnel roles, lines of authority and communication
- Safe distances and places of refuge
- Site security and control
- Evacuation routes and procedures
- Emergency medical treatment and first aid
- Emergency alerting and response procedures
- Critique of response and follow-up
- PPE and emergency equipment

Training. Training for emergency employees must be completed before they are called upon to perform in real emergencies. The training must include the elements of the emergency response plan, standard operating procedures, the PPE to be worn, and procedures for handling emergency incidents.

Procedures for Handling Emergency Incidents. The following must be included in emergency plans:

- Site topography, layout, and prevailing weather conditions
- Procedures for reporting incidents to local, state, and federal agencies
- Coordination of the plan with disaster, fire, and/or emergency response plans of local, state, and federal agencies
- A periodic review of the plan
- Installation of an alarm system
- Evaluation of the incident

Emergency Response to Hazardous Substance Releases. This section covers employees engaged in emergency response no matter where it occurs. It does not cover employees engaged in operations as described in the previous section under emergency response.

An emergency response plan must be developed that includes the following:

- Pre-emergency planning and coordination with outside parties
- Personal roles, lines of authority, training, and communication
- Emergency recognition and prevention
- Safe distances and places of refuge
- Site security and control
- Evacuation routes and procedures
- Decontamination
- Emergency medical treatment and first aid
- Emergency alerting and response procedures
- Critique of response and follow-up procedures
- PPE and emergency equipment

Procedures for Handling Emergency Response. The senior emergency response official responding to an emergency shall become the individual in charge of a site-specific incident command system (ICS).

Skilled Support Personnel. Skilled support is personnel, not necessarily the employer's own employees, are skilled in the operation of certain equipment.

Specialist Employees. Specialist employees are trained in the hazards of specific substances and will be called upon to provide technical assistance.

Training of Responders. Training shall be based on the duties and function of each responder.

First responder awareness-level individuals are people who are likely to witness or discover a hazardous substance release. They notify the proper authorities. They take no further action.

First responder operations-level individuals are people who respond to releases or potential releases of hazard substances. They take defensive action to prevent the release from contaminating the environment. They must receive at least eight hours of training.

Hazardous material technicians respond to releases or potential releases for the purpose of stopping the release. They assume a more aggressive role than the first responder. They must receive at least twenty-four hours of training.

Hazardous material specialists respond with and provide support to hazardous material technicians. Their duties are similar to those of hazardous material technicians. They must have a more specific knowledge of the hazardous substances.

The on-scene incident commander assumes control of the incident beyond the first responder awareness level. These commanders must receive at least twenty-four hours of training.

Trainers who teach all these personnel must have completed an approved training course.

All responder employees must take refresher training annually.

Medical Surveillance and Consultation. Members of HAZMAT teams and hazardous material specialists must have baseline physical examinations.

Any emergency response employees who show signs or symptoms as a result of exposure must be provided with medical consultation.

RESOURCE CONSERVATION AND RECOVERY ACT (RCRA)

RCRA is enforced by the Environmental Protection Agency (EPA) and encompasses the protection of the environment. This legislation was passed in 1976 by the U.S. Government to protect the environment from hazardous waste. It describes a "cradle to grave" accountability for the disposal of this waste. The law also provides for fines and criminal penalties for noncompliance. The sections that allied health will be concerned with are 40 CFR 261, 262, and 263.

EPA 40 CFR 261 Categories of Hazardous Waste

The categories of hazardous waste are as follows (the letters in parentheses following the waste category are hazardous codes assigned by the EPA to the waste):

1. *Ignitable (I)*
   - It is ignitable if it is a liquid (not an aqueous solution) containing less than 24% alcohol by volume and has a flash point less than 60°C (140°F).

- It is not a liquid and is capable under standard temperature and pressure of causing a fire.
- It is an ignitable compressed gas.
- It is an oxidizer.
- It is a solid waste that is ignitable.

2. *Corrosive (C)*
   - It is an aqueous solution with a pH less than or equal to 2 or greater than 12.5.
   - It is a liquid that corrodes steel at a rate greater than 6.35 mm (0.25 in.) per year at a temperature of 55°C (130°F).

3. *Reactive (R)*
   - It is normally unstable and undergoes violent change without being detonated.
   - It reacts violently with water.
   - It forms a potentially explosive mixture with water.
   - When mixed with water, it generates toxic gases, vapors, or fumes in quantities that cause a danger to health or the environment.
   - It is a cyanide- or sulfide-bearing waste when exposed to pH conditions between 2 and 12.5, and it can generate toxic gases, vapors, or fumes in quantities that cause a danger to health or the environment.
   - It can cause detonation or explosive decomposition if subjected to a strong initiating source or if heated under confinement.
   - It is capable of detonation or explosive decomposition or reaction at standard temperature and pressure (STP).
   - It is a forbidden explosive determined by 49 CFR 173.51, 53, or 88.

4. *Toxic Characteristic (E)*
   - This is the list of wastes described in Table I of 40 CFR 261.24. The table describes the toxic substance causing the waste to be hazardous.

5. *Acute Toxic Waste (H)*
   - This is the list of wastes described in Subpart D 40 CFR 261.33 that are assigned "P" numbers. These wastes are very toxic to health and the environment.

6. *Toxic Waste (T)*
   - This is the list of wastes described in Subpart D 40 CFR 261.31 (waste from nonspecific sources) that are assigned "F" numbers
   - The list of wastes described in 261.32 (waste from specific sources) that are assigned "K" numbers
   - The list of wastes described in 261.33 that are assigned "U" numbers

EPA 40 CFR 262 Standards Applicable to Generators of Hazardous Waste

A generator who generates less than 100 kilograms (220 pounds) of hazardous waste or less than one kilogram (2.2 pounds) of an acute hazardous waste in a calendar month is a *conditionally exempt small quantity generator*. They do not have to comply with certain parts of the RCRA law providing that they identify their waste, don't accumulate more than 1,000 kilograms (2,200 pounds) on-site, and transport the waste to an approved disposal facility.

A generator who generates greater than 100 kilograms (220 pounds) but less than 1,000 kilograms (2,200 pounds) of hazardous waste or no more than one kilogram (2.2 pounds) of acute hazardous waste in a calendar month is a *small quantity generator*. They may accumulate hazardous waste on-site for 180 days or less without a permit or without having interim status provided that they comply with the following:

- The quantity of waste accumulated on-site never exceeds 6,000 kilograms (13,200 pounds)
- At all times there is at least one employee either on the premises or on call with the responsibility for coordinating all emergency response measures.
- Information is posted next to the telephone that includes the name and telephone number of the emergency coordinator, location of fire extinguishers, spill control material, and fire alarm if installed.
- Have the telephone number of the fire department posted.
- Ensure that all employees are familiar with proper waste-handling procedures during normal operations and emergencies.

- In the event of a fire, call the fire department or attempt to extinguish it using a fire extinguisher.
- In the event of a spill, contain the flow of hazardous waste to the extent possible, and as soon as practicable clean up the waste and any contaminated materials or soil.
- In the event of a fire or explosion, or other release that could threaten human health outside the facility, or when the generator has knowledge that a spill has reached surface water, the generator immediately notifies the National Response Center.

A generator who generates greater than 1,000 kilograms of hazardous waste or more than one kilogram (2.2 pounds) of acute hazardous waste in any one calendar month is a *large quantity generator*. They have the same requirements as a small quantity generator, except they cannot accumulate more than 1,000 kilograms (2,200 pounds) on-site for more than ninety days without getting a permit.

General Requirements for All Generators.
Generators must comply with the following:

- Mark all containers as hazardous waste and affix the EPA required label that prohibits improper disposal.
- Identify all hazardous waste.
- Obtain an identification number from the EPA
- Inspect containers every week and put leaking containers in salvage drums in accordance with 49 CFR 173.3 (c) and 173.28.
- Ensure that storage is in a secure area.
- Make every effort to reduce the volume and toxicity of hazardous waste generated (this can be done through thermal, chemical, or physical means).

EPA 40 CFR 263 Standards Applicable to Transporters of Hazardous Waste

These standards apply to persons transporting hazardous waste within the United States if the transportation requires a manifest. These requirements must be met whether the generator transports his/her own waste or uses an outside transporter.

Transporters cannot accept hazardous waste from a generator unless it is accompanied by a manifest signed by the generator.

Before transporting the hazardous waste, the transporter must sign and date the manifest acknowledging acceptance of the hazardous waste from the generator. The transporter must return a signed copy to the generator before leaving the generator's property.

The transporter must ensure that the manifest accompanies the hazardous waste.

If a transporter delivers hazardous waste to another transporter or to the designated facility on the manifest, he/she must retain one copy of the manifest and give the remaining copies to the accepting transporter or designated facility.

General Requirements for All Transporters.
Transporters must have sufficient liability insurance in case of spills on public roads (the generator is held equally liable with the transporter if an accident should occur); must have transporters trained in emergency procedures when a spill or accident occurs. This would involve contacting the appropriate agencies to control the incident; and trucks must have the proper placards bearing the UN (United Nations) or NA (North American) number for the waste in accordance with Department of Transportation (DOT) requirements.

EPA Forms 8700-22 and 8700-22A Uniform Hazardous Waste Manifest

The manifest must be completed and must accompany the waste during transport. Before the carrier leaves the premises, the manifest must be signed by both the generator and the transporter. The transporter must have a USEPA identification number.

The generator must receive a signed copy of the manifest from the treatment, storage, or disposal facility (TSD) within fifteen days of shipment. If it is not received within that interval, the generator must notify the TSD and find out why it has not been received. If it goes to twenty days, then the generator must notify the EPA and the state environmental agency.

EPA 40 CFR 22 AND 259 STANDARDS FOR THE TRACKING AND MANAGEMENT OF MEDICAL WASTE (RMW)

Medical waste is any solid waste that is generated in the diagnosis, treatment, or immunization of human beings or animals, in research pertaining thereto, or in the production or testing of biologicals. The term does not include any hazardous waste identified or listed under RCRA, or any household waste. RMW includes culture and stocks of infectious agents and associated biologicals; cultures from biological, medical, and pathological laboratories; cultures and stocks from research and industrial laboratories; discarded live and attenuated vaccines; culture dishes and devices used to transfer, inoculate, and mix cultures; pathological wastes, including tissues, organs, and body parts removed during surgery or autopsy; waste human blood or products of blood, including serum, plasma, and other blood components; sharps that have been used in patient care or in medical, research, or industrial laboratories, including hypodermic needles, syringes, pasteur pipettes, broken glass, and scalpel blades; contaminated animal carcasses, body parts, and bedding that was exposed to infectious agents; waste from surgery or autopsy that were in contact with infectious agents; laboratory wastes from medical, pathological, pharmaceutical, or other research, commercial, or industrial laboratories that were in contact with infectious agents; dialysis wastes that were in contact with the blood of patients undergoing hemodialysis; discarded medical equipment and parts that were in contact with infectious agents; biological waste and discarded materials contaminated with blood, excretion, exudates, or secretion from human beings or animals who are isolated to protect others from communicable diseases.

Medical waste generators include hospitals, physician's offices, dental offices, veterinary practices, funeral homes, research laboratories that perform health-related analyses or services, nursing homes, and hospices.

General Packaging Requirements. In all cases, regulated medical waste (RMW) intended for trans-

port off-site must be placed in a single container or a combination of containers that is rigid and leakproof (this could include approved plastic bags). If untreated regulated medical waste is packaged in a plastic bag, the bag must be red in color or display the universal biohazard symbol. The bag must prevent tearing or breaking and must be sealed securely to prevent leaking.

When treated regulated medical waste, other than sharps and fluids, is packaged in plastic bags, it must be packaged the same as untreated regulated medical waste, except that the bags do not need to be labeled. Reusable containers that hold treated medical waste may be used as long as they are not subject to undue mechanical stress or compaction.

Sharps and Fluids Packaging. All sharps, including those that contain residual fluids, must be placed in rigid, leak-resistant, and puncture-resistant containers. If the container cannot be sealed to prevent leakage, it must be placed in a plastic bag or other leak-resistant container that can be sealed to prevent leakage.

Storage of RMW. RMW must be stored in such a way that it is segregated so that handlers, workers, and the public are protected from exposure.

Segregation of RMW. Generators must segregate medical waste to the extent practicable. It is generally necessary to segregate sharps, including sharps containing residual fluids, and fluids in quantities greater than 20 cubic centimeters from other medical wastes.

Mixing of RMW. When regulated medical waste cannot be segregated from other waste, the generator must ensure that the waste is packaged and marked accordingly. If untreated waste or refuse is mixed with treated waste, the package and tracking form must indicate untreated waste.

Decontamination Standards. Any rigid container that is reused must be decontaminated if the container is visibly contaminated. If the container cannot be decontaminated it must be considered RMW and must be treated, handled, and disposed of as such. Containers must be free of any visible signs of contamination before use.

Labeling Requirements. Each package containing untreated medical waste must have a label with the words "**Infectious Waste**" or "**Medical Waste**" or the universal biohazard symbol.

When a red bag is used as a container, however, the color red is recognized as an indicator that the bag contains untreated medical waste and serves the same function as the label. However, a label is always required on the outer surface of an untreated regulated medical waste package, regardless of the color of the package.

RMW categorized as treated waste does not require a label.

Marking Requirements. Generators that ship RMW off-site must have containers identified to show the generator and transporter. The identification must show the generator's name and state permit or identification number.

When RMW is handled by more than one transporter, each transporter must affix an additional tag indicating the name, address, and state identification number of the transporter.

Generators. Small quantity generators who generate less than 50 pounds of RMW in a calendar month are not required to complete tracking forms for each shipment, but they are responsible for proper packaging, labeling, and marking of waste and must use a log to record when waste is transported off-site. The transporter's log must contain the following information: generator's name, generator's state permit or identification number, quantity of waste by category (treated or untreated), and date of shipment. They may personally transport their own RMW.

All shipments of 50 pounds or more of RMW from a large quantity generator must be accompanied by a tracking form that has been filled out by the generator and signed by both the generator and the transporter. They must use an outside transporter.

The generator shall contact the destination facility if tracking forms are not returned to the generator from the destination facility within thirty-five days from date of shipment. The generator shall contact the EPA and state environmental agency if the form is not received after forty-five days from date of shipment.

Recordkeeping. Generators who are required to use a tracking form must keep a copy of each tracking form for at least three years from date of acceptance of the shipment by the transporter.

The generators must also keep a copy of the tracking form signed by the destination facility for three years from the date of acceptance of the shipment by the transporter.

CHAPTER REVIEW

Multiple Choice

Select the best answer from the choices provided.

1. The hazardous waste emergency response plan must include
   a. prior planning and coordination with outside agencies
   b. decontamination of the site
   c. medical and first aid treatment for the injured
   d. a, b, and c

2. Monitoring of employees at uncontrolled hazardous waste sites must be done
   a. before entry to the site
   b. during cleanup
   c. to ensure that conditions are not present that are dangerous to life and health
   d. a, b, and c

3. A large quantity generator generates
   a. between 100 and 499 kilograms of hazardous waste in any month
   b. between 500 and 999 kilograms of hazardous waste in any one month
   c. 1,000 kilograms or more of hazardous waste in any one month
   d. 1,500 kilograms or more of hazardous waste in any one month

4. Leaking containers of hazardous waste must
   a. have the leaks plugged
   b. be put into salvage drums
   c. be emptied into another container
   d. have the contents disposed of at an approved site

5. Small quantity generators of regulated medical waste generate
   a. less than 50 pounds of RMW per month
   b. 50 pounds or more of RMW per month
   c. 100 pounds or more of RMW per month
   d. less than 30 pounds of RMW per month

True/False

Indicate whether the statement is true or false by circling T or F.

6. T   F   Hazardous waste and hazardous material are one and the same.

7. T   F   Skilled support personnel are not directly involved in hazardous waste cleanup.

8. T   F   Acute toxic waste is listed by "U" numbers under RCRA requirements.

9. T   F   Generators are equally liable with transporters for highway accidents involving hazardous waste.

10. T   F   Hypodermic needles are considered regulated medical waste.

Matching

Match the terms in column 1 with the definitions in column 2.

Column 1		*Column 2*	
11.	Emergency response plan	a.	Hazardous waste containers
12.	Acute hazardous waste	b.	Regulated medical waste
13.	Needs USDOT approval	c.	Waste minimization processes
14.	Thermal, chemical, or physical	d.	Part of the safety and health plan
15.	Infectious waste	e.	"P" number listing under RCRA

Short Answer

Briefly but thoroughly answer each statement.

16. List some of the associated OSHA standards that apply to hazardous waste operations.

17. How would you handle a small spill or leak in a hospital laboratory?

18. Explain when a hazardous substance becomes a hazardous waste.

19. What are some ways you can reduce the quantity and toxicity of the hazardous waste you generate?

20. Describe what might be regulated medical waste in your area of operations.

Ethylene Oxide

After studying this chapter, you should be able to

➤ Discuss the OSHA requirements concerning EtO exposure.
➤ Describe how it is used that causes exposure.
➤ List the chemical properties of EtO.
➤ Describe the hazard it poses.
➤ List the various synonyms by which it is also known.

WHERE AND HOW IT IS USED

Ethylene oxide (EtO) is a gas sterilizing agent used in hospitals and other health care facilities to disinfect medical equipment. The sterilizer is purged of air and replaced with ethylene oxide. In the past, such sterilizing agents as chlorine, ozone, sulfur dioxide, and formaldehyde were used. These agents presented health and safety problems because they are corrosive and toxic. Ethylene oxide is safer and more efficient (although still very hazardous). Synonyms for EtO include: oxirane, dihydrooxirene, dimethylene oxide, epoxyethane, 1,2-epoxyethane, oxacyclopropane, and oxidoethane.

EtO is also used in the manufacture of monoethylene, diethylene, triethylene, and polyethylene glycols, ethylene glycol ethers, ethanolamine, and ethoxylation products of fatty alcohols, fatty amines, alkyl phenols, cellulose, and polypropylene glycol. These compounds are constituents of products ranging from antifreezes and heat transfer liquids to solvents, deicers, and pharmaceuticals.

Chemical formula: C_2H_4O

HAZARDS AND HOW EXPOSURE OCCURS

Ethylene oxide is a toxic and volatile chemical compound. It is a colorless gas at room temperature, has a melting point of –112°F, and a normal boiling point of 51°F. Its liquid specific gravity of .875 indicates that it is lighter than water, and its **density** of .8711 indicates that it is lighter than air. The gas rises rather than stays along the floor.

Its flash point is less than 0°F, which makes it very dangerous if a source of ignition, such as a spark, flame, or heated surface comes in contact with the gas. It self-ignites at 804°F (**autoignition temperature**). This indicates that it creates its own heat through an exothermic reaction and bursts into flame or explodes at that temperature.

The **lower explosive limit (LEL)** is 2.6% by volume, and the **upper explosive limit (UEL)** is 100% by volume. When the gas concentration in air by volume is between these limits, it is an ignition or explosion hazard when a source of ignition is present. If it is below the LEL, the concentration is too lean to burn; if above the UEL, it is too rich to burn.

It reacts with acids and bases, alcohols, aluminum chloride, aluminum oxide, ammonia, copper, iron chlorides, iron oxide, magnesium perchlorate, mercaptans, potassium, and tin chlorides to create a dangerous fire hazard.

It decomposes at 450°F to form carbon monoxide, methane, ethane, hydrogen, carbon, and acetaldehyde. It also has a tendency to polymerize. This indicates that its molecules combine with other molecules to form longer molecular chains, making the resulting compound more unstable.

It is toxic by the oral and inhalation routes and is a **carcinogen** (cancer causing agent) and **mutagen** (agent that causes genetic mutations).

Exposure can occur if the sterilizing equipment leaks or if there is a leak in any of the pipelines leading to the sterilizer from a **manifold** or compressed gas tank.

OSHA 29 CFR 1910.1047 ETHYLENE OXIDE

Permissible Exposure Limits

The permissible exposure limits (PEL) are the maximum concentrations of a toxic substance that employees can be exposed to over a designated period of time.

The **time weighted average (TWA)** for EtO is one part per million (1.0 ppm). During an eight-hour day, employees cannot be exposed as averaged over the eight hours to more than 1.0 ppm.

The **excursion limit** is 5 ppm. This means that during any fifteen-minute period, employees cannot be exposed to more than 5 ppm as averaged over a sampling period of fifteen minutes.

The **action level** is 0.5 ppm. This level requires employee monitoring and medical surveillance.

Employee Monitoring for Exposure

Determinations of exposure must be done by representative air samples at the employee's breathing zone. These samples must consist of an eight-hour TWA and fifteen-minute exposure.

Initial Monitoring. Every employee who is exposed to EtO must be initially monitored to determine his/her exposure level.

Monitoring Frequency. If monitoring shows employee exposure at or above the action level, but at or below the eight-hour TWA, monitoring must be repeated at least every six months.

If monitoring shows employee exposure above the eight-hour TWA, monitoring must be repeated at least every three months.

The monitoring schedule may be altered from quarterly to semiannually when two consecutive measurements, taken at least seven days apart, indicate that exposure has decreased to, or below, the eight-hour TWA.

If monitoring shows exposure above the fifteen-minute excursion limit, monitoring must be repeated at least every three months, and more often as necessary, to evaluate the employee's short-term exposure.

Termination of Monitoring. When initial monitoring shows exposure below the action level of 0.5 ppm, TWA monitoring may be discontinued for those employees whose exposures are determined by the initial monitoring.

When periodic monitoring shows employee exposure, as indicated by at least two consecutive measurements taken at least seven days apart, below the action level, TWA monitoring may be discontinued for those employees whose exposure is determined by this monitoring.

When initial monitoring shows employee exposure to be at or below the excursion limit, excursion limit monitoring may be discontinued for those employees whose exposures are determined by this monitoring.

When periodic monitoring shows employee exposure, as indicated by at least seven days apart, is at or below the excursion limit, excursion limit monitoring may be discontinued for those employees whose exposures are determined by this monitoring.

Additional Monitoring. Monitoring requirements must also be instituted when there is a change in the production, process, control equipment, personnel, or work practices that may result in new or additional exposures to EtO, or when the employer has a reason to suspect that a change may result in new or additional exposures.

Monitoring Accuracy. Monitoring must be accurate to a confidence level of 95 percent, to within plus or minus 25 percent for airborne concentrations of EtO at the 1.0 ppm TWA, and to within plus or minus 35 percent for airborne concentrations of EtO at the action level of 0.5 ppm. Monitoring must be accurate to a confidence level of 95 percent, to within plus or minus 35 percent for airborne concentrations of EtO at the excursion limit of 5 ppm.

Monitoring Results Notification. Within fifteen working days of receiving the results of any monitoring required by this standard, the employer must let the affected employee know the results in writing either individually or by posting in a location that is accessible to employees.

The written notification must indicate the corrective action that is being taken to bring exposure to or below the TWA and/or excursion limit if these limits have been exceeded.

Observation of Monitoring. The employer must give affected employees, or their designated representatives, the opportunity to observe monitoring methods used to detect EtO.

If observation of monitoring involves going to an area where protective clothing or equipment is required, the observer must be required to use this clothing and equipment and must comply with all applicable safety and health procedures.

Regulated Areas

Regulated areas (areas that require controls because exposure, or potential exposure, may be above mandated limits) must be established where concentrations of EtO may, or do, exceed the TWA or excursion limit. These areas are limited to authorized persons and must be set up to minimize the number of employees within the area.

Engineering and Work Practice Controls

Engineering and work practice controls, whenever feasible, must be used to keep exposure levels at or below the TWA and the excursion limit. Engineering controls are required where OSHA demonstrates they are feasible. If these controls are not sufficient to reduce EtO to safe levels (at or below the TWA or excursion limit), they must still be used and employees must additionally wear respirators. Engineering controls refer to local or general exhaust ventilation systems that remove the contaminant at its source, or dilute room air to below the TWA or excursion limit. Work practice controls refer to reducing the time employees are exposed so that the exposure

averaged over an eight-hour day, or exposure averaged over fifteen minutes, is below the TWA or excursion limit, whichever applies. Employee rotation is not permitted as a means of reducing exposure to, or below, the TWA or excursion limit.

Engineering controls are usually not feasible for collecting of quality assurance sampling from sterilized materials, removal of biological indicators from sterilized materials, loading and unloading of tank cars, changing of ethylene tanks on sterilizers, and vessel cleaning. Other controls must be implemented if exposure exceeds the TWA or excursion limit during these operations. These controls can be real-time monitors. If they are used, it is important to properly set the alarm level.

Compliance Program

When the TWA or excursion limit is exceeded, the employer must establish and implement a written program to reduce exposure to or below the TWA or excursion limit by means of engineering and work practice controls. This also includes the wearing of respirators, when required.

The compliance program must also indicate a schedule for periodic leak detection surveys and a written plan for emergency situations.

Written plans must be reviewed every twelve months and updated as necessary when significant changes occur that alter the compliance program.

Respiratory Protection

When respirators are required to be worn by employees, the employer must supply the proper respirators and ensure that they are worn.

Respirators must be worn in the following situations:

1. During the time necessary to install or implement feasible engineering and work practice controls.
2. When engineering and work practice controls are not feasible, such as maintenance and repair activities and vessel cleaning.
3. When feasible engineering and work practice controls are not sufficient to reduce exposure to or below the TWA or excursion limit.
4. In emergencies.

Respirator Selection. When respirators are required, the employer must provide the proper respirator at no cost to the employee and ensure that he/she wears it. The respirator must be for protection against EtO and jointly approved by the **Mine Safety and Health Administration (MSHA)** and the National Institute for Occupational Safety and Health (NIOSH). Both are federal agencies that set the standards for respiratory protection and certification.

Respirator Program. When respirators are required, the employer must institute a respirator program that complies with OSHA 29 CFR 1910.134 (see Chapter 16).

Protective Clothing and Equipment

When employees are exposed to skin or eye contact with liquid EtO or EtO solutions, the employer must provide, at no cost to the employee, appropriate protective clothing or other equipment that meets OSHA requirements (29 CFR 1910.132 and 133). The employer has to ensure that the employees wear the protective clothing and equipment that is provided.

Emergency Situations

The employer must have a written plan that addresses emergencies, and employees must be made aware of this plan.

Written Plan. A written plan must be developed when there is the possibility that an emergency may occur upon release of EtO. The plan must indicate that employees involved in responding to and correcting the emergency, must wear an appropriate respirator that protects against EtO. The plan must also include those elements that OSHA requires in emergency plans (see Chapter 6).

Employee Alert. When there is the possibility of employee exposure to EtO due to an emergency, a procedure must be developed that alerts potentially affected employees of the emergency as soon as possible. Affected employees must be immediately evacuated from the area.

Medical Surveillance

All employees who are or may be exposed to EtO at or above the action level (regardless of the wearing of respirators) for at least thirty days, must be included in a **medical surveillance** program.

Medical examinations must also be given to employees who were exposed during an emergency.

Physician's Examinations. All examinations must be conducted by licensed physicians, provided at no cost to the employee, without loss of pay, and at a reasonable time and place.

Examination and Consultation Schedule. Examinations and consultations must be given as follows:

1. Before assignment where the exposure may be at or above the action level for at least thirty days per year.
2. At least annually where exposure was at or above the action level during the past year.
3. At termination or reassignment to an area where exposure to EtO is not at or above the action level for at least thirty days per year.
4. For any employee, where appropriate, who was exposed due to an emergency.
5. As soon as possible when an employee notifies the employer that he/she has developed signs or symptoms that indicate possible overexposure, or when the employee wishes medical advice concerning the effects of past or present exposure to EtO on the ability to have a healthy child.
6. If the examining physician determines that the examinations should be provided more frequently than specified, the employer must provide examinations to employees on the physician's recommended frequency.

Examination Content. The examination must include

1. A medical and work history with emphasis on symptoms related to pulmonary, hematologic, neurologic, and reproductive systems and to the skin.

2. A complete blood count that includes a red, white, and **differential cell count, hematocrit**, and **hemoglobin**. Differential cell count is the determination of the number of each variety of cell in one milliliter of blood. Hematocrit is an evaluation of the iron-containing pigment of the red blood cells by using a centrifuge to separate the solids from the plasma in the blood. It is also the volume of **erythrocytes** (red blood cells) packed by centrifugation in a given volume of blood. Hemoglobin is the iron-containing pigment of the red blood cells.

3. Any other tests that the examining physician finds necessary by good medical practice.

The content of these examinations will be determined by the examining physician, and will include pregnancy testing or laboratory evaluation of fertility when requested by the employee and found necessary by the physician.

Information Given to the Physician

The following information must be given to the examining physician by the employer when employees are examined because of EtO exposure:

1. A copy of the EtO standard.
2. A copy of Appendix A (Substance Safety Data Sheet for Ethylene Oxide).
3. A copy of Appendix B (Substance Technical Guidelines for Ethylene Oxide).
4. A copy of Appendix C (Medical Surveillance Guidelines for Ethylene Oxide). These appendices are nonmandatory but will give the examining physician detailed information concerning the hazards of EtO as well as methods to protect against exposure.
5. A description of the employee's duties as they relate to exposure.
6. The employee's representative.
7. The expected exposure level.
8. A description of any personal protective equipment used, or to be used.
9. Information from previous examinations of the employee that is not otherwise available to the examining physician.

Physician's Written Opinion

The employer must obtain a written opinion from the examining physician that should indicate

- Whether the employee has any detected medical conditions resulting from exposure to EtO that require further explanation or treatment.
- Any recommended limitations concerning the use of personal protective equipment.
- A statement that the employee has been informed by the physician of the results of the examination and of any medical conditions resulting from exposure that require further explanation or treatment.

The employer must tell the physician that any findings or diagnoses *unrelated* to EtO exposure cannot be included in the written opinion.

A copy of the written opinion must be given to the employee by the employer within fifteen days of receipt.

Communicating Hazards to Employees

Signs and labels must be used to communicate the hazards of ethylene oxide.

Signs. Legible signs must be posted and maintained indicating regulated areas, entrances, or accessways to regulated areas that have the following legend:

> **Danger. Ethylene Oxide. Cancer and Reproductive Hazard. Authorized Personnel Only. Respirators And Protective Clothing May Be Required To Be Worn In This Area.**

Labels. Labels must be put on all containers of EtO that can cause employee exposure at or above the action level, or at or above the excursion limit. The labels must remain on the containers when they leave the workplace. Reaction vessels, storage tanks, pipes, and piping systems are not considered containers, so they do not require labels.

The labels must comply with OSHA 29 CFR 1910.1200 Hazard Communication. They must have the following legend:

1. **Danger. Contains Ethylene Oxide. Cancer and Reproductive Hazard.**
2. A warning statement against breathing airborne concentrations of EtO.

Information and Training

Employees who are exposed to EtO at or above the action level or excursion limit must be provided with information and training on EtO on initial assignment and at least annually thereafter.

Information must include the following:

1. The requirements of the standard with an explanation of its contents, including Appendixes A and B.
2. Work area operations where EtO is present.
3. Availability of the written EtO final rule and where it is located. The final rule is the latest OSHA standard concerning EtO.
4. The medical surveillance program required by the standard and an explanation of Appendix C.

Training must include the following:

1. Methods and observations used to detect EtO in the work area (monitoring and monitoring devices used).
2. The physical and health hazards of EtO.
3. Measures employees can take to protect against exposure. These include specific methods implemented by the employer such as work practices, controls, emergency procedures, and personal protective equipment
4. Details of the hazard communication program developed by the employer, including an explanation of the labeling system and how employees can and use appropriate hazard information.

Recordkeeping

Exposure measurements and medical surveillance records concerning EtO exposure must be maintained.

Exposure Measurements. Accurate records of employee exposure measurements must be kept and must contain the following information:

1. Date of the measurement
2. The operation that involves the exposure to EtO that is being monitored
3. The sampling and analytical methods used and evidence of their accuracy
4. Number, duration, and results of samples taken
5. Protective devices worn, if any
6. Name, social security number, and exposure level of the employee

Records must be maintained for at least thirty years in accordance with OSHA requirements for the retention of exposure and medical records (see Chapter 5).

Medical Surveillance. Accurate records must be kept for employees subject to medical surveillance. This record must contain the following information:

1. The name and social security number of the employee
2. Physician's written opinions
3. Any employee medical complaints related to EtO exposure
4. A copy of the information provided to the physician

These records must be retained for the duration of employment plus thirty years, in accordance with the OSHA requirements for the retention of exposure and medical records (see Chapter 5).

Availability of Records. Upon written request, exposure and medical records must be made available to the affected employee, the employee's authorized representative, and to OSHA. This is in accordance with OSHA regulations 29 CFR 1910.1020 (see Chapter 5).

Transfer of Records. OSHA must be notified by the employer at least ninety days prior to disposal of records when he/she ceases to do business and there is no successor. The records must be sent to OSHA where a determination will be made as to disposition.

CHAPTER REVIEW

Multiple Choice

Select the best answer from the choices provided.

1. EtO is also known as
    a. perchloroethylene
    b. styrene monomer
    c. oxidoethane
    d. proponal

2. The action level for EtO is
    a. 0.1 ppm   c. 0.2 ppm
    b. 0.5 ppm   d. 0.3 ppm

3. EtO is
    a. lighter than air
    b. the same density as air
    c. heavier than air
    d. none of the above

4. EtO decomposes at
    a. 450°F   c. 600°F
    b. 500°F   d. 200°F

5. The autoignition temperature of EtO is
    a. 100°F   c. 500°F
    b. 200°F   d. 804°F

True/False

Indicate whether the statement is true or false by circling T or F.

6. T F   In health care facilities, EtO is used as a gas sterilizing agent.

7. T F   The time weighted average for EtO is 5 parts per million.

8. T F   An EtO compliance program must be reviewed every fifteen months.

9. T F   The medical examination for employees exposed to EtO above the action level can be performed by a health technician.

10. T F   Its main health hazard is that EtO sensitizes the skin upon contact.

Matching

Match the terms in column 1 with the definitions in column 2.

Column 1		*Column 2*
11. EtO excursion limit		a. Part of a complete blood count
12. EtO explosive limits		b. Red blood cells
13. Hematocrit		c. EtO specific gravity
14. Erythrocytes		d. 5 ppm
15. .875		e. 2.6% to 100%

Short Answer

Briefly but thoroughly answer each statement.

16. Explain the employee monitoring requirements under the EtO standard.

17. Describe the engineering and work practice controls that are used to protect against exposure to EtO and what control is not permitted.

18. List the required parts of an employee examination for those exposed to EtO.

19. Describe the content of an employee training program for those exposed to EtO.

20. List the operations in your facility where exposure to EtO may occur.

CHAPTER 29

Formaldehyde

OBJECTIVES

After studying this chapter, you should be able to

- ➤ Describe the OSHA requirements for controlling exposure to formaldehyde (OSHA 29 CFR 1910.1048).
- ➤ List the various solutions of formaldehyde.
- ➤ Discuss the hazards of this chemical.
- ➤ Determine the respiratory protection required for various levels of exposure.
- ➤ Describe the required medical surveillance of employees who are exposed.

HOW IT IS USED

Formaldehyde is covered under OSHA 29 CFR 1910.1048. It is a pungent, colorless, irritant gas that is made by oxidation of methyl alcohol. A 10 percent solution is used as an astringent and for sterilizing feces, urine, and sputum, and a 5–10 percent solution is used for sterilizing clothing and towels. A 1 or 2 percent solution is used for cleaning dishes, instruments, or fabrics. This concentration acts as a germicidal agent but usually takes twenty to thirty minutes to be effective. Formaldehyde solution that contains 37 percent is used for medicinal purposes. Methanol is usually added to this solution. Formaldehyde hardens tissues, which makes it a very effective preservative.

EXPOSURE OCCURRENCES

Employees working in histology laboratories may become exposed to formaldehyde solutions as well as workers in laundry and housekeeping operations.

Exposure may cause skin irritation and irritation of the eyes, nose, mouth, throat, respiratory tracts, gastrointestinal tracts, and central nervous system. Abdominal pain, convulsions, unconsciousness, and kidney damage are also possible from exposure. Harmful effects depend upon the level and duration of exposure and whether it is local or systemic. Local refers to one spot in the body, and systemic refers to exposure throughout the body.

OSHA 29 CFR 1910.1048 FORMALDEHYDE

OSHA has specific requirements concerning exposure to formaldehyde. Employers must protect employees who are exposed to this chemical.

Exposure Limits

Exposure limits are the maximum concentration of formaldehyde that employees can be exposed to over designated periods.

Employees cannot be exposed to more than 0.75 parts per million (ppm) airborne concentrations. This is an eight-hour time weighted average (TWA) or PEL. This means that as averaged over an eight-hour day, employees cannot be exposed to above 0.75 ppm.

Employees cannot be exposed to more than 2 parts per million (2 ppm) airborne concentrations, which is a fifteen-minute **short-term exposure limit (STEL)**. This means that during the fifteen-minute period, the 2 ppm exposure limit cannot be exceeded at any time during the eight-hour work shift. This is required even though the eight-hour TWA may be within the PEL.

The action level is 0.5 ppm TWA. This means that when this level is exceeded as averaged over an eight-hour day, the employer has to start certain programs as defined in the standard.

Monitoring

Where there is exposure to formaldehyde, the employer must monitor airborne concentrations to determine levels of exposure.

> *Note:* The fritted bubbler is effective in determining airborne levels of formaldehyde. The bubbler is comprised of fritted glass (fused glass with small porous openings). Air is drawn through the bubbler, which is submerged in an absorbing solution or reagent (sodium bisulfite). Collection efficiency is 95 percent. The sample is then analyzed by instrumentation to determine the concentration of formaldehyde.

Estimates of airborne concentrations can also be obtained by using a colorimetric indicating tube for formaldehyde. This is a bellows device that draws a measured volume of air into the tube after the tube end tips are broken off. The tube contains a granular agent such as silica gel or aluminum oxide that has been impregnated with xylene vapor in the conversion layer and sulphuric acid in the indicating layer. A pink stain appears, and the length of the stain on the tube determines the airborne concentration (read directly on the tube in ppm). The concentration is about plus or minus 10 percent of the actual airborne concentration.

Initial Monitoring. The employer has to identify all employees who may be exposed at or above the action level or the STEL and accurately determine the level of exposure.

The initial monitoring must be done whenever there is a change in production, equipment, process, personnel, or control measures that can result in new or additional exposure.

When the employer receives reports of signs or symptoms that include respiratory or dermal conditions that indicate formaldehyde exposure, he/she must promptly monitor the affected employee's exposure.

Periodic Monitoring. If employees are exposed at or above the action level or STEL as determined by initial monitoring, the employer must conduct periodic monitoring to accurately determine levels.

If the most recent monitoring results show employee exposure at or above the action level, the employer must repeat monitoring at least every six months.

If the most recent monitoring results show employee exposure at or above the STEL, the employer must repeat monitoring at least once a year under worst conditions.

Monitoring Termination. Periodic monitoring can be discontinued when the results from two consecutive sampling periods taken at least seven days apart indicate exposure below the action level and STEL. These results must be statistically representative and consistent with the employer's knowledge of the job and work operation.

Monitoring Accuracy. Monitoring must be accurate at the 95 percent confidence level, to within plus or minus 25 percent for airborne concentrations at the TWA and STEL and to within plus or minus 35 percent at the action level.

Monitoring Results Notification. The employer must notify affected employees within fifteen days of the results of exposure monitoring required under this standard. The notification has to be in writing by either distributing copies of the results to employees or by posting the results. If exposure is over the PEL, the employer must develop and implement a written plan that reduces exposure to below the PELs. The plan must have a description of the action being taken to decrease exposure to below the PELs, and employees must be notified of the plan.

Monitoring Observation. Affected employees or their designated representatives have the right to observe any monitoring required under this standard.

When observation requires entry into an area where protective clothing or equipment is required, the employer must furnish the necessary clothing or equipment and require that it be worn or used. The employer must also make sure that the observer complies with all applicable safety and health procedures.

Regulated Areas

Regulated areas are areas that require controls because exposure to hazardous substances are or may be above mandated limits.

Where airborne concentrations of formaldehyde exceed the TWA or STEL, all entrances and access ways must have signs that indicate:

Danger
Formaldehyde
Irritant and Potential Cancer Hazard
Authorized Personnel Only

Only authorized persons who have been trained to recognize the hazards of formaldehyde can have access to regulated areas.

Compliance Methods

Employers must use engineering and work practice controls to reduce and keep exposures at or below the TWA and STEL.

When engineering and work practice controls are not feasible to reduce levels to or below the TWA or STEL, the employer must use these controls to whatever extent possible to reduce these levels and supplement engineering and work practices with respirators that satisfy the standard.

Respiratory Protection

When respirators are required, they will be provided at no cost to the employee. The employer must make sure that they are properly used. The respirators must comply with this standard and reduce concentrations inhaled to at or below both the TWA and STEL.

Respirators will be used only

1. During the interval necessary to install or implement feasible engineering and work practice controls.

2. In maintenance and repair activities or vessel cleaning when it is determined that engineering and work practice controls are not feasible.
3. In situations when engineering and work practice controls cannot reduce levels to or below the PELs.
4. In emergencies.

Respirator Selection. Respirators must be selected as described in this standard and must be approved by the National Institute for Occupational Safety and Health (NIOSH) and the Mine Safety and Health Administration (MSHA). Both are federal agencies that approve and certify respirators, among other safety and health responsibilities.

Powered air purifying respirators (PAPRs) must be made available to any employee who experiences difficulty wearing a negative pressure respirator to reduce exposure to formaldehyde.

Respirator Use. Respirators, when assigned, must comply with 29 CFR 1910.134 (see Chapter 16).

Quantitative or qualitative fit tests must be done for employees who must wear negative pressure respirators. These tests must be at the time of the initial fitting and at least annually thereafter.

Respirators chosen must be from those exhibiting the best face piece fit. (See Table 29-1.) Respirators cannot be selected that permit employees to inhale formaldehyde at concentrations in excess of either the TWA or PEL.

Replacement of Cartridges and Canisters. Respirator cartridges in air purifying respirators must be replaced after three hours of use or at the end of the work shift, whichever is sooner, unless the cartridge has a NIOSH-approved end-of-service indicator.

Respirator canisters used in atmospheres up to 7.5 ppm ($10 \times$ PEL) must be replaced every four hours, and industrial sized canisters used in atmospheres up to 75 ppm ($100 \times$ PEL) must be replaced every two hours or at the end of the work shift, whichever is sooner, unless the canister has a NIOSH-approved end-of-service indicator.

TABLE 29-1 Minimum Requirements for Respiratory Protection Against Formaldehyde	
Condition of Use or Formaldehyde Concentration	Minimum Respirator Required[1]
Up to 7.5 ppm (10 × PEL)	Full face piece with cartridges or canisters specifically approved for protection against formaldehyde[2]
Up to 75 ppm (100 × PEL)	Full face mask with chin style or chest or back mounted type, with industrial size canister specifically approved for protection against formaldehyde
	Type C supplied air respirator, demand type, or continuous flow type, with full face piece, hood, or helmet
Above 75 ppm or unknown (emergencies) (100 × PEL)	Self-contained breathing apparatus (SCBA) with positive pressure full face piece
Fire fighting	SCBA with positive pressure in full face piece
Escape	SCBA in demand or pressure demand mode. Full face mask with chin style or front or back mounted type industrial size canister specifically approved for protection against formaldehyde

[1] Respirators specified for higher concentrations may be used for lower concentrations.

[2] A half-mask respirator with cartridges specifically approved for protection against formaldehyde can be substituted for the full face piece respirator providing that effective gas proof goggles are provided and used in combination with the half-mask respirator.

Protective Clothing and Equipment

Employers must provide protective equipment and clothing in accordance with 29 CFR 1910.132 and 133. Protective devices must be provided at no cost to the employee, and the employer must ensure that the employee wears them.

Protective clothing and equipment is to be selected based upon the form of the formaldehyde, conditions of use, and the hazard to be controlled.

Contact of the eyes and skin with liquids containing one percent or more formaldehyde must be prevented by the use of formaldehyde impervious protective clothing and the use of other personal protective equipment, such as appropriate face shields and goggles.

A face shield and goggles are required when there is the danger of formaldehyde reaching the eyes.

Full body protection must be worn for entry into areas where the concentration exceeds 100 ppm and for emergency reentry into areas of unknown concentration.

Maintenance of Clothing and Equipment. Clothing that has become contaminated with formaldehyde must be cleaned or laundered before reuse.

When formaldehyde contaminated clothing and equipment are ventilated, the employer must establish a storage area to minimize employee exposure. Containers for contaminated clothing and equipment and storage areas must have labels and signs as follows:

Danger
Formaldehyde Contaminated
Clothing/Equipment
Avoid Inhalation and Skin Contact

Only persons trained to recognize formaldehyde hazards can remove contaminated material from storage areas for cleaning, laundering, or disposal.

Protective equipment and clothing must be repaired or replaced by the employer to maintain its effectiveness.

People who launder, clean, or repair clothing and equipment must be informed of formaldehyde's potentially harmful effects and of procedures to safely handle items.

Hygiene Protection

Change rooms must be provided, as described in 29 CFR 1910.141, for employees required to change from work clothing into protective clothing to prevent skin contact.

Safety showers have to be provided in convenient locations for those workers whose skin may come in contact with solutions containing 1 percent or more of formaldehyde. Proper eyewash stations must be provided in the immediate work area when employees' eyes can come in contact with solutions containing 0.1 percent or greater formaldehyde.

Housekeeping

There has to be a program to detect leaks and spills of formaldehyde liquids or gas. This includes regular visual inspections.

Preventative maintenance has to be conducted at regular intervals.

In areas where spillage is possible, provisions must be made to contain the spill, decontaminate the work area, and dispose of the waste.

Leaks must be repaired and spills cleaned up promptly by employees wearing proper protective equipment and who are trained in proper cleanup and decontamination.

Formaldehyde contaminated waste resulting from leaks and spills must be placed in sealed containers that have labels indicating the presence of formaldehyde and its hazards.

Emergencies

When there is the possibility of an emergency involving formaldehyde, the employer must make sure that appropriate procedures are adopted to minimize injury and loss of life.

Medical Surveillance

Medical surveillance programs have to be instituted for all employees exposed to formaldehyde at or above the action level or STEL.

Medical surveillance must also be made available to those employees who develop signs and symptoms of overexposure and to those exposed because of an emergency.

Physician's Examination. All medical procedures and the administering of medical disease questionnaires must be done by or under the supervision of a licensed physician. This is provided without cost or loss of pay to the employee and at a reasonable time and place.

Based on an evaluation of the medical disease questionnaire, the physician will determine whether an employee, who is not required to wear a respirator under this standard to reduce exposure, must have a medical examination.

Medical examination. Medical examinations have to be given to any employee who the physician feels, based on the medical disease questionnaire, may be at risk from exposure to formaldehyde. The examination must also be given at the time of initial assignment at least annually thereafter to all employees required to wear a respirator to reduce exposure. The examination must include

1. A physical examination that includes evidence of irritation or sensitization of the skin and respiratory system, shortness of breath, or eye irritation.
2. A laboratory examination for respirator wearers that includes a baseline and annual pulmonary function test. The tests, as a minimum, must consist of **forced vital capacity (FVC)**, **forced expiratory volume in one second (FEV-1)**, and **forced expiratory flow (FEF)**. FVC is the volume of air forcibly expelled from the lungs following full inspiration. FEV-1 is the volume of air forcibly expelled from the lungs in one second following full inspiration. FEF is a method to determine the condition of the lungs by measuring the expulsion of the air when it is forcibly breathed out.

3. Any other test necessary to complete the written opinion.
4. Counseling of employees who have medical conditions that would be worsened by exposure to formaldehyde.

Examination of employees exposed due to an emergency. The employer has to make examinations available as soon as possible to employees exposed because of an emergency.

The examination has to include a medical and work history with emphasis on evidence of upper and lower respiratory problems, allergic conditions, skin reaction or hypersensitivity, and any evidence of eye, nose, or throat irritation.

Further examination must consist of those points considered appropriate by the examining physician.

Information Given to the Physician by the Employer. For examinations given to employees, the employer must provide the following to the physician:

1. A copy of the formaldehyde standard and Appendixes A, C, D, and E.
2. A description of the employee's job duties as they relate to the exposure.
3. The representative exposure level for the employee's job assignment.
4. The personal protective equipment and respiratory protection used or to be used by the employee.
5. Information from previous examinations that can be provided by the employer.
6. Whether it is a nonroutine examination because of an emergency exposure. If so, the employer must provide to the physician as soon as possible a description of how the emergency occurred and the exposure the employee may have received.

Physician's Written Opinion. For examinations required under this standard, the employer has to obtain a written opinion from the examining physician. The opinion must indicate the results of the examination except that it cannot reveal specific findings or diagnoses not related to occupa-

tional exposure to formaldehyde. The written opinion must include

1. Whether the employee has any medical condition that would place him/her at increased risk from exposure to formaldehyde.
2. Recommendations on limitations concerning the employee's exposure or changes in use of personal protective equipment, which includes respirators.
3. A statement that the employee has been informed of any medical conditions that could be worsened by exposure to formaldehyde. The exposure may have resulted from past or emergency exposure. The physician must also indicate whether there is a need for further examination or treatment.

The employer has to retain the results of the medical examination and any tests conducted by the physician.

A copy of the physician's written opinion must be provided to the affected employee by the employer within fifteen days after the employer receives it.

Medical Removal. Medical removal, as described in this standard, applies when an employee reports significant irritation of the mucosa of the eyes or upper airways, respiratory sensitization, dermal irritation, or dermal sensitization because of workplace exposure. Medical removal does not apply when dermal irritation or sensitization is the result of being exposed to less than 0.05 percent formaldehyde concentration products.

The employee's report of signs or symptoms of possible overexposure must be evaluated by a physician chosen by the employer, pursuant to this standard. If the physician determines that a medical examination is not needed, as described in the standard, there must be a two-week evaluation and remediation period so that the employer can determine whether the signs and symptoms subside without treatment or with the use of creams, gloves, first aid treatment, or personal protective equipment. Industrial hygiene measures that limit the exposure to formaldehyde can also be implemented during this period. If the signs or symptoms worsen prior to the end of the two-week period, the employee must be immediately referred to a physician. Earnings, seniority, and benefits cannot be altered during the two-week period because of the report.

If the signs or symptoms have not subsided or been remedied by the end of the two-week period, or earlier if signs or symptoms warrant, the employee must be examined by a physician selected by the employer. The physician must presume, in the absence of other evidence, that the employee's dermal irritation or dermal sensitization are not caused by exposure to formaldehyde products to which the affected employee is exposed that contain less than 0.1 percent formaldehyde.

If the physician finds that significant irritation of the mucosa of the eyes or upper airways, respiratory sensitization, dermal irritation, or dermal sensitization result from exposure in the workplace and recommends restrictions or removal, the employer must promptly comply with the restrictions or removal recommendation. When the recommendation is for removal, the employer must remove the affected employee from the current exposure, and if possible, transfer the employee to work where there is no exposure or significantly less exposure.

When the employee is removed pursuant to the standard, the employer has to transfer the employee to comparable work for which the employee is qualified or can be trained in a short period (up to six months). This work must be where formaldehyde exposures are as low as possible, but not higher than the action level. The employee's current earnings, seniority, and other benefits have to be maintained. If no such work is available, the employer must maintain the employee's current earnings, seniority, and other benefits until work becomes available, or until the employee is determined to be unable to return to workplace exposure, or until the employee is determined to be able to return to his/her original job, or for six months, whichever comes first.

The employer must arrange for a follow-up examination within six months after the employee is removed pursuant to this paragraph. The examination will determine if the employee can return to his/her job, or if removal is to be permanent. The physician must make a determination within six months from the date the employee was removed as to a return or permanent removal.

The employee's earnings, seniority, and other benefits may be reduced for the extent the employee receives compensation from a publicly or employer funded compensation program or from employment with another employer.

Multiple Physicians' Review. After the employer selects the initial physician to conduct a medical examination to determine if medical removal or restriction is appropriate, the employee may designate a second physician to review any findings, determinations, or recommendations of the initial physician. The second physician may conduct examinations, consultations, and laboratory tests deemed necessary to evaluate the effects of formaldehyde exposure.

The employer has to notify the employee of his/her right to a second examination and consultation after being examined by the initial physician to determine the need for medical removal or restriction.

If the second physician's findings, determinations, or recommendations differ from that of the initial physician, the employee and employer must get the two physicians together to agree to a resolution. If the two physicians cannot agree to a determination, then the employee and employer, through their respective physicians, must designate a third physician who is a specialist in the field under review.

The employer must act based upon the findings, determinations, and recommendations of the third physician, unless the employer and employee reach an agreement that is in accordance with the recommendations of at least one of the three physicians.

Hazard Communication

The hazards of formaldehyde must be communicated to employees in accordance with the requirements of this paragraph and 29 CFR 1910.1200 Hazard Communication.

Minimum information concerning health hazards to be conveyed to employees include the following:

- It is a cancer hazard.
- It is an irritant and sensitizer of the skin and respiratory system.

- It is an eye and throat irritant.
- It is an acutely toxic substance.

Labels

The employer must have warning labels affixed to all formaldehyde containers, complying with 29 CFR 1910.1200(f) Hazard Communication.

Label Information. All containers containing formaldehyde materials capable of releasing formaldehyde at levels of 0.1 ppm to 0.5 ppm must carry labels having the following information:

1. Indicating that the material contains formaldehyde.
2. A listing of the responsible party.
3. A statement that physical and health hazard information is available from the employer and the material safety data sheets.

For materials capable of releasing formaldehyde at levels above 0.5 ppm, the labels must address all hazards as defined in 29 CFR 1910.1200(d) and 29 CFR 1200 Appendixes A and B, including respiratory sensitizer, and must have the words "Potential Cancer Hazard."

The label must identify the contents, have the name and address of the manufacturer, and identify the health hazards—namely the target organs the material may affect if either inhaled, ingested, or touched to the skin.

Material Safety Data Sheet

Material safety data sheets must be available at all times and updated as necessary in accordance with 29 CFR 1910.1200.

Written Hazard Communication Program

The employer must develop, implement, and maintain a written hazard communication program for formaldehyde exposure. It must include as a minimum

1. How the requirements for labels and other forms of warning will be met.
2. How the requirements for material safety data sheets will be met.

3. How employee information and training will be met.

Information and Training

The employer has to provide training for all employees who have exposure to formaldehyde at or above 0.1 ppm.

The information and training must be given at the time of initial assignment and whenever there is a new exposure in the workplace. This training must be done at least annually.

Training Program. The training has to be presented in a manner that the employee will understand and must include

1. A discussion of this regulation and the information on the material safety data sheet.
2. The purpose for and a description of the medical surveillance program, which includes a description of the health hazards, the signs and symptoms of exposure, and the requirement to immediately report to the employer any adverse signs or symptoms that may be the cause of formaldehyde exposure.
3. An explanation of operations where formaldehyde is present and the safe work practices to be used to limit exposure.
4. The purpose and need, including its limitations, of personal protective equipment.
5. How to handle spills, emergencies, and cleanup.
6. The importance of engineering and work practice controls for protection and instruction in the use of these controls.
7. A review of emergency procedures and specific duties and assignments of each employee if an emergency occurs.

Access to training materials. The employer must tell affected employees of the location of written training materials and must make these materials available without cost.

Upon request by OSHA, the employer must provide all employee training materials.

Recordkeeping

Records must be kept concerning exposure monitoring, exposure determinations, medical surveillance, respirator fit testing, and medical examinations.

Exposure Measurements. An accurate record has to be established and maintained of all monitoring results that indicate employee exposure to formaldehyde.

The record must include the following:

1. Date of measurement
2. Operation being monitored
3. Methods used to sample and analyze along with the evidence of their accuracy and precision
4. Number, durations, time, and results of samples taken
5. Protective devices worn
6. Names, job classifications, social security numbers, and exposure estimates of employees whose exposures are indicated by the monitoring results

Exposure Determinations. If the employer has determined that monitoring is not required under the regulation, he/she must maintain a record of the data relied upon that supports this determination that no employee is exposed at or above the action level.

Medical Surveillance. An accurate record must be established and maintained for each employee included in medical surveillance.

This record has to include the following:

1. Name and social security number of the employee
2. Physician's written opinion
3. A list of any health complaints that may be related to formaldehyde exposure

4. A copy of the results of the medical examination, including medical disease questionnaires and results of medical tests required by the formaldehyde standard or examining physician

Respirator Fit Testing. An accurate record must be established and maintained for employees who must be negative pressure respirator fit tested as required by the standard.

This record must include the following:

1. A copy of the protocol used for fit testing
2. A copy of fit test results
3. Size and manufacturer of respirator types available for selection
4. Date of the most recent fit test, name and social security number of each fit tested employee, and the respirator type and face piece selected

Records Retention. Records required by this standard must be retained as follows:

1. Exposure records and determinations must be kept for at least thirty years.
2. Medical records must be kept for the duration of employment plus thirty years.
3. Respirator fit tests must be kept until updated by the most recent test.

Records Availability. Upon request by OSHA, the employer must make all records required by this standard available for examination and copying.

The employer must make exposure records, including estimates made from representative monitoring, and medical records available upon request for examination and copying to the employee, or former employee, or to anyone who has written consent of the employee or former employee.

This availability will be in conformance with 29 CFR 1910.1020 Access To Exposure and Medical Records.

Multiple Choice

Select the best answer from the choices provided.

1. Exposure to formaldehyde can cause
   a. skin, eye, and respiratory irritation
   b. abdominal pain
   c. kidney damage
   d. a, b, and c

2. The STEL for formaldehyde is
   a. 1 ppm   c. 3 ppm
   b. 2 ppm   d. 0.75 ppm

3. Exposure above 75 ppm requires
   a. an air purifying respirator
   b. a Type C supplied air respirator
   c. a SCBA
   d. none of the above

4. Cartridges in air purifying respirators used to protect against formaldehyde must be replaced every
   a. hour   c. three hours
   b. two hours   d. four hours

5. Training must be given to all employees exposed to formaldehyde at or above
   a. 0.4 ppm   c. 0.5 ppm
   b. 0.3 ppm   d. 0.1 ppm

True/False

Indicate whether the statement is true or false by circling T or F.

6. T   F   The time weighted average for formaldehyde is 0.75 ppm.

7. T   F   You can use a Type C supplied respirator for concentrations of 0 ppm to 75 ppm.

8. T   F   Medical removal protection does not apply to formaldehyde exposure—only to lead exposure.

9. T   F   The physician's opinion concerning employees exposed to formaldehyde must be given within ten days by the employer to the employee.

10. T   F   Regulated areas are required by OSHA when employees work in excessively hot or cold environments.

Matching

Match the terms in column 1 with the definitions in column 2.

Column 1
11. Formaldehyde action level
12. Fritted bubbler
13. FEF
14. 7.5 ppm
15. 0.1 ppm to 0.5 ppm release

Column 2
a. Part of pulmonary function test
b. When labels on containers are required
c. 0.5 ppm
d. Measures formaldehyde concentrations in air
e. Maximum concentration when air purifying respirators can be used

Short Answer

Briefly but thoroughly answer each statement.

16. List and describe the areas in your health care facility where there may be exposure to formaldehyde.

17. How would you set up a regulated area for employees exposed to formaldehyde?

18. Discuss the personal protective equipment required to protect against exposure.

19. Explain the content of the medical examination required of employees.

20. How would you test for concentrations of airborne formaldehyde?

CHAPTER 30

Benzene

After studying this chapter, you should be able to

➤ Discuss the OSHA benzene standard requirements (OSHA 29 CFR 1910.1028).
➤ State how benzene is used and how exposure occurs.
➤ Describe the medical surveillance requirements for employees exposed to benzene.
➤ List the type of respirator required for the various airborne concentrations.
➤ Discuss the medical removal requirements concerning employee exposure.

WHERE AND HOW IT IS USED

The OSHA standard for occupational exposure to **benzene** is 29 CFR 1910.1028.

Benzene is an aromatic hydrocarbon that is an organic intermediate (middle step in a series of chemical reactions). It is derived from coal or petroleum.

Benzene is a major constituent of most fuels, notably gasoline and other motor fuels. It is present in either the liquid or gaseous state. The OSHA standard includes benzene contained in liquid mixtures and the vapors released by these liquids. It does not include trace amounts of unreacted benzene contained in solid materials.

HOW EXPOSURE OCCURS

Every time there is a dispensing of fuel, either from gasoline pumps or from dispensing cans, benzene vapors become airborne and are inhaled.

OSHA 29 CFR 1910.1028 BENZENE

Health care workers may think that they are not exposed to benzene because it is a chemical not found in medical settings. It is a hydrocarbon that has widespread use in various fuels. The chances of exposure are high, particularly when exposed to gasoline engine and space heater vapors.

Exposure Limits

The exposure limits are the maximum concentration of a toxic substance that employees can be exposed to over a designated period of time.

The time-weighted average (TWA) or permissible exposure limit (PEL) for benzene is 1 part per million (1 ppm). This means no worker can be exposed to more than this concentration averaged over an eight-hour day.

The short-term exposure limit (STEL) is 5 parts per million (5 ppm). This means a worker cannot be exposed to more than this concentration as averaged over any fifteen-minute period over the eight-hour day.

The action level (AL) is 0.5 part per million (0.5 ppm). This is the level averaged over an eight-hour day that, if exceeded, requires that affected employees be monitored for exposure levels and undergo medical surveillance.

Regulated Areas

A regulated area is an area that has required controls because exposure to hazardous substances are or may be above mandated limits.

Regulated areas have to be established when the airborne concentration of benzene exceeds or can be expected to exceed either the eight-hour time-weighted average of 1 ppm or the short-term exposure limit of 5 ppm for fifteen minutes.

Only authorized persons may have access to regulated areas.

The regulated area must be situated so that the number of employees in the area exposed to benzene is kept to a minimum.

Exposure Monitoring

Exposure must be made from breathing zone samples that represent each employee's average exposure to airborne benzene.

Representative eight-hour exposure is to be determined by taking one sample or samples representing the full-shift exposure for each job classification in each work area.

To determine compliance with the STEL exposure, fifteen-minute breathing zone samples are to be made at operations where there is reason to believe exposures are high. The employer may use objective data, such as measurements from brief-period measuring devices, to determine where STEL monitoring is required.

Except for initial monitoring, which is required, if the employer can document that one shift will consistently have higher exposures, then only the operation on the higher-exposure shift is required to be monitored.

Initial Monitoring. Initial monitoring has to be completed within thirty days after benzene is introduced in the workplace.

Periodic Monitoring and Frequency. If monitoring indicates employee exposure at or above the action level but below the TWA, the employee must be monitored at least every year.

If monitoring indicates employee exposure above the TWA, monitoring must be done every six months.

The monitoring schedule can be altered from every six months to yearly when two consecutive measurements taken at least seven days apart indicate that the employee exposure has decreased to the TWA or below but is above the action level.

STEL monitoring must be repeated as necessary to evaluate exposures of employees who are exposed to short-term concentrations.

Termination of Monitoring. When initial monitoring indicates employee exposure below the action level, the employer may discontinue monitoring for that employee except when there is a new or additional exposure to benzene.

Additional Monitoring. Exposure monitoring, as required by the standard, has to be done when there has been a change in the production process, control equipment, personnel, or work practices that could result in new or additional exposure, or when the employer has any reason to suspect that a change could result in a new or additional exposure.

When spills, leaks, ruptures, or other breakdowns occur that may lead to exposure, the employer must monitor, by using area or personal sampling, after cleanup or repair to make sure that exposures have returned to the level that existed before the incident.

Employee Notification of Monitoring Results. Within fifteen days after receiving the results of any monitoring under this standard, the employer must notify the employee of the results in writing either informally or by posting in an area accessible to affected employees.

When the PELs are exceeded, the written notification must indicate the corrective action taken by the employer to reduce exposure to or below the PEL, or shall refer the employee to a document that indicates the corrective action taken.

Monitoring Observation. The employer must provide the opportunity for employees or their designated representatives to observe the measuring and monitoring of exposure to benzene conditions in accordance with this standard.

When observation requires entry into areas where the use of protective clothing or equipment is required, the employer must provide the observer with personal protective clothing and equipment or respirators. The respirators must be the same as those required to be worn by employees working in the area. The employer must also ensure use of the clothing and equipment or respirators and require the observer to comply with all required safety and health procedures.

Compliance Methods

Engineering and work practice controls are to be used to reduce employee exposure to at or below the TWA, except to the extent the employer can establish that these controls are not feasible.

When engineering and work practice controls are not feasible, the employer must utilize these controls and supplement them with the use of respiratory protection that complies with the requirements of this standard.

If the employer can document that benzene is used in the workplace less than a total of thirty days per year, the use of engineering and work practice controls or respiratory protection or any combination of these controls is required to be used to reduce exposure to or below the PELs. The exception is that employers must use engineering and work practice controls to reduce exposure to or below 10 ppm as an eight-hour TWA, if possible.

Compliance Program

When exposures exceed the PELs, the employer must establish and implement a written program that reduces employee exposure to or below the PEL. This is to be done primarily through engineering and work practice controls required by this standard.

The written program must include a schedule for development and implementation of the engineering and work practice controls. The plans must be reviewed and revised, as necessary, based on the most recent exposure monitoring data that reflect the current status of the program.

These plans are required to be sent to OSHA, affected employees, and designated employee representatives when requested for examination and copying.

Respiratory Protection

The employer must supply respirators, and ensure that they are used, when required by this standard. Respirators must be used as follows:

1. During the time necessary to install or implement engineering or work practice controls.
2. In operations where the employer establishes that engineering and work practice controls alone cannot reduce exposure to or below the TWA or STEL.
3. In operations where engineering and work practice controls are not yet sufficient or are not required because of the thirty-day-or-less exposure exception as indicated under "Compliance Methods" to reduce exposure to or below the PELs.
4. In emergencies.

Respirator Selection. When respirators are required under this standard, the employer has to select and provide, at no cost to the employee, the proper respirator as indicated in the respirator table. The employer must also ensure that the employee uses the respirator.

The respirators selected are required to be approved by the National Institute for Occupational Safety and Health (NIOSH) and the Mine Safety and Health Administration (MSHA) under the provisions of 30 CFR Part 11. Both federal agencies are responsible for approving and certifying respirators, among other responsibilities. Negative pressure respirators must have filter elements approved by MSHA/NIOSH for organic vapors or benzene.

Employees who cannot wear a negative pressure respirator are to be given the option of wearing a respirator with less breathing resistance such as a powered air purifying (PAPR) or supplied air respirator.

Respirator Program. The respirator program is required to comply with OSHA 29 CFR 1910.134 Respiratory Protection.

Respirator Use. When air purifying respirators are used, the employer must replace the air purifying element at the expiration of its service life or at the beginning of each shift where it is used, whichever comes first.

If the air purifying element has an end-of-useful-life indicator for benzene approved by MSHA/NIOSH, the element can be used until the indicator shows the end of useful life.

Employees who wear respirators are to be permitted to leave regulated areas to wash their faces and respirator face pieces in order to prevent skin irritation associated with respirator use. They must also be permitted to leave to change filter elements of air purifying respirators when they detect a change in breathing resistance or chemical vapor breakthrough.

Respirator Fit Testing. The employer must perform and certify the quantitative or qualitative fit test results at the time of initial fit testing and at least annually thereafter for each employee who wears a negative pressure respirator. (See Table 30-1.)

Protective Clothing and Equipment

Protective clothing and equipment are required to be worn where appropriate to prevent eye contact and to limit skin exposure to benzene. This clothing and equipment are to be provided at no cost to the employee, and the employer must ensure its use when necessary. Eye and face protection must comply with OSHA 29 CFR 1910.133.

Medical Surveillance

Medical surveillance must be made available to employees who

1. Are or may be exposed to benzene above the action level thirty days or more per year.
2. Are or may be exposed to benzene at or above the PELs ten days or more per year.
3. Have been exposed to more than 10 ppm of benzene for thirty or more days in a year prior to the effective date of the standard when employed by their present employer.

TABLE 30-1 Respiratory Protection for Benzene

Airborne Concentration of Benzene or Condition of Use	Minimum Respirator Required
Less than or equal to 10 ppm	Half-mask air purifying respirator with organic vapor cartridge
Less than or equal to 50 ppm	Full face piece respirator with organic vapor cartridges Full face piece gas mask with chin style canister[1]
Less than or equal to 100 ppm	Full face piece powered air purifying respirator with organic vapor canister[1]
Less than or equal to 1,000 ppm	Supplied air respirator with full face piece in positive pressure mode
Greater than 1,000 ppm or unknown concentration	Self-contained breathing apparatus with full face piece in positive pressure mode Full face piece positive pressure supplied air respirator with auxiliary self-contained air supply
Escape	Any organic vapor gas mask or any self-contained breathing apparatus with full face piece
Fire fighting	Full face piece self-contained breathing apparatus in positive pressure mode

[1] Canisters must have a minimum service life of four hours when tested at 150 ppm benzene, at a flow rate of 64 LPM, 25°C, and 85% relative humidity for nonpowered air purifying respirators. The flow rate must be 115 LPM for tight fitting and 170 LPM for loose fitting powered air purifying respirators.

4. Are involved in tire-building operations where they use solvents containing greater than 0.1 ppm benzene.

Medical examinations are to be conducted by licensed physicians, and laboratory tests are to be done by accredited laboratories.

The employer must make sure that if other than licensed physicians conduct pulmonary function tests, those persons must have completed a training course in spirometry sponsored by an appropriate governmental, academic, or professional institution.

All examinations must be at no cost to the employee and at a reasonable time and place.

Initial Examination. Employees must have an initial examination within sixty days of the effective date of this standard, or before initial assignment. The examination must include

1. A detailed occupational history that includes past work exposure to benzene or any other hematological toxins.
2. A family history of blood diseases, including hematological neoplasms.
3. A history of blood diseases, including genetic hemoglobin and bleeding abnormalities, and abnormal function of formed blood elements.
4. A history of renal or liver dysfunction.
5. A history of routinely taken drugs.
6. A history of previous exposure to ionizing radiation.
7. A history of exposure to marrow toxins outside the present work situation.
8. A complete physical examination.
9. Laboratory tests which includes a complete blood count including a **leukocyte count with differential**, a **quantitative thrombocyte count**, hematocrit, hemoglobin, erythrocyte count and **erythrocyte indices** (MCV, MCH, MCHC). A leukocyte count is a count of the white blood corpuscles. A quantitative thrombocyte count is a count of blood platelets. A hematocrit is an evaluation of the iron-containing pigment of the blood cells by using a centrifuge to separate solids from the plasma in the blood. Hemoglobin is the iron-containing pigment of the red blood cells. An erythro-

cyte count is the counting of mature red blood cells or corpuscles. Erythrocyte indices are reference points for evaluation of the red blood cells. The results of these tests must be reviewed by an examining physician.

10. Additional tests as necessary in the opinion of the examining physician, based on alterations to the components of the blood or other signs that may be related to benzene exposure.
11. For all workers required to wear respirators for at least thirty days a year, the physical examination must include the cardiopulmonary system and a pulmonary function test.

An initial examination is not required if the employer can show adequate records that the employee has been examined in accordance with the procedures of this standard within twelve months prior to the effective date of the standard.

Periodic Examinations. Employees required to be included in the medical surveillance under this standard must be provided with an examination annually following the previous examination. The examination must include the following:

1. A brief history regarding any new exposure to potential marrow toxins, changes in medicinal drug use, and the appearance of physical signs relating to blood disorders.
2. A complete blood count including a leukocyte count with differential, quantitative thrombocyte count, hemoglobin, hematocrit, erythrocyte count, and erythrocyte indices (MCV, MCH, MCHC).
3. Appropriate additional tests as necessary in the opinion of the examining physician when there are alterations in the blood components or other signs that may be related to benzene exposure.

When an employee develops signs and symptoms associated with exposure to benzene, the employer must provide the employee with an additional medical examination that includes those elements considered appropriate by the examining physician.

When respirators are required to be worn for at least thirty days a year, a pulmonary function test must be performed every three years. An evaluation of the cardiopulmonary system must be done at the time of the pulmonary function test.

Employees Exposed in Emergency Situations. In emergency situations, in addition to the required medical surveillance under this standard, the employer must have the exposed employee provide a urine sample at the end of the shift and have a urinary phenol test performed on the sample within seventy-two hours. The urine **specific gravity** must be corrected to 1.024.

If the result of the urinary phenol test is below 75 mg phenol/L of urine, no further testing is required.

If the result of the urinary phenol test is equal to or greater than 75 mg phenol/L of urine, the employee must be provided with a complete blood count including an erythrocyte, leukocyte and differential, and thrombocyte count at monthly intervals for a duration of three months following the emergency exposure.

If any conditions specified under "Additional Examinations and Referrals" exist, then the additional requirements of the section must be met and the employer, in addition, must provide employees with periodic examinations if indicated by the physician.

Additional Examinations and Referrals. When the results of the complete blood count required for the initial and periodic examinations indicate any of the following abnormal conditions, the blood count must be repeated within two weeks:

- The hemoglobin level or the hematocrit falls below the normal limit which is outside the 95% confidence interval (CI) as determined by a laboratory for the particular geographic area and/or these indices show a persistent downward trend from the person's preexposure norms (provided these cannot be explained by other medical reasons).
- The thrombocyte (platelet) count varies more than 20 percent below the employee's most re-

cent values or falls outside the normal limit (95% CI) as determined by the laboratory.
- The leukocyte count is below 4,000 per mm^3, or there is an abnormal differential count.

If the abnormality persists, the examining physician must refer the employee to a hematologist or an internist for further evaluation unless the physician believes that such a referral is not necessary.

The employer must provide the hematologist or internist with the information and medical record required to be supplied the physician under this standard.

The hematologist or internist must make a determination as to the need for further tests. If the tests are required, the employer must provide these tests for the employee.

Information provided to the physician. The following information is to be provided to the physician:

- A copy of the standard and its Appendixes
- A description of the employee's duties as they relate to exposure
- The employee's actual or representative exposure level
- A description of any personal protective equipment used or to be used
- Information from previous employment-related examinations that is not available to the examining physician

Physician's Written Opinion. For each examination required under this standard, the employer must provide the employee with a copy of the physician's written opinion within fifteen days of the examination.

The written opinion is required to be limited to the following:

1. The pertinent occupational results of the medical examination and tests.
2. The physician's opinion as to whether the employee has any detected medical conditions that place the employee at greater risk or impairment because of exposure to benzene.
3. The physician's recommended limitations concerning the employee's exposure to ben-

zene or the employee's use of protective clothing, equipment, and respirators.

4. A statement that the employee has been informed by the physician of the results of the medical examination and any medical conditions resulting from benzene exposure that require further explanation and treatment.

The written opinion cannot reveal specific records, findings, and diagnoses that do not relate in any way to the employee's ability to work in a workplace where there is exposure to benzene.

Medical Removal

Medical removal is the temporary removal of an employee from a hazardous exposure in order to reduce the exposure when other methods cannot.

When a physician makes a referral to a hematologist/internist as required under this standard, the employee must be removed from areas where exposure may exceed the action level until the physician makes a determination as described in the next paragraph.

After the examination and evaluation by the hematologist/internist, the physician must consult with the hematologist/internist and a decision is required to be made as to whether the employee is to be removed from areas where benzene exposure is above the action level. The employer and employee must be informed of this decision in writing. If the employee is removed, the physician is required to state the probable duration of removal from occupational exposure above the action level. The physician must also indicate the requirements for future medical examinations to review the decision.

If the employee is removed in accordance with the above paragraph, the employer has to provide for a follow-up examination. The physician, in consultation with the hematologist/internist, must make a decision within six months of the date the employee was removed as to whether the employee must be returned to the usual job or should be removed permanently.

Temporary Removal. When an employee is temporarily removed from exposure in accordance with this standard, the employer must transfer the employee to a comparable job for which he/she is qualified or one for which he/she can be trained in a short period. The employee may also be transferred to a job where the exposure to benzene is as low as possible but in no event higher than the action level. The current wage rate, seniority, and other benefits are required to be maintained by the employer. If no such job is available, the employer must provide medical protection benefits until such job becomes available or for six months, whichever comes first.

Permanent Removal. When an employee is permanently removed from exposure based on a physician's recommendation in accordance with this standard, the employee must be given the opportunity to transfer to another position that is available or becomes available later for which he/she is qualified or can be trained in a short period. The employee may also be transferred to a job where exposure to benzene is as low as possible but in no event higher than the action level. The employer must ensure that the employee will not suffer a reduction in current wage rate, seniority, or other benefits because of the transfer.

Medical Removal Protection Benefits. The employer must provide six months of medical removal protection benefits immediately following the removal of an employee because of hematological findings pursuant to this standard. The exception is if the employee is transferred to a comparable job where benzene exposures are below the action level.

The requirement that an employer provide medical removal protection benefits means that the employer must maintain the current wage rate, seniority, and other benefits as though the employee was never removed.

The medical protection benefits to a removed employee are required to be reduced to the extent that the employee receives compensation for earnings lost during the period of removal either from a publicly or employer-funded compensation program, or from employment with another employer made possible by the removal.

Communication of Benzene Hazards

Signs and labels are required to warn employees of the hazards of benzene exposure.

Signs and Labels. Regulated areas must have the following sign:

Danger. Benzene. Cancer Hazard. Flammable—No Smoking. Authorized Personnel Only.

The employer must make sure that containers are properly labeled. The labels must conform to the requirements of OSHA 1910.1200 Hazard Communication. Pipes do not have to be labeled. Container labels must include the following legend:

Danger. Contains Benzene. Cancer Hazard.

Material Safety Data Sheets

The employer must obtain or develop a material safety data sheet (MSDS) for benzene that complies with OSHA 29 CFR 1910.1200 Hazard Communication.

Information and Training

The employer must train employees and provide information at the time of initial assignment to the work area where benzene is present. If exposures are above the action level, information and training must be provided at least annually.

Training must be in accordance with OSHA 1910.1200 Hazard Communication and must include specific information on benzene for each category of information included in this standard.

In addition to the information required under 29 CFR 1910.1200, the employer must

1. Provide an explanation of the contents of this standard, including Appendixes A and B, and indicate where the standard is available.
2. Describe the medical surveillance program required in this standard and explain the information contained in Appendix C.

Recordkeeping

Exposure and medical records must be kept on all employees exposed to benzene.

Exposure Measurement Records. The employer must establish and maintain an accurate record of all measurements required by this standard and in accordance with OSHA 29 CFR 1910.1020 Access to Employee Exposure and Medical Records (Chapter 5).

The record must include

1. Dates, number, and results of each sample taken, including a description of the procedure used to determine representative employee exposures.
2. A description of the sampling and analytical methods used.
3. A description of the types of respirators worn, if any.
4. Name, social security number, job classification, and exposure levels of the employee monitored and all other employees whose exposure the measure is intended to represent.

This record must be maintained for at least thirty years in accordance with OSHA 29 CFR 1910.1020.

Medical Surveillance Record. This record must include the following:

1. Name and social security number of the employee.
2. The employer's copy of the physician's written opinion on the initial, periodic, and special examinations, including results of medical examinations and all tests, opinions, and recommendations.
3. Any employee medical complaints related to exposure.
4. A copy of the information provided to the physician as required by this standard.
5. A copy of the employee's medical and work history related to exposure to benzene or any other hematologic toxins.

The employer must maintain this record for the duration of employment plus thirty years in accordance with OSHA 1910.1020.

Records Availability. The employer must make all records available to OSHA upon request for examination and copying.

Employee monitoring records required by this standard must be provided upon request for examination and copying to employees, employee representatives, and OSHA in accordance with 1910.1020.

Employee medical records required by this standard must provided upon request for examination and copying to the employee, to anyone having a specific written consent of the employee, and to OSHA.

Records Transfer. The employer must comply with the requirements of OSHA 29 CFR 1910.1020 when records are transferred.

If the employer stops doing business and there is no successor employer to receive and retain the records for the required period, the employer must notify OSHA at least three months prior to disposal, and send them to OSHA if required by them within that period.

CHAPTER REVIEW

Multiple Choice

Select the best answer from the choices provided.

1. Benzene is a(n)
   a. halogen
   b. hydrocarbon
   c. polymer
   d. acid

2. A regulated area is required to control benzene airborne concentrations when the
   a. TWA of 1 ppm is exceeded
   b. STEL of 5 ppm is exceeded
   c. action level of 0.5 ppm is exceeded
   d. a and b

3. Medical examinations are to be conducted by
   a. medical technicians
   b. physicians
   c. nurses
   d. a, b, and c

4. Benzene is mainly a
   a. cancer hazard
   b. skin hazard
   c. ingestion hazard
   d. eye hazard

5. Benzene exposure records of employees must be made available to
   a. NIOSH
   b. EPA
   c. OSHA
   d. DOT

True/False

Indicate whether the statement is true or false by circling T or F.

6. T F The time weighted average for benzene is 2 ppm.

7. T F Respirators used for benzene exposure must be approved by OSHA.

8. T F Medical removal is required when the benzene action level is or may be exceeded.

9. T F Airborne concentrations less than or equal to 1,000 ppm benzene require a half-mask air purifying respirator with vapor cartridge to be worn.

10. T F Only licensed physicians can conduct pulmonary function tests.

Matching

Match the terms in column 1 with the definitions in column 2.

Column 1

11. 0.5 ppm
12. Thirty days after benzene introduced
13. More than 1,000 ppm concentration
14. History of renal or liver dysfunction
15. Duration of employment plus thirty years

Column 2

a. Part of clinical examination
b. Medical record retention
c. Action level
d. Monitoring required
e. SCBA respirator required

Short Answer

Briefly but thoroughly answer each statement.

16. Explain how employees can be exposed to benzene vapors.

17. Describe where there is exposure to benzene in your health care facility.

18. Describe how exposure to benzene can be controlled.

19. Explain the monitoring requirements when employees are exposed to benzene vapors.

20. Describe the medical removal protection requirements for employees exposed to benzene.

CHAPTER 31

Lead

After studying this chapter, you should be able to

➤ Describe the OSHA lead standard requirements.
➤ State how lead affects the body.
➤ List the engineering and work practice controls used to control lead exposure.
➤ Describe the medical examination and medical removal protection procedures required for employees exposed to lead.

Employees who are exposed to lead are covered under OSHA 29 CFR 1910.1025 Lead. Employees in the construction trades are covered under OSHA 29 CFR 1926.62 Lead (construction standards), which follows the lead general industry standards.

Lead exposure can cause anemia, kidney damage, paralysis, coma, and death.

OSHA 29 CFR 1910.1025 LEAD

OSHA has specific requirements that the employer must follow to control employee lead exposure.

Definitions

Action level refers to employee exposure, without regard to the use of respirators, to an airborne concentration of lead of 30 micrograms per cubic meter of air ($30\,\mu g/m^3$) averaged over an eight-hour period.

Lead means metallic lead, all inorganic lead compounds, and organic lead soaps. Excluded from the definition are all other organic lead compounds.

Permissible exposure limit (PEL). The employer shall assure that no employee is exposed to lead concentrations greater than 50 micrograms per cubic meter of air ($50\,\mu g/m^3$) averaged over an eight-hour period.

If an employee works more than eight hours a day, the formula to determine exposure limit is 400 divided by the number of hours worked (400/hrs. worked).

Employer Lead Control

The employer must conform to specific requirements concerning lead exposure.

Exposure Monitoring. Employee exposure is the exposure that would occur if the employee were not using a respirator.

The employer shall collect full-shift (for at least seven continuous hours) personal samples including at least one sample for each shift for each job classification in each work area.

Full-shift personal samples shall be representative of the monitored employee's regular, daily exposure to lead.

The employer shall monitor employee exposures and base initial determinations on the employee exposure monitoring results and any of the following relevant considerations:

• Any information, observations, or calculations that would indicate employee exposure to lead
• Any previous measurements of airborne lead
• Any employee complaints of symptoms that may be attributable to lead exposure

If the initial determination or subsequent monitoring reveals employee exposure to be at or above the action level but below the permissible exposure limit, the employer shall repeat monitoring every six months.

If the initial monitoring reveals that employee exposure is above the permissible exposure limit, the employer shall repeat monitoring quarterly. The employer shall continue monitoring at the required frequency until at least two consecutive measurements, taken seven days apart, are below the PEL but at or above the action level, at which time the employer shall repeat monitoring for the employee at least every six months.

Whenever there is a production, process, control, or personnel change that may result in new or additional exposures to lead, or whenever the employer has any other reason to suspect a change that may result in new or additional exposures to lead, additional monitoring shall be conducted in accordance with this paragraph.

Within five working days after receipt of monitoring results, the employer shall notify each employee in writing of the results that represent that employee's exposure.

Whenever the results indicate that the representative employee exposure, without regard to the use of respirators, exceeds the permissible exposure limit, the employer shall include in the written notice a statement that the permissible exposure limit was exceeded and a description of the corrective action taken or to be taken to reduce exposure to or below the permissible exposure limit.

Methods of Compliance. Where any employee is exposed to lead above the permissible exposure limit for more than thirty days per year, the employer must implement engineering and work practice controls (including administrative controls) to reduce employee exposure to lead, except to the extent that the employer can demonstrate that such controls are not feasible. Wherever the engineering and work practice controls that can be instituted are not sufficient to reduce employee exposure to or below the permissible exposure limit, the employer shall nonetheless use them to reduce exposures to the lowest feasible level and shall supplement them by the use of respiratory equipment that complies with this section.

When any employee is exposed to lead above the permissible exposure limit, but for thirty days or less per year, the employer shall implement engi-

neering controls to reduce exposures to 200 µg/m^3, but thereafter may implement any combination of engineering and work practice (including administrative) to reduce and maintain concentrations below 50 µg/m^3.

When engineering and work practice controls do not reduce employee exposure to or below the 50 µg/m^3 permissible exposure limit, the employer must supplement these controls with respirators in accordance with this paragraph.

Compliance Program. Each employer shall establish and implement a written compliance program to reduce exposures to or below the permissible exposure limit, and interim levels, if applicable, solely by means of engineering and work practice controls.

Written plans for these compliance programs must include at least the following:

- A description of each operation in which lead is emitted
- A description of the specific means that will be used to achieve compliance
- A report of the technology considered in meeting the permissible exposure limit
- Air-monitoring data that documents the source of lead emissions
- A detailed schedule for implementation of the program
- A work practice program that includes items required in the regulation
- An administrative control schedule required by the regulation
- Other relevant information.

Written programs must be revised and updated at least every six months to reflect the current status of the program.

Mechanical Ventilation. When ventilation is used to control exposure, measurements that demonstrate the effectiveness of the system in controlling exposure, such as capture velocity, duct velocity, or static pressure, shall be made at least every three months. Measurements of the system's effectiveness in controlling exposure shall be made within five days of any change in production, process, or control that might result in a change in employee exposure to lead.

If air from the exhaust ventilation system is recirculated into the workplace, the employer must assure that the system has both a high-efficiency filter with reliable backup filter and controls that monitor the concentration of lead in the return air and that bypass the recirculation system automatically if it fails. These devices must be installed, operating, and maintained.

Administrative Controls. If administrative controls are used as a means of reducing employee TWA exposure to lead, the employer shall establish a job rotation schedule that includes name and identification number of each affected employee, duration and exposure levels at each job or workstation where each affected employee is located, and any other information that may be useful in assessing the reliability of administrative controls to reduce exposure to lead.

Respiratory Protection

Where the use of respirators is required under this section, the employer shall provide (at no cost to the employee) and assure the use of respirators that comply with the requirements of this paragraph. Respirators shall be used in the following circumstances:

- During the time period necessary to install or implement engineering or work practice controls, except no employer shall require an employee to wear a negative pressure respirator longer than 4.4 hours per day
- In work situations in which engineering and work practice controls are not sufficient to reduce exposures to or below the permissible exposure limit
- Whenever an employee requests a respirator

Where respirators are required, the employer shall select the appropriate respirator or combination of respirators as shown in Table 31-1.

The employer shall provide a powered, air purifying respirator in lieu of the respirator specified whenever an employee chooses to use this type of respirator and the respirator will provide adequate protection to the employee.

The employer shall assure that the respirator issued to the employee exhibits minimum face piece leakage and that the respirator is fitted properly.

Employers shall perform either quantitative or qualitative face fit tests at the time of initial fitting and at least every six months thereafter for each employee wearing negative pressure respirators.

TABLE 31-1 Respiratory Protection for Lead Aerosols	
Airborne Concentration of Lead or Condition of Use	**Minimum Respirator Required[1]**
Not in excess of 0.5 mg/m^3 ($10 \times$ PEL)	Half-mask, air purifying respirator equipped with HEPA filters[2]
Not in excess of 2.5 mg/m^3 ($50 \times$ PEL)	Full face piece, air purifying respirator with HEPA filters
Not in excess of 50 mg/m^3 ($1,000 \times$ PEL)	(1) Powered air purifying respirator with HEPA filters or (2) Half-mask supplied air respirator operated in positive pressure mode
Not in excess of 100 mg/m^3 ($2,000 \times$ PEL)	Supplied air respirator with full face piece, hood, helmet, or suit, operated in positive pressure mode
Greater than 100 mg/m^3, unknown concentrations, or fire fighting	Full face piece, self-contained breathing apparatus operated in positive pressure mode

[1] Respirators specified for high concentrations of lead can be used for lower concentrations, and if lead aerosols cause eye or skin irritation where half-masks are specified, a full face piece is required.
[2] High-efficiency particulate air (HEPA) filters trap 99.97% of particles 0.3 microns or larger.

If an employee exhibits difficulty in breathing during the fitting test or during use, the employer shall make available to the employee an examination to determine whether the employee can wear a respirator while performing the required duty.

The employer shall institute a respiratory protection program in accordance with 29 CFR 1910.134.

The employer shall permit each employee who uses a filter respirator to change the filter elements whenever an increase in breathing resistance is detected and shall maintain an adequate supply of filters for this purpose.

Employees who wear respirators shall be permitted to leave work areas to wash their face and respirator whenever necessary to prevent skin irritation associated with respirator use.

Protective Work Clothing and Equipment.
If an employee is exposed to lead above the PEL, without regard to the use of respirators, or where the possibility of skin or eye irritation exists, the employer shall provide (at no cost to the employee) and assure that the employee uses appropriate protective work clothing and equipment such as, but not limited to, coveralls or similar full-body work clothing; gloves, hats, and shoes or disposable shoe coverlets; and face shields, vented goggles, or other appropriate protective equipment.

The employer shall provide the protective clothing in a clean and dry condition at least weekly, and daily to employees whose exposure levels, without regard to respirators, are over 200 µg/m^3 of lead as an eight-hour TWA.

The employer shall provide for the cleaning, laundering, or disposal of protective clothing.

The employer shall repair or replace required protective clothing and equipment as needed to maintain effectiveness.

The employer shall assure that protective clothing is removed at the completion of the work shift only in change rooms provided for this purpose.

The employer shall assure that contaminated protective clothing that is to be cleaned, laundered, or disposed of is placed in a closed container in the change room. That container must prevent dispersion of lead outside the container.

The employer shall inform in writing any person who cleans or launders protective clothing or equipment of the potentially harmful effects of exposure to lead.

The employer shall assure that the containers of contaminated protective clothing and equipment are labeled: **"Caution: Clothing Contaminated With Lead. Do Not Remove Dust By Blowing Or Shaking. Dispose Of Lead Contaminated Wash Water In Accordance With Applicable Local, State, Or Federal Regulations."**

Housekeeping

All surfaces shall be maintained as free as practicable of accumulations of lead.

Where vacuuming methods are selected, the vacuums shall be used and emptied in a manner that minimizes the re-entry of lead into the workplace.

Hygiene Facilities and Practices

Hygiene facilities and practices must be maintained to control lead exposure to persons other than lead workers.

Change Rooms. The employer must provide clean change rooms for employees who work in areas where their airborne exposure to lead is above the PEL, without regard to the use of respirators.

Change rooms shall be equipped with separate storage facilities for protective work clothing and equipment and for street clothes. This separation prevents cross-contamination.

Showers. The employer shall assure that employees who work in areas where their airborne exposure to lead is above the PEL, without regard to the use of respirators, shower at the end of the work shift. Shower facilities must be provided by the employer.

The employer shall assure that employees who are required to shower do not leave the workplace wearing clothing or equipment worn during the work shift.

Lunchrooms. The employer shall provide lunchroom facilities for employees who work in areas where their airborne concentrations to lead are above the PEL, without regard to the use of respirators.

The employer shall assure that employees who work in areas where airborne exposure to lead is above the PEL, without regard to the use of respirators, wash their hands and face prior to eating, drinking, smoking, or applying cosmetics.

The employer shall assure that employees do not enter lunchroom facilities with protective work clothing or equipment unless surface lead dust has been removed by downdraft booth or other cleaning method.

Medical Surveillance. The employer must institute a medical surveillance program for all employees exposed above the action level for more than thirty days per year.

The employer shall assure that all medical examinations and procedures are performed by or under the supervision of a licensed physician.

The employer shall provide the required medical surveillance, including multiple physician review, without cost to the employee and at a reasonable time and place.

Biological Monitoring. The employer shall make available biological monitoring in the form of blood sampling and analysis for lead and **zinc protoporphyrin test (ZPP)** levels to each employee exposed above the action level for more than thirty days per year on the following schedule (zinc protoporphyrin is a test that determines the effects of lead on the body):

- At least every six months for each employee covered under this section.
- At least every two months for each employee whose blood lead level is at or above 40µg/100 g of whole blood. This frequency must continue until two consecutive blood samples and analyses indicate a blood lead level below 40 µg/100 g of whole blood.
- At least monthly during the removal period of each employee removed from exposure to lead due to an elevated blood level.

Within five working days after receipt of biological monitoring results, the employer shall notify in writing each employee whose blood lead level exceeds 40 µg/100 g.

The employer must make available medical examinations and consultations to each employee exposed above the action level for more than thirty days per year. The examinations must be done prior to assignment to areas where concentrations are above the action level, as soon as possible when an employee develops signs or symptoms associated with lead poisoning, or when an employee experiences difficulty in breathing during a respirator fit test.

The examination must consist of a detailed work history and medical history; a thorough physical examination; a blood pressure measurement; a blood sample and analysis that determines blood lead level and **hemoglobin** (the iron-containing pigment of the red blood cells) and **hematocrit** (an evaluation of the red blood cells using a centrifuge); zinc protoporphyrin; blood urea nitrogen; serum creatinine; routine urinalysis; any laboratory or other test that the examining physician deems necessary by sound medical practice.

The employer shall promptly notify an employee of the right to seek a second medical opinion after each occasion that an initial physician conducts a medical examination or consultation.

If the findings, determinations, or recommendations of the second physician differ from those of the initial physician, then the employer and the employee shall assure that efforts are made for the two physicians to resolve any disagreement.

Information Provided to Examining and Consulting Physicians. The employer shall provide an initial physician conducting a medical examination or consultation under this section with the following information:

- A copy of this regulation for lead, including all appendices
- A description of the employee's duties
- The employee's level or anticipated exposure to lead or any other toxic substance
- A description of any personal protective equipment used
- Prior blood lead determinations
- All prior written medical opinions concerning the employee in the employer's possession or control

The employer shall obtain and furnish the employee with a copy of written medical opinions from each examining or consulting physician that contains the following information:

- The physician's opinion as to whether the employee has a detected medical condition that would place the employee at risk
- Any recommended special protective measures
- Any recommended limitation upon the use of respirators
- The results of the blood lead determinations

Medical Removal Protection (MRP). Medical removal is the temporary removal of an employee from a hazardous exposure in order to reduce the exposure when other methods cannot. The employer shall remove any employee from work having an exposure to lead at or above the action level on each occasion that the average of the last three blood sampling tests conducted indicates that the employee's blood lead level is at or above 50μg/100 g of whole blood; provided, however, that an employee need not be removed if the last blood sampling test indicates a blood lead level at or above 40μg/100 g of whole blood.

The employer must remove any employee from work having an exposure to lead at or above the action level on each occasion that a final medical determination, or opinion that the employee has a detected medical condition that places the employee at increased risk of material impairment to health from exposure to lead.

The employer shall return an employee to his or her former job status according to the following guidelines:

- For an employee removed due to a blood lead level at or above 80 μg/100 g, when two consecutive blood sampling tests indicate that the employee's blood lead level is at or below 60 μg/100 g of whole blood
- For an employee removed due to a blood lead level at or above 70 μg/100 g, when two consecutive blood sampling tests indicate that the employee's blood lead level is at or below 50 μg/100 g of whole blood

- For an employee removed due to a blood lead level at or above 60 μg/100 g, or when two consecutive blood sampling tests indicate that the employee's blood lead level is at or below 40 μg/100 g of whole blood
- For an employee removed due to a final medical determination, when a final medical determination results in a medical finding, determination, or opinion that the employee no longer has a detected medical condition that places the employee at increased risk of material impairment to health from exposure to lead.

The employer shall provide to an employee up to eighteen months of medical removal protection. The employer shall maintain the earnings, seniority, and other employment rights and benefits of the employee as though the employee had not been removed from normal exposure to lead or otherwise limited.

The employer shall take the following measures with respect to any employee removed from exposure to lead due to an elevated blood lead level whose blood lead level has not declined within the past eighteen months of removal so that the employee has been returned to his or her former job status:

- The employer shall make available to the employee a medical examination.
- The employer shall assure that the final medical determination obtained indicates whether or not the employee may be returned to his or her former status, and if not, what steps should be taken to protect the employee's health
- Where the final medical determination indicates that the employee may not be returned to his or her former job status, the employer shall continue to provide medical removal protection benefits to the employee until a final determination is made
- Where the employer acts pursuant to a final medical determination that permits the return of the employee to his or her former job status despite what would otherwise be an unacceptable blood lead level, later questions concerning removing the employee shall again be decided by a final medical determination.

Where an employer, although not required to do so, removes an employee from exposure to lead or otherwise places limitations on an employee due to effects of lead exposure on the employee's medical condition, the employer shall provide medical removal protection benefits to the employee.

Employee Information and Training. The employer shall institute a training program for and assure the participation of all employees who are subject to exposure to lead at or above the action level or for whom the possibility of skin or eye irritation exists.

The training program shall be repeated at least annually for each employee.

The employer shall assure that each employee is informed of the following:

- Content of the lead standard and appendices
- The specific nature of the operations that could result in exposure to lead above the action level
- The purpose, proper selection, fitting, use, and limitations of respirators
- The purpose and description of the medical surveillance program including information concerning the adverse health effects associated with excessive exposure to lead (with particular attention to adverse effects specific to males and females)
- The engineering controls and work practices associated with the employee's job assignment
- The contents of the compliance plan in effect
- Instructions to employees that chelating agents should not be routinely used to remove lead from their bodies and should not be used at all except under the direction of a licensed physician

The employer shall make readily available to all affected employees a copy of this standard and its appendices.

Signs. The employer shall post the following warning signs in each work area where the PEL is exceeded: **Warning—Lead Work Area—Poison—No Smoking Or Eating**.

Recordkeeping. The employer shall establish and maintain an accurate record of all monitoring required. This record must include the following:

- The date(s), number, duration, location, and results of each of the samples taken, including a description of the sampling procedure used
- A description of the sampling and analytical methods used
- The type of respiratory protective devices worn, if any
- Name, social security number, and job classification of the employee monitored
- The environmental variables that could affect the measurement of employee exposure

The employer shall maintain these monitoring records for at least forty years or for the duration of employment plus twenty years, whichever is longer.

The employer shall establish and maintain an accurate record for each employee subject to medical surveillance. This record must include the name, social security number, and description of duties of the employee; a copy of the physician's written opinions; results of any airborne monitoring; and any employee complaints related to exposure to lead.

The employer shall keep, and assure that the examining physician keeps, the following medical records: a copy of the medical examination results, a description of the laboratory procedures, and a copy of the results of biological monitoring.

The employer shall maintain or assure that the physician maintains those medical records for at least forty years or for the duration of employment plus twenty years, whichever is longer.

The employer shall establish and maintain an accurate record of each employee removed from current exposure to lead. Each record shall include the name and social security number of the employee, the date on each occasion the employee was removed from the current exposure to lead, a brief explanation of how each removal was or is being accomplished, and a statement indicating whether or not the removal was for an elevated blood lead level.

The employer shall maintain each medical removal record for at least the duration of the employee's employment.

Observation of Monitoring. Whenever observation of the monitoring of employee exposure to lead requires entry in an area where the use of respirators, protective clothing, or protective equipment is required, the employer shall provide the observer with and assure the use of such respirators, clothing, and equipment and shall require the observer to comply with all applicable safety and health procedures.

Without interfering with the monitoring, observers shall be entitled to receive an explanation of the measurement procedures, observe all steps related to the monitoring of lead, and record the results obtained or receive copies of the results when returned by the laboratory.

CHAPTER REVIEW

Multiple Choice

Select the best answer from the choices provided.

1. The time weighted average for lead exposure is

    a. $25 \, \mu g/m^3$
    b. $30 \, \mu g/m^3$
    c. $50 \, \mu g/m^3$
    d. $60 \, \mu g/m^3$

2. A full facepiece, self-contained breathing apparatus operated in the positive pressure mode can be used for concentrations greater than

    a. $2.5 \, mg/m^3$
    b. $50 \, mg/m^3$
    c. $100 \, mg/m^3$
    d. a, b, and c

3. HEPA filters trap 99.97% of particles

    a. 0.1 microns or larger
    b. 0.3 microns or larger
    c. 0.5 microns or larger
    d. 0.8 microns or larger

4. The action level starts

    a. monitoring
    b. cleaning
    c. signage
    d. MRP
    e. ZPP test

5. When employees are exposed to lead in concentrations exceeding the action level, the employer must institute

    a. monitoring
    b. medical surveillance
    c. training and education
    d. a, b, and c

True/False

Indicate whether the statement is true or false by circling T or F.

6. T F Engineering controls are to be used before work practice controls in controlling lead exposure.

7. T F A powered air purifying respirator with HEPA filter and half-mask supplied air respirator operated in the positive pressure mode are to be worn for concentrations not exceeding $100 \, mg/m^3$.

8. T F Industrial-type vacuum cleaners can be used to vacuum up lead particles.

9. T F The effects of lead on the body are determined by the ZPP test.

10. T F An employer can voluntarily put an employee on MRP.

Short Answer

Briefly but thoroughly answer each statement.

11. Describe some of the symptoms that would indicate that an employee has lead poisoning.

12. List some of the personal protective equipment (PPE) you would issue employees exposed to lead. PPE must conform to what OSHA standard?

13. Describe some of the training elements for employees exposed to lead.

14. Explain how you would control airborne concentrations of lead.

CHAPTER 32

Asbestos

After studying this chapter, you should be able to

➤ Discuss the OSHA requirements of the asbestos standard.
➤ Describe the required respirator for the airborne concentration.
➤ Describe the required training for employees exposed to asbestos.
➤ List the content of the medical surveillance program.
➤ State the requirements for regulated areas.

The OSHA general industry standard for asbestos is 29 CFR 1910.1001. It covers all employees exposed to asbestos who are not involved in construction activities. The OSHA standard for construction employees is 29 CFR 1926.1101—not discussed here because health care personnel will generally not get involved with this type of work. Allied health personnel will be covered under the general industry standard.

OSHA 29 CFR 1910.1001 ASBESTOS

The asbestos standard covers occupational exposure.

Definitions

Asbestos is a hydrated magnesium silicate in the form of a fiber.

Asbestos-containing material (ACM) refers to any material containing more than 1 percent asbestos.

High-efficiency particulate air (HEPA) filter is a filter capable of trapping and retaining at least 99.97 percent of 0.3 micrometer diameter mono-dispersed particles.

Presumed asbestos-containing material (PACM) refers to thermal insulation sprayed on or troweled on surfacing material and debris in work areas where such material is present.

Regulated area is an area established by the employer to demarcate where airborne concentrations of asbestos exceed or there is a reasonable possibility they may exceed the permissible exposure limit (maximum concentration of a toxic substance employees can be exposed to over a designated period of time).

Permissible Exposure Limits (PELs). The employer shall ensure that no employee is exposed to an airborne concentration of asbestos of 0.1 fiber per cubic centimeter of air as an eight-hour time weighted average (TWA).

The employer shall ensure that no employee is exposed to an airborne concentration of asbestos in excess of 1.0 fiber per cubic centimeter of air as averaged over a sampling period of thirty (30) minutes. This is the **excursion limit**.

Monitoring. Initial monitoring must be done when employees are, or may reasonably be expected to be, exposed to airborne concentrations at or above the TWA permissible exposure limit and/or excursion limit.

After initial monitoring, samples shall be of such frequency and pattern as to represent with reasonable accuracy the level of exposure of employees. In no case shall sampling be at intervals greater than six months.

When monitoring determines that employees are exposed below the TWA or excursion limit, the employer may discontinue monitoring.

The employer shall, within fifteen working days after receipt of the results of any monitoring, notify the affected employees of the results. The written notification shall contain the corrective action being taken to reduce employee exposure to or below the TWA and/or excursion limit whenever monitoring results indicate that the TWA and/or excursion limit has been exceeded.

Regulated Areas. Regulated areas must be established whenever airborne concentrations of asbestos and/or PACM are in excess of the TWA and/or excursion limit.

Regulated areas must be demarcated from the rest of the workplace and access limited to authorized persons.

Each person entering a regulated area shall be supplied with and required to use the proper respirator.

Employees must not be allowed to eat, drink, smoke, chew tobacco or gum, or apply cosmetics in regulated areas.

Engineering Controls and Work Practices. Engineering and work practice controls must be used to reduce exposure to or below the TWA and/or excursion limit. If these controls do not reduce exposure to or below the TWA and/or excursion limit, they must be used to reduce levels as low as possible, and then the employer must supplement these controls with respirators.

Insofar as practicable, asbestos shall be wetted down whenever it is handled, cut, scored, or otherwise worked.

Sanding of asbestos-containing flooring is prohibited.

Compliance Program. Where the TWA and/or excursion limit is exceeded, the employer shall establish and implement a written program to reduce employee exposure to below the TWA and excursion limit. This must be done through the use of engineering and work practice controls and by the use of respiratory equipment where required.

The written program must be reviewed and updated as necessary.

The employer cannot use employee rotation as a means of compliance with the TWA and/or excursion limit.

Respirator Program. The employer must supply respirators (see Table 32-1) in the following circumstances:

- During the interval necessary to install or implement engineering and work practice controls
- In work operations, such as maintenance and repair, for which engineering and work practice controls are not feasible
- In work situations where feasible engineering and work practice controls are not yet sufficient to reduce exposure to or below the TWA and/or excursion limit
- In emergencies

Each employee who uses a filter respirator must be permitted to change filter elements whenever an increase in breathing resistance is detected.

Employees who wear respirators shall be permitted to leave the regulated area to wash their faces and respirator facepieces whenever necessary to prevent skin irritation.

For each employee wearing negative pressure respirators, employers shall perform either **qualitative** or **quantitative fit testing** when the employee is first issued the respirator and at least every six months thereafter. Qualitative fit testing is a pass/fail test that tests the adequacy of the fit by relying on a response to a test agent; quantitative fit testing numerically assesses the adequacy of the fit by measuring the amount of leakage in the face piece.

Protective Work Clothing. If an employee is exposed to asbestos above the TWA and/or excursion limit, or where the possibility of eye irritation exists, the employer shall provide (at no cost to the employee) appropriate protective clothing.

The employer must assure that employees remove protective work clothing in change rooms provided for this purpose.

TABLE 32-1 Respiratory Protection for Asbestos Fibers

Airborne Concentration of Asbestos or Conditions of Use	Minimum Respirator Required
Not in excess of 1 f/cc (10 × PEL), or otherwise as required independent of an exposure pursuant to (h)(2)(iv) of the standard	Half-mask air purifying respirator other than a disposable respirator, equipped with a high-efficiency filter.
Not in excess of 5 f/cc (50 × PEL)	Full face piece air purifying respirator equipped with high-efficiency filter.
Not in excess of 10 f/cc (100 × PEL)	Any powered air purifying respirator equipped with high-efficiency filter or any supplied air respirator operated in the continuous flow mode.
Not in excess of 100 f/cc (1,000 × PEL)	Full face piece supplied air respirator operated in the pressure demand mode.
Greater than 100 f/cc (1,000 × PEL) or unknown concentration	Full face piece supplied air respirator operated in the pressure demand mode, equipped with an auxiliary positive pressure self-contained breathing apparatus.

Notes:
- Respirators that are listed for high concentrations may be used at lower concentrations, or when respirator use is independent of concentration.
- A high-efficiency filter will filter out at least 99.97 percent of dispersed particles 0.3 micrometers or larger in diameter.
- Employees must be permitted to change filters whenever a resistance to breathing is experienced when wearing a filter respirator. They must also be permitted to leave regulated work areas to wash their face and respirator face piece whenever necessary to prevent skin irritation.

Work clothing is not permitted to be taken out of the change room.

Contaminated work clothing must be placed and stored in closed containers to prevent dispersion of asbestos.

The employer shall clean, launder, repair, or replace protective clothing and equipment to maintain effectiveness. Clean clothing and equipment must be supplied at least weekly.

Laundering must be done to prevent the release of airborne fibers. When contaminated clothing is given to another to clean, that person must be informed to prevent release of fibers in excess of permissible exposure limits. The person must also be informed of the harmful effects of asbestos.

Contaminated clothing shall be transported in sealed, permeable bags or other closed containers.

Hygiene Facilities. Clean change rooms must be provided when employees are exposed to levels above the TWA and/or excursion limit. Provision must be made to separate work clothes from street clothes.

Employees exposed to levels above the TWA and/or excursion limit must be provided with showers.

Lunchrooms must have a positive pressure filtered air supply.

The employer must make sure that employees wash their hands and faces prior to eating, drinking, smoking, or applying cosmetics.

Employees cannot enter lunchroom facilities with work clothing unless surface asbestos has been removed by vacuuming or other method that removes dust without causing it to become airborne.

Employees in work areas are not permitted to smoke in these areas.

Building and Facility Owners. Employers and building and facility owners must inform employees about the presence and location of ACM and PACM. Records must be maintained concerning the presence and location of ACM and PACM.

Building and facility owners and employers must inform employees who will perform housekeeping activities in areas that contain ACM and PACM of the presence and location of ACM and/or PACM.

Warning Signs. Warning signs must be posted at each regulated area. The sign must bear the following information:

Danger
Asbestos
Cancer and Lung Disease Hazard
Authorized Personnel Only
Respirators and Protective
Clothing are Required In This Area

Warning labels shall be affixed to all raw materials, mixtures, scrap, waste, debris, and other products containing asbestos fibers or to their containers. The label shall read:

Danger
Contains Asbestos Fibers
Avoid Creating Dust
Cancer and Lung Disease Hazard

Employee Information and Training. The employer shall institute a training program for all employees who are exposed to airborne concentrations at or above the TWA and/or excursion limit.

Training must be provided at the time of initial assignment and at least annually thereafter.

The training shall include the following:

- The health effects associated with asbestos exposure
- The relationship between smoking and asbestos producing lung cancer

- The nature of operations that can result in asbestos exposure
- The engineering and work practice controls associated with the employee's job assignment
- The specific procedures implemented to protect employees from exposure
- The purpose, proper use, and limitations of respirators and protective clothing
- The purpose and description of the medical surveillance program
- The content of the standard
- The names, addresses, and phone numbers of public health organizations that provide information on smoking cessation
- The requirement of posting signs and labels

The employer must also train employees who perform housekeeping operations in a facility that contains ACM or PACM on asbestos awareness. The course must include:

- Health effects of asbestos
- Locations of ACM and PACM
- Recognition of damaged ACM and PACM
- Proper response to fiber release episodes

These employees must be trained at least once a year.

Housekeeping. All surfaces shall be maintained as free as practicable of accumulation of dusts and waste asbestos.

All spills and sudden releases of material containing asbestos shall be cleaned up as soon as possible.

Surfaces contaminated with asbestos may not be cleaned by the use of compressed air.

HEPA-filtered vacuuming equipment must be used and emptied in a manner that minimizes the re-entry of asbestos into the workplace. A HEPA filter is a high-efficiency particulate air filter that traps 99.97 percent of particles 0.3 microns or larger.

Shoveling, dry sweeping, and dry cleanup may only be used when vacuuming or wet cleaning is not feasible.

Waste asbestos must be put in sealed impermeable bags or closed impermeable containers.

Medical Surveillance. The employer must institute a medical surveillance program for all employees exposed or who will be exposed at or above the TWA and/or excursion limit.

Medical examinations must be done by a licensed physician or under the supervision of a licensed physician.

Persons other than a licensed physician who administer the pulmonary function test shall complete a training course in spirometry.

Before an employee is assigned to an occupation exposed to asbestos fibers at or above the TWA and/or excursion limit, a preplacement examination must be provided. The examination must include a medical and work history; a complete examination of all systems with emphasis on the respiratory system, cardiovascular system, and digestive tract; completion of the respiratory disease standardized questionnaire in Appendix D, Part 1; a chest roentgenogram; pulmonary function test that includes forced vital capacity and forced expiratory volume at one second; and any additional tests deemed necessary by the physician.

Periodic examinations shall be made available annually.

The employer shall provide, or make available, a termination of employment examination for any employee exposed to fibers of asbestos at or above the TWA and/or excursion limit.

The employer must provide the physician the following information for examinations: a copy of the OSHA standard and Appendices D and E; a description of the employee's duties; the employee's exposure level or anticipated level; a description of any personal protective and respiratory equipment used; and information from previous examinations.

The physician must provide the employer a written opinion containing the results of the medical examination. This includes the following:

- The physician's opinion as to whether the employee has any detected medical conditions that would place the employee at risk of health impairment from exposure to asbestos
- Any limitations on the use of personal protective equipment or respirators
- A statement that the employee has been informed by the physician of the results of the medical examination resulting from asbestos exposure that require further treatment
- A statement that the employee has been informed of the increased risk of lung cancer from the combined effect of smoking and exposure to asbestos

A copy of the physician's written opinion must be given to the employee within thirty days from its receipt.

Recordkeeping. Records of exposure measurements must kept and maintained. They must include the date of measurement; the operation involving exposure to asbestos that was monitored; sampling and analytical methods used; number, duration, and results of samples taken; type of respiratory devices worn, if any; and name, social security number, and exposure of the employee. The record must be maintained for at least thirty years.

The employer shall establish and maintain an accurate record of each employee subject to medical surveillance. The record must include the name and social security number of the employee; physician's written opinions; any employee medical complaints relating to asbestos exposure; and a copy of the information provided to the physician.

This record must be kept for the duration of employment plus thirty years.

Training records shall be maintained for one year beyond the last date of employment of the employee.

Exposure and medical records must be made available to employees upon request.

CHAPTER REVIEW

True/False
Indicate whether the statement is true or false by circling T or F.

1. T F The excursion limit for asbestos is 1.0 fiber per cubic centimeter.

2. T F Employee rotation may be used as a means to reduce exposure below the time weighted average.

3. T F A full face piece supplied air respirator operated in the pressure demand mode can be used for concentrations greater than 100 fibers per cubic centimeter.

4. T F Employees exposed above the time weighted average or excursion limit need not wear PPE such as enclosed suits as long as they are wearing the proper respirator.

5. T F Asbestos-containing material (ACM) may be removed by compressed air only if there is a enclosed ventilation system

Matching
Match the terms in column 1 with the definitions in column 2.

Column 1
6. Asbestos time weighted average
7. Part of the training program
8. Part of exposure measurements
9. Access to only authorized persons
10. Part of medical surveillance program

Column 2
a. Respirator type worn
b. FVC and FEV-1
c. Regulated areas
d. Location of ACM and PACM in the building
e. 0.1 fiber per cubic centimeter

Short Answer
Briefly but thoroughly answer each statement.

11. Where do you think asbestos-containing materials may be present in your facility?

12. Explain why HEPA vacuuming is preferred over other methods for cleaning up fibers.

13. Explain the employer's responsibilities when employees are exposed above the excursion limit or time weighted average.

14. Describe engineering and work practice controls that can be implemented to reduce asbestos exposure.

15. Explain when the proper respirator for the exposure can be worn by employees.

CHAPTER 33

Air Contaminants

After studying this chapter, you should be able to

➤ Describe the OSHA air contaminant standard.
➤ State the terms used to define exposure limits for contaminants.
➤ Identify the equations used to calculate eight-hour time weighted averages for single and multisubstance exposures.
➤ Describe the hazards of nitrous oxide, **methyl methacrylate**, and glutaraldehyde.
➤ Identify the **Z tables** and the substances listed on each.

OSHA 29 CFR 1910.1000 AIR CONTAMINANTS

Air contaminants are covered under OSHA Subpart Z, which includes the requirements for determining exposure levels of regulated air contaminants as well as the requirements for controlling exposure to specific substances.

This section describes 29 CFR 1910.1000 Air Contaminants, which includes calculations to determine exposure levels for specific contaminants.

The section describes the Z-1, Z-2, and Z-3 tables, which list the permissible exposure limits for over 500 hazardous substances. In order to understand what the contaminant levels signify in these tables, an understanding of some terms is necessary.

There are approximately 500 substances on the OSHA list of regulated chemicals and particulates. It is the responsibility of the employer to determine if employees are being exposed to levels above regulated limits.

Definitions

The permissible exposure limit (PEL) for a contaminant can be defined as its time weighted average (TWA), ceiling limit (C), and/or short-term exposure limit (STEL). Particular standards also refer to action limits (AL) and excursion limits that trigger monitoring, training, and medical surveillance.

The time weighted average (TWA) is the concentration of contaminant above which the employee cannot be exposed to as averaged over an eight-hour day of a forty-hour work week.

The ceiling concentration (C) is the concentration of contaminant a worker cannot be exposed to at any time during the work day. If instantaneous monitoring cannot be done, the ceiling is then assessed as a fifteen-minute time weighted average exposure that cannot be exceeded at any time during the work day.

The acceptable ceiling concentration is the concentration that cannot be exceeded during the eight-hour work day except for a time period and up to a concentration not exceeding the maximum duration and concentration allowed by Table Z-2.

The short-term exposure limit (STEL) is a fifteen-minute average concentration that cannot be exceeded at any time during the eight-hour work shift. This is required even though the eight-hour TWA is within the PEL.

Calculations

When employees are exposed to different concentrations of a substance during the eight-hour work day, the eight-hour TWA can be determined as follows:

$$E = (C_a T_a + C_b T_b + \ldots C_n T_n) \div 8$$

E is the equivalent exposure for the work shift.

C is the concentration during any period of time *T* where the concentration remains constant.

T is the duration in hours of the exposure at the concentration *C*.

Example

An employee is exposed to ethyl benzene, which has a TWA of 100 ppm (parts per million). The employee is exposed for two hours at 150 ppm, two hours at 75 ppm, and four hours at 50 ppm.

Substituting in the formula:

$(2 \times 150) + (2 \times 75) + (4 \times 50) \div 8 =$ 81.25 ppm

The 81.25 ppm is less than the 100 ppm TWA allowed for ethyl benzene. The exposure is acceptable.

When employees are exposed to a mixture of substances during the eight-hour work day, the following formula is used:

$$E_m = (C_1/L_1 + C_2/L_2) + \ldots (C_n/T_n)$$

E_m is the equivalent exposure for the mixture.

C is the concentration for a particular contaminant.

L is the exposure limit for that substance as listed in the subpart Z tables.

Example

An employee is exposed to perchloroethylene at 75 ppm (50 ppm TWA); methylamine at 5 ppm (10 ppm TWA); and chlorobromomethane at 300 ppm (200 ppm TWA).

Substituting in the formula:

$E_m = 75/50 + 5/10 + 300/200 =$
1.5 + .5 + 1.5 = 3.5

Because E_m exceeds 1 (unity), the employee's concentration of mixtures is exceeded and the employer must take immediate steps to reduce the concentration.

Table Z-1

This table lists over 500 hazardous substances and denotes their TWAs, STELs, and ceiling concentrations. The PELs are listed in parts per million (ppm) and/or milligrams per cubic meter (mg/m^3).

Table Z-2

This table lists substances that have TWAs, acceptable ceiling concentrations, and acceptable maximum peaks above the acceptable ceiling concentration for an eight-hour shift.

The PELs are listed in ppm and/or mg/m^3.

Table Z-3

This table lists mineral dusts, and the PELs are denoted by million particles per cubic foot (mppcf) and milligrams per cubic meter (mg/m^3).

SPECIFIC AIR CONTAMINANTS RELATING TO ALLIED HEALTH

There are a number of chemicals that are exposed to allied health professionals in the course of their activities. Three important chemicals described here are nitrous oxide, methyl methacrylate, and gluataraldehyde. This is in addition to formaldehyde, ethylene oxide, and benzene, which are described in separate chapters because they have specific standards. Of the three just identified here, methyl methacrylate is specifically listed in the OSHA Z-1 Table.

Nitrous Oxide

Permissible Exposure Limit. Nitrous oxide is not regulated by OSHA, but it does have properties that can be harmful.

Union Carbide Corporation, who manufactures nitrous oxide, has established their own exposure limit of 25 ppm.

Use. It is used primarily as an anesthetic in operating rooms and dental and medical offices. It is also known as dinitrogen monoxide, nitrogen oxide, hyponitrous acid anhydride, and laughing gas. The anesthetic grade is composed of 80% nitrous oxide and 20% oxygen.

Physical Characteristics. It is a colorless gas at normal temperature and pressure. Its vapor is heavier than air, so it gravitates to the floor. It is also slightly soluble in water, and the solution is acidic.

Health Hazard Information. It is not regulated by OSHA, but the American Conference of Governmental Industrial Hygienists (ACGIH) has a recommended exposure limit (REL). The ACGIH is a private agency that is responsible for establishing threshold limit values (TLVs) for toxic substances. An REL is a limit of exposure for a toxic substance that is recommended based on studies of the substance. The REL exposure should not exceed 25 ppm as averaged over a ten-hour day or forty-hour week. The TLV is a recommended limit established by the ACGIH, but these are in most cases the same as the OSHA PELs.

Short-term exposure. Inhalation may cause dizziness and difficulty breathing. Exposure may also cause headaches, nausea, fatigue, and irritability. Oxygen deficiency in the air could be the result of high concentrations.

The liquid may cause frostbite and freezing burns on the skin. The vapors do not irritate. When ingested, the liquid may cause frostbite and freezing burns of the mouth and throat.

Long-term exposure. There may be incidences of liver, kidney, and neurological disease, and spontaneous abortion. It has been responsible for birth defects in rats. Chronic exposure to anesthetic concentrations has resulted in metabolic injury to the nervous system. Long-term exposure can also cause numbness, tingling of hands and legs, loss of feeling in the fingers, and muscular weakness.

Overexposure. Prolonged overexposure to high concentrations may suppress the body's immunological defenses when administered as an anesthetic.

First Aid. Persons should be moved to fresh air if nitrous oxide is inhaled. If required, give artificial respiration and get medical attention.

Soak affected parts in luke warm water for frostbite and seek medical attention, if it is necessary.

Medical attention should also be sought if nitrous oxide is ingested.

Fire and Explosion Information. Nitrous oxide is not flammable but could make fires more intense.

A dry powder, halon, or carbon dioxide extinguisher should be used to extinguish fires that involve nitrous oxide.

Reactivity Information. Reactivity is the ability of a substance to undergo a chemical reaction that may produce another substance that could be corrosive, be toxic, explode, or burn.

Nitrous oxide can form explosive mixtures in air in the presence of ammonia, carbon monoxide, hydrogen, hydrogen sulfide, and phosphine.

Decomposition occurs when heated above 650°C (1,202°F). It forms toxic vapors and oxygen, which can increase fire severity.

Protective Handling Information. Nitrous oxide should be stored in a cool, ventilated area in containers that are fireproof.

A local exhaust ventilation system or scavenging system should be employed when nitrous oxide is used as an anesthetic.

Rubber gloves, safety eyewear, and protective clothing should be worn when handling nitrous oxide.

High concentrations require wearing a self-contained breathing apparatus. Note that engineering and work practice controls should always be put into use first before using respirators.

Spill and Leak Information. When there is a spill or leak, the area should be evacuated. When removing the leaking cylinder, appropriate protective equipment should be worn and the area ventilated. The leaking cylinder should be brought out of doors to a safe location.

Methyl Methacrylate

Methyl methacrylate is regulated by OSHA concerning employee exposure. The employer should determine the exposure concentrations and institute controls, if necessary.

Permissible Exposure Limits. Methyl methacrylate has an OSHA time weighted average (TWA) of 100 parts per million (100 ppm) and 410 milligrams per cubic meter (410 mg/m^3).

Use. It is a constituent in bone cement used in orthopedic procedures. It is also known as acrylic acid, methyl ester, diakon, methyl methacrylate monomer, methyl alpha-methacrylate, 2-methyl-2-propenoic acid methyl ester, mme, and monocite methacrylate monomer.

Physical Information. It is a colorless liquid slightly soluble in water. It has a vapor density greater than air, so its vapors gravitate to the floor.

Health Hazard. Methyl methacrylate has both short-term (acute) and long-term (chronic) exposure.

Short-term exposure. It is toxic if ingested, inhaled, or absorbed through the skin. The vapor or mist is an eye irritant. Contact with the skin can cause irritation.

Exposure symptoms can include a burning feeling, headache, nausea, and vomiting. It also can cause allergic respiratory and skin reactions.

Long-term exposure. Chronic exposure can cause prolonged narcotic effects to the nose, liver, and kidneys.

First Aid. If there is contact with the eyes or skin, immediately flush with copious amounts of water for at least fifteen minutes. Remove contaminated clothing and shoes while flushing.

If it is inhaled, get to fresh air. Give artificial respiration, if necessary. Give oxygen if breathing is difficult.

Wash out the mouth with water if it is swallowed and call a physician immediately.

Contaminated clothing should be removed and washed as soon as possible. Contaminated shoes should be discarded.

Fire and Explosion Information. It is a fire and explosion hazard. It has an autoignition temperature of 815°F. This is the temperature at which it will self-ignite due to its exothermic reaction. Its lower explosive limit (LEL) is 1.7%, and its upper explosive limit (UEL) is 8.2%. The LEL is the lowest percentage of the chemical in air that will ignite or explode when a source of ignition is introduced, and the UEL is the highest percentage of the chemical in air that will ignite or explode when a source of ignition is introduced. The range between the LEL and UEL is the flammable range.

The vapor can travel a long distance to a source of ignition and flash back. Containers may explode under fire conditions. When fighting fires involving methyl methacrylate, containers should be kept cool with a water spray and self-contained breathing apparatus and protective clothing should be worn.

Methyl methacrylate may undergo autopolymerization. It will react violently with benzoyl peroxide. **Polymerization** occurs in a substance when two or more of its molecules form a larger chain of molecules that contain the structure of the original molecules. This causes the substance to become unstable, which causes it to release energy.

Carbon dioxide or dry chemical fire extinguisher should be used to fight fires involving methyl methacrylate.

Reactivity Information. It is incompatible with oxidizing agents, peroxides, bases, acids, reducing agents, amines, halogens, and heat. It may polymerize when exposed to light.

Upon decomposition, it may release carbon monoxide and carbon dioxide.

Protective Handling Information. Heavy rubber gloves, chemical safety goggles, and a face shield should be worn when it is handled. A proper respirator should also be worn when concentrations might exceed the PEL (engineering or work practice controls should always be used first).

Wash thoroughly after handling.

Keep container lids on tight and keep container away from sources of heat, sparks, or open flame. The chemical should also be refrigerated in an explosion-proof refrigerator.

Spill and Leak Information. The area should be evacuated and ignition sources shut off. Self-contained breathing apparatus should be worn along with heavy rubber boots and gloves.

The chemical can be covered with an activated carbon absorbent and then placed in a closed container. The container should then be removed to the outdoors.

The area should be ventilated and washed down after the material is removed. It may be burned in an incinerator with an afterburner, but make sure that all applicable federal, state, and local laws are complied with before disposing of the waste.

Glutaraldehyde

Glutaraldehyde is being proposed for regulation but currently does not have OSHA exposure PELs. The employer should control exposure and refer to the proposed limits.

Proposed Permissible Exposure Limits (PELs).
Glutaraldehyde has an OSHA proposed ceiling limit (C) of 0.2 part per million (0.2 ppm) and 0.8 milligram per cubic meter (0.8 mg/m^3).

The American Conference of Governmental Industrial Hygienists (ACGIH) established the ceiling limit as 0.2 ppm and 0.7 mg/m^3.

Use. It is a constituent of cold sterilents and is also known as cidex, 1,5-pentanedione, 1,5-pentanedial, glutaral, potentiated acid glutaraldehyde, sonacide, glutaric dialdehyde, O-2957, G-151, and ACC10421.

Physical Information. It is a colorless to pale yellow liquid. It is soluble in water and has a vapor density greater than air. This means that its vapors gravitate to the floor.

Health Hazard Information. Glutaraldehyde has both acute and chronic exposure hazards. Employers must be aware of the airborne concentrations and institute controls, if required.

Acute exposure. Inhalation can cause nose and upper respiratory tract irritation. Severe exposure can cause coughing, shortness of breath, headache, dizziness, drowsiness, and central nervous system depression.

Skin contact can cause irritation. Previously exposed persons could develop a sensitized dermatitis. The chemical can be absorbed through the skin and affect the central nervous system. Headache, dizziness, and drowsiness can also result.

Eye contact can cause severe irritation along with redness, pain, and corneal burns.

If swallowed, it can cause stomach irritation, abdominal pain, nausea, and it may affect the central nervous system.

Chronic exposure. Inhalation can cause irritation to the mucous membrane.

Skin exposure can cause sensitization dermatitis.

Eye contact can cause conjunctivitis.

Swallowing may affect the reproductive organs and may cause fetal developmental abnormalities.

First Aid Information. For inhalation, remove the person from the area into fresh air. Perform artificial respiration if breathing has stopped. Keep the person warm and rested. Get medical attention immediately.

For skin contact, remove contaminated clothing and shoes immediately. Wash the affected area with soap or mild detergent and copious amounts of water. After there is no evidence that the chemical is still on the person, call for medical help immediately.

For eye contact, immediately flush with copious amounts of water. Occasionally lift the upper and lower lids until you no longer see any evidence of the chemical. Continue irrigating with a normal saline solution until the pH has returned to normal. Cover the eye with a sterile bandage and get medical attention immediately.

If swallowed, and the person is conscious and not convulsing, induce emesis by giving syrup of ipecac followed by water. Repeat in twenty minutes if emesis is not induced. Give activated charcoal. If the person has depressed respiration or if emesis is not produced, perform gastric lavage cautiously. Gastric lavage should be performed only by qualified medical personnel. Get medical attention immediately. Gastric lavage is the washing out of the stomach with a sterile water or normal saline solution by inserting a stomach tube or catheter.

Fire and Explosion Information. It is not a severe threat if exposed to heat or flame. A dry chemical, carbon dioxide, or halon extinguisher should be used to fight fires involving glutaraldehyde. For larger fires use water spray, fog, or foam.

If possible, remove containers from the fire area. Do not scatter spilled material with high-pressure hose streams. Dike the water used on the fire for proper disposal. Avoid breathing the vapors and try to stay upwind when fighting the fire.

Reactivity Information. Glutaraldehyde is stable under **normal temperature and pressure (NTP)**. NTP is a temperature of 70°F and a pressure of 29.92 inches of Hg (mercury) or 14.7 psi. It is incompatible with oxidizers (with which it can react violently), reducing agents, acids, and alkalies. Thermal decomposition can release toxic and hazardous gases.

The chemical can undergo slow, nonhazardous polymerization when stored for long periods of time at ambient temperatures.

Protective Handling Information. Local exhaust or enclosure in a fume hood should be used to keep airborne levels below the PEL. Local exhaust captures the contaminant near its source. It is comprised of a hood, duct system, fan, and filter.

The respirator worn depends upon the airborne concentration and must be approved by MSHA and NIOSH.

Protective clothing and gloves must be worn to prevent skin contact.

Chemical-type safety goggles and face shield must be worn to prevent face and eye contact.

When employees' skin or eyes are exposed to the chemical, an eyewash fountain and deluge shower should be available within the area.

Spill and Leak Information. Shut off sources of ignition and attempt to stop the leak, if possible. Use water spray to reduce the vapors. Small spills can be absorbed with sand or other absorbent. Material should be placed in containers for disposal. Dike larger spills and containerize for future disposal.

Prohibit flame, flares, and smoking in the spill or leak area. Allow only authorized persons in the area and isolate the area.

CHAPTER REVIEW

Multiple Choice

Select the best answer from the choices provided.

1. The Z-1 table lists approximately
   a. 100 substances
   b. 200 substances
   c. 300 substances
   d. 500 substances
   e. 1,000 substances

2. When calculating exposure for a mixture of substances, if E_m is less than unity
   a. the exposure is hazardous
   b. the exposure is safe
   c. the exposure cannot be determined
   d. the exposure level has to be recalculated

3. Reactivity is the ability of a substance to become
   a. toxic
   b. corrosive
   c. an explosive
   d. a, b, and c

4. Nitrous oxide at high concentrations requires wearing
   a. an air purifying respirator
   b. a supplied air respirator
   c. a SCBA
   d. no respirator because it is not an OSHA regulated substance

5. Glutaraldehyde is also known as
   a. sonacide
   b. nitrogen oxide
   c. acrylic acid
   d. a, b, and c

True/False

Indicate whether the statement is true or false by circling T or F.

6. T F The same formula can be used to determine exposure from a single substance and exposure from several substances.

7. T F Table Z-3 lists hazardous mineral dusts and their PELs in mppcf and mg/m^3.

8. T F Nitrous oxide is regulated by OSHA.

9. T F Methyl methacrylate is not regulated by OSHA.

10. T F The ACGIH has established legal limits for glutaraldehyde.

Matching

Match the terms in column 1 with the definitions in column 2.

Column 1
11. Excursion limit
12. Ceiling concentration
13. STEL
14. Anesthetic
15. Constituent in bone cement

Column 2
a. Nitrous oxide
b. Triggers monitoring and training
c. Methyl methacrylate
d. Exposure not permitted at anytime
e. Average fifteen-minute concentration that cannot be exceeded

Short Answer

Briefly but thoroughly answer each statement.

16. Explain the differences between TWA, STEL, C, and excursion limit.

Note: For questions 17 and 18, you have to refer to 29 CFR 1910.1000 Z-1 Table.

17. What is the exposure of an employee exposed to cyclohexane at 400 ppm for 3 hours, 150 ppm for 2 hours, and 200 ppm for 3 hours? Is the exposure below or above the TWA?

18. What is the equivalent exposure of an employee exposed to diethylamine at 10 ppm for 2 hours, ethyl formate at 175 ppm for 3 hours, and heptane at 600 ppm for 3 hours? Is the equivalent exposure less or more than 1?

19. Explain where methyl methacrylate is used in your facility.

20. Explain where nitrous oxide is used in your facility.

CHAPTER 34

Ionizing Radiation

OBJECTIVES

After studying this chapter, you should be able to

➤ Describe the OSHA ionizing radiation standard.

➤ Identify the various types of ionizing radiation.

➤ Define the terms used for ionizing radiation exposure.

➤ List the requirements for radiation areas.

➤ List the employee records required and when exposure notification is required.

Occupational exposure to **ionizing radiation** is included in OSHA 29 CFR 1910.96, General Industry Standards.

OSHA 29 CFR 1910.96 IONIZING RADIATION

This standard covers occupational exposure to ionizing radiation.

Definitions

Radioactive material is any material that emits, by spontaneous nuclear disintegration, particular or electromagnetic emanations.

Restricted area is an area controlled to prevent employee exposure to radiation or radioactive materials.

Dose refers to the quantity of ionizing radiation per unit of body mass.

Rad (radiation absorbed dose) is a measure of dose of any ionizing radiation to body tissue in terms of the energy absorbed per unit of mass of the tissue.

Rem (roentgen equivalent man) is a measure of dose of any ionizing radiation to body tissues.

Exposure of Individuals to Radiation in Restricted Areas. Individuals in restricted areas cannot receive in any period of one calendar quarter a dose in excess of the following:

- Whole body: head and trunk, active blood-forming organs; lens of eyes; or gonads—$1\frac{1}{4}$ rems per calendar quarter
- Hands and forearms; feet and ankles—$18\frac{3}{4}$ rems per calendar quarter
- Skin of whole body—$7\frac{1}{2}$ rems per calendar quarter

An employer may permit an individual in a restricted area to receive doses to the whole body greater than those permitted so long as

- During any calendar quarter the dose to the whole body shall not exceed 3 rems.
- The dose to the whole body when added to the accumulated dose to the whole body shall not exceed $5 (N - 18)$ rems, where N equals the individual's age in years at his/her last birthday.
- The employer maintains past and current exposure records that show that the addition of such a dose will not exceed the authorized amount. Dose to the whole body shall include any dose to the whole body, gonads, active blood-forming organs, head, trunk, or lens of the eye.

No employee who is under 18 years of age can receive in any period of one calendar quarter a dose in excess of 10 percent of the limits described earlier.

Exposure to Airborne Radioactive Materials.
Employees in restricted areas cannot be exposed to airborne radioactive materials in average concentrations in excess of the limits specified in Table I of Appendix B to 10 CFR Part 20.

Employees under 18 years of age in restricted areas cannot be exposed to airborne radioactive materials in an average concentration in excess of the limits specified in Table I of Appendix B to 10 CFR Part 20.

Precautionary Procedures and Personal Monitoring. Surveys must be made that evaluate radiation hazards.

Employees must be supplied with personnel monitoring equipment such as film badges, pocket chambers, dosimeters, and film rings.

Each employee who enters a restricted area who receives or is likely to receive a dose in any calendar quarter in excess of 25 percent of the limits allowed must be equipped with personnel monitoring equipment.

Each employee under 18 years of age who enters a restricted area and receives or is likely to receive a dose in any calendar quarter in excess of 5 percent of the limits specified must be equipped with personnel monitoring equipment.

Each employee who enters a high-radiation area must be equipped with personnel monitoring equipment.

A radiation area is any area where radiation exists at such levels that a major portion of the body could receive in any one hour a dose in excess of 5 **millirem**, or in any five consecutive days a dose in excess of 100 millirem. A millirem is 1/1,000 rem.

A high-radiation area is any area where radiation exists at such levels that a major portion of the body could receive in any one hour a dose in excess of 100 millirem.

Caution Signs, Labels, and Signals. Radiation symbols shall use the conventional radiation caution colors (magenta or purple on yellow background). This is the conventional three bladed design.

Radiation areas must be posted with a sign or signs that bear the radiation symbol and the words: **Caution: Radiation Area**.

High-radiation areas must be posted with a sign or signs bearing the radiation symbol and the words: **Caution: High-Radiation Area**.

High-radiation areas must be equipped with control devices that cause the level of radiation an individual might receive to be reduced to a dose of 100 millirems or less in one hour upon entry or shall energize an alarm. Control devices are not required if the high-radiation area is established for thirty days or less.

Airborne Activity Areas. Airborne activity areas are rooms, enclosures, or operating areas in which airborne radioactive materials exist in concentrations in excess of the amounts specified in column 1 of Table 1 of Appendix B to 10 CFR Part 20 or exist in concentrations that, averaged over the number of hours in any week during which individuals are in the area, exceed 25 percent of the amounts specified in column 1 of Table 1 of Appendix B to 10 CFR Part 20.

Airborne radioactivity areas must be conspicuously posted with a sign or signs bearing the radiation caution symbol and the words: **Caution: Airborne Radioactivity Area**.

Evacuation Warning Signals. A sufficient number of signals must be installed so that individuals can make immediate and rapid evacuation.

The signal shall sound automatically and be equipped with an emergency power supply. Signal components must be protected against damage.

Periodic tests, inspections, and checks must be made of the signaling system to ensure that it is operating properly.

Exceptions from Posting Requirements. A room or area is not required to be posted with the caution sign because of a sealed source provided that the radiation level 12 inches from the surface of the source container does not exceed 5 millirem.

Rooms or other areas in on-site medical facilities are not required to be posted with caution signs because of the presence of patients containing radioactive materials, provided there are personnel in attendance who shall take precautions to prevent exposure to any individual in excess of the provisions stated in the standard.

Caution signs are not required to be posted at areas or rooms containing radioactive materials for less than eight hours provided that precautions are taken to prevent exposure in excess of the limits established in this standard and that the area or room is under the employer's control.

Instruction of Personnel. Individuals working in or frequenting any portion of a radiation area must be informed of the materials. They must be instructed in safety problems associated with exposure and in precautions and devices to minimize exposure. They must be instructed in the requirements of this standard that protect against exposure and be advised of radiation exposure reports.

Copies of the standard provisions and operating procedures must be posted in a conspicuous place.

Storage of Radioactive Materials. Radioactive materials stored in nonradiation areas must be secured against unauthorized removal.

Waste Disposal. Applicable state and federal laws must be observed when disposing of radioactive materials.

Notification of Incidents. OSHA must be immediately notified when exposure to the whole body of an individual is 25 rems or more; exposure to the skin of the whole body is 150 rems or more; or exposure to the feet, ankles, hands, or forearms is 375 rems or more; or there is a release in concentrations that, if averaged over a period of twenty-four hours, would exceed 5,000 times the limit specified in Table II of Appendix B to 10 CFR Part 20.

OSHA must be notified within twenty-four hours when exposure to the whole body is 5 rems or more; exposure to the skin of the whole body is 30 rems or more; or exposure of the feet, ankles, hands, or forearms is 75 rems or more.

Records. Radiation exposure records of employees must be maintained for those employees requiring personnel monitoring.

At the request of a former employee, an employer must furnish a report of the employee's exposure to radiation. The report must be furnished within thirty days from the time the request was made and must cover each calendar quarter of the individual's employment involving exposure to radiation or such lesser period as may be requested by the employee. The report must also include the results of any calculations or analyses of radioactive materials deposited in the body.

APPENDIX

This appendix describes the various forms of ionizing radiation.

Ionizing Radiation

Ionizing radiation is radiation that has the ability to "ionize" tissue it strikes. This means that it has the power to cause electrons to be released from their orbits around the nuclei. When ionizing radiation penetrates the body, the ionizing process causes a tissue change, which can lead to cancer among other illnesses. The higher the energy level, the more its ability to penetrate tissue.

Alpha, beta, and **neutron radiation** are called particle radiation because they are atomic particles. Alpha radiation can be stopped by the skin or a sheet of paper, beta by ½-inch aluminum, and neutron by several inches of lead. Alpha and beta radiation become harmful when inhaled or swallowed (internal hazard).

Gamma and **X radiation** are wave or electromagnetic radiation with extremely high frequencies and very short wavelengths. Gamma radiation can be stopped by several inches of lead and X radiation by concrete or lead. The thickness of the shield depends upon the energy level. Gamma and X radiation are both internal and external hazards.

CHAPTER REVIEW

True/False
Indicate whether the statement is true or false by circling T or F.

1. T F Gamma and X radiation is particle radiation.

2. T F High-radiation areas require alarms.

3. T F Emergency signals must be properly maintained.

4. T F Employers must notify the local OSHA office when an employee has whole body exposure of 25 rems or more.

5. T F When a former employee requests in writing his/her exposure data, the employer must furnish this information within sixty days.

Matching
Match the terms in column 1 with the definitions in column 2.

Column 1
6. Alpha radiation
7. Neutron radiation
8. X radiation
9. Radioactive exposure
10. Absorbed dose

Column 2
a. Rem
b. Internal hazard
c. Rads
d. Stopped by concrete or lead
e. Stopped by several inches of lead

Short Answer
Briefly but thoroughly answer each statement.

11. Explain the various types of radiation and what can be used to stop each.

12. Describe the term "ionizing radiation."

13. Describe the instruments you have at your facility to measure radiation levels. What types of radiation do they monitor?

14. Describe how your facility disposes of radioactive waste.

15. Explain how radioactive sources are controlled at your facility.

CHAPTER 35

Non-Ionizing Radiation

OBJECTIVES

After studying this chapter, you should be able to

➤ Describe the OSHA non-ionizing radiation standard.

➤ Describe the construction industry OSHA standard for lasers.

➤ Identify the terminology used for non-ionizing radiation.

Non-ionizing radiation is covered under OSHA 29 CFR 1910.97 General Industry. Lasers are covered under OSHA 29 CFR 1926.54 Construction.

Non-ionizing radiation does not have the penetrating power of ionizing radiation. Its major hazard is its ability to heat body tissue (soft tissue). It has longer wavelengths and less frequency than electromagnetic radiation. Its frequencies and wavelengths are in the radio frequency range.

OSHA 29 CFR 1910.97 NON-IONIZING RADIATION

This standard covers occupational exposure to non-ionizing radiation.

Definitions

Electromagnetic radiation is restricted to that portion of the spectrum commonly defined as the radio frequency region, which for the purposes of this specification shall include the microwave frequency region.

Partial body radiation pertains to the case in which part of the body is exposed to the incident electromagnetic energy.

Radiation protection guide is the radiation level that should not be exceeded without careful consideration for doing so.

Whole body irradiation pertains to the case in which the entire body is exposed to the incident electromagnetic energy or in which the cross section of the body is smaller than the cross section of the incident radiation beam.

Radiation Protection Guide. For normal environmental conditions and for incident electromagnetic energy of frequencies from 10 MHz to 100 GHz, the radiation protection guide is 10 mw/cm^2 as averaged over any possible 0.1 hour period. This means power density of 10 mw/cm^2 for periods of 0.1 hour or more; energy density of 1 mw/cm^2 during any 0.1 hour period.

This applies whether the radiation is continuous or intermittent.

These recommendations pertain to both whole body irradiation and partial body irradiation.

Warning Symbol. The warning symbol for radio frequency radiation hazards shall consist of a red isosceles triangle above an inverted black isosceles triangle separated and outlined by an aluminum color border. The words **Warning—Radio Frequency Radiation Hazard** must appear in the upper triangle.

OSHA 29 CFR 1926.54 LASERS

Only qualified and trained employees shall be assigned to install, adjust, and operate laser equipment. Proof of qualification of the laser equipment operator must be available and in possession of the operator at all times.

Employees when working in areas in which a potential exposure to direct or reflected laser light is greater than 0.005 watts (5 milliwatts), they shall be provided with antilaser eye protection as specified in Table 35-1.

TABLE 35-1 Selecting Laser Safety Glasses

Intensity, CW Maximum Power Density in Watts/cm^2	Attenuation	
	Optical Density (OD)	Attenuation Factor
10^{-2}	5	$10-5$
10^{-1}	6	$10-6$
1.0	7	$10-7$
10.0	8	$10-8$

Areas where lasers are used shall be posted with standard laser warning placards.

Beam shutters or caps must be utilized, or the laser turned off, when laser transmission is not actually required.

When the laser is left unattended for a substantial period, it must be turned off.

Only mechanical or electronic means shall be used as a detector for guiding the internal alignment of the laser.

The laser shall not be directed at employees.

Laser equipment shall bear a label to indicate maximum output.

Employees shall not be exposed to light densities above direct staring of one microwatt per square centimeter (1 µw/cm^2); incidental observing of 1 mw/cm^2; and diffused reflected light of 2.5 w/cm^2.

Laser unit in operation should be set up above the heads of the employees, whenever possible.

Employees cannot be exposed to microwave power densities in excess of 10 mw/cm^2.

CHAPTER REVIEW

True/False

Indicate whether the statement is true or false by circling T or F.

1. T F Non-ionizing radiation in comparison to ionizing radiation has a much higher frequency and shorter wavelength.

2. T F Non-ionizing radiation's hazard is that it heats up body tissue.

3. T F Eye protection is not required for employees working with lasers at certain exposure levels as long as they do not look into the beam.

4. T F When a laser is not being used, it must be turned off and caps put in place.

5. T F The exposure limit for non-ionizing radiation is 10 mw/cm^2 at frequencies from 10 MHz to 100 GHz.

Short Answer

Briefly but thoroughly answer each statement.

6. Explain the difference between ionizing and non-ionizing radiation.

7. Describe the hazards of non-ionizing radiation.

8. Describe the hazards of lasers.

9. Where in your facility is there possible exposure to non-ionizing radiation and lasers?

10. Explain how you would measure non-ionizing radiation.

CHAPTER 36

Multiple Chemical Sensitivity

After studying this chapter, you should be able to

➤ Discuss multiple chemical sensitivity (MCS) and how it relates to the workplace and home.
➤ Identify the symptoms and causes of MCS.
➤ Explain employer responsibilities concerning MCS.

Multiple chemical sensitivity (MCS) is an illness that occurs to people who are hypersensitive to chemicals or other contaminants that may be present in the air, water, ground, or in the various products, materials, and food to which they are exposed.

It can strike people anywhere and at anytime. Concentrations of contaminants do not have to be high to affect these people. In fact, the contaminants may be barely detectable. Multiple chemical sensitivity can occur to people when they are at home, at work, or merely walking down the street. They may experience a sudden onset of eye irritation, breathing problems, skin rash, atrial or ventricular fibrillation, and/or pain to joints or muscles, and so forth. In some cases as the symptoms progress, the person may become seriously ill. In rare cases, the affliction can be fatal, such as if an airway became obstructed because of swelling of the trachea.

People may become affected because they live in areas that have poor air quality or because they happen to live near toxic burial sites, and so forth. They can become affected because of off-gassing of chemicals and **volatile organic compounds (VOC)** that may be present in their homes or at work. VOCs are organic liquid compounds that have the ability to vaporize very rapidly. People could be sensitive to paint vapors or to the preservatives in food products or to tobacco smoke. These are just a few of the agents that cause reactions.

People have been forced to move out of their homes because of this sensitivity. Other people have been forced to get rid of all their furnishings and live in spartan surroundings to avoid being affected by off-gassing from carpets and furniture. Some of the off-gassing contaminants in the home include formaldehyde, which is found in carpets, wall paneling, and other home construction materials, and volatile organic compounds. Volatile organic compounds are found in numerous products.

Some people have faced financial ruin because of the costs involved in fighting their illness.

People may become affected at work because of exposure to copy machine toners, correction fluid, organic cleaners, and so forth.

Persons can suffer symptoms once and maybe never become ill again. Other people may suffer constant symptoms. Others may suffer symptoms intermittently. The degree of sensitivity depends upon many factors. Reactions of persons who suffer from multiple chemical sensitivity will vary in many different ways. The severity will depend upon the person's sensitivity level and duration of the exposure as well as the person's natural defenses in fighting the illness.

Physicians and other health care professionals are beginning to recognize multiple chemical sensitivity as an illness that requires treatment. Various diagnostic and treatment methods have been developed that are helping people who suffer from MCS.

Employers are required in some instances under the Americans with Disabilities Act (ADA), to provide for reasonable accommodations for employees who suffer from multiple chemical sensitivity. Reasonable accommodations could be as simple as keeping work areas clean of dust or chemicals, opening windows to dilute contaminants, or substituting copy machine toners, organic cleaners, and so forth that contain sensitizing chemicals with those that do not.

The Social Security Administration in some cases will grant disability benefits to sufferers of MCS if they cannot work because of their hypersensitivity. Each case is evaluated based upon medical information, testing, and severity of symptoms.

The people who are sensitive to most everything are at greatest risk of severe illness. They virtually have to live in a contaminant-free environment and cannot work in any place where there is the slightest degree of sensitizing materials. In the real world this can be extremely difficult.

As more and more chemicals are introduced in the products we use, at work, and in the surrounding community, an increasing number of people are beginning to suffer the symptoms of multiple chemical sensitivity.

The output of workers is also being affected because of this problem. This is costing business and industry millions of dollars in lost productivity.

To help solve this problem, products can and are being produced that do not contain chemicals that can cause health problems in sensitive people. Integrated pest management (IPM) can be used to control insects instead of using insecticides and herbicides. Heating and ventilating systems (HVAC) can be maintained to control building contaminants. The HVAC system comprises the heating, ventilation, and air-conditioning systems that maintain air quality and comfort. These are just a few of the means that can be implemented to reduce the amount of toxics in the environment.

The problems of multiple chemical sensitive people are slowly being addressed. It is being understood that they have a right to live and work in environments that will not incapacitate them.

CHAPTER REVIEW

Multiple Choice

Select the best answer from the choices provided.

1. Symptoms of MCS can vary
   a. only one way
   b. many ways
   c. two ways
   d. three ways

2. MCS can strike
   a. only in the home
   b. only at work
   c. anywhere
   d. only outdoors

3. Financial losses to business and industry due to lost time related to MCS amounts to
   a. hundreds   c. millions
   b. thousands   d. billions

True/False

Indicate whether the statement is true or false by circling T or F.

4. T F The Social Security Administration recognizes MCS as a disabling illness in certain cases.

5. T F Formaldehyde exposure is one cause of MCS.

CHAPTER 37

Exposure to Laboratory Hazardous Chemicals

OBJECTIVES

After studying this chapter, you should be able to

➤ Describe the attributes that make a substance hazardous.
➤ Describe the OSHA standard that covers laboratory hazardous chemicals.
➤ State the requirements for a chemical hygiene plan.
➤ Identify the elements to be included in employee training.
➤ List the requirements for employee medical consultation and examinations.

HAZARDOUS CHEMICALS

Occupational exposure to hazardous laboratory chemicals is covered by OSHA 29 CFR 1910.1450. OSHA defines a laboratory as a facility where use of hazardous chemicals occurs in which relatively small quantities of the chemicals are used on a non-production basis. This means that chemical handling is carried out on a "laboratory scale," multiple chemical procedures or chemicals are used, the procedures are not part of a production process, and protective laboratory practices and equipment are available and in common use to minimize the potential for employee exposure.

A hazardous chemical is a chemical about which there is significant evidence that acute exposure (exposure that lasts for a short period of time) or chronic exposure (exposure that is prolonged or repeated) effects may occur in exposed employees.

This includes chemicals that are carcinogens (cancer causing agents), toxic or highly toxic agents, **reproductive toxins** (a poison or toxic material injurious to tissue of the reproductive system), irritants, corrosives, sensitizers, **hepatotoxins** (toxic to the liver), **nephrotoxins** (toxic to the kidney), **neurotoxins** (toxic to nerve cells), agents that act on the **hematopoietic systems** (blood-making organs such as bone marrow and lymph nodes), and agents that damage the lungs, skin, eyes, or mucous membranes.

This standard is a performance standard, which allows the employer flexibility in methods used to comply as long as the standard requirements are met.

OSHA 29 CFR 1910.1450 EXPOSURE TO LABORATORY HAZARDOUS CHEMICALS

The employer is responsible for ensuring that laboratory workers are not exposed to chemical airborne concentrations above the permissible exposure limits (PELs). The PEL is the maximum concentration of a toxic substance that employees can be exposed to over a designated period of time.

OSHA Regulated Substances

When substances are used in the laboratory that are listed in OSHA 29 CFR 1910, subpart Z, the employer must make sure that exposures do not exceed the PELs.

249

Employee Exposure Initial Monitoring

Employers must measure the employee's exposure to any substance regulated by a standard by monitoring. The OSHA PELs must not be exceeded for chemicals regulated by OSHA. If the chemical is not OSHA regulated, the employee must be made aware of the recommended exposure level (REL). The American Conference of Governmental Industrial Hygienists (ACGIH) threshold limit values (TLVs) are used as recommended levels when an OSHA PEL is not established. The ACGIH is a private agency responsible for establishing the TLVs and making recommendations concerning industrial hygiene in the workplace. The TLV is the recommended maximum allowable exposure to toxic substances over designated periods as determined by the ACGIH.

Periodic Monitoring

If initial monitoring shows that the level of exposure is over the action level (AL), or the PEL if the substance has no listed action level, the employer must periodically monitor. The action level is the time weighted exposure averaged over an eight-hour day that triggers monitoring and medical surveillance.

Monitoring Results Notification

Employers must let employees know of monitoring results within fifteen working days after receipt of the results. The notification can be in writing or posted in a location accessible to employees.

Chemical Hygiene Plan

The employer must develop a written chemical hygiene plan for the laboratory. The plan must

1. Address the protection of employees from health hazards associated with exposure to hazardous chemicals.
2. Be capable of keeping exposures below the PELs.
3. Contain the following elements:
   a. Standard operating procedures to be followed when exposed to hazardous chemicals.
   b. Situations when the employer will require use of engineering controls, personal protective equipment, and hygiene practices.

Extremely hazardous substances will require special attention.
   c. The requirement that fume hoods and other protective equipment are working properly and that the equipment is periodically checked.
   d. Provisions made for employee training and information.
   e. The circumstances when a particular laboratory operation will require the approval of the employer or his/her designee before it is implemented.
   f. Provisions for medical consultation and examinations.
   g. The designation of the person(s) responsible for the chemical hygiene plan and designation of the chemical hygiene officer. The chemical hygiene officer must have the expertise to implement the chemical hygiene plan. A chemical hygiene committee may be formed if deemed appropriate by the employer.
   h. Provisions for employee protection when handling extremely hazardous substances such as select carcinogens, reproductive toxins, and substances with a high degree of toxicity.

The chemical hygiene plan must be reviewed at least annually and updated as required.

Extremely Hazardous Substances

These substances should be considered to be put in designated areas; put in fume hoods or glove boxes; have procedures in place for their safe removal when they become waste; and have decontamination procedures in place for employees who work with these substances.

Employee Information and Training

Employees must be made aware of the hazards in their work area. This information must be given when the employee is first assigned to areas where hazardous chemicals are present and prior to new assignments where exposure occurs. The frequency of training is determined by the employer.

Information. Information must include the contents of the standard and its appendices, the location of the chemical hygiene plan, the PELs for OSHA regulated substances or other limits if a PEL does not apply, signs and symptoms of exposure to hazardous chemicals, and the location of reference material on the safe handling, storage, and disposal of hazardous chemicals found in the laboratory (this may be material safety data sheets [MSDSs] as well as other reference material). The MSDS is written or printed material concerning a hazardous chemical that describes information required by OSHA's hazard communication standard.

Training. Training must include the following:

1. Methods and observations used to detect the presence of hazardous chemicals (monitoring devices, odor, and the like)
2. The physical and health hazards of chemicals in the work area
3. Measures employees can take to protect themselves, which includes specific procedures the employer has developed
4. Details of the chemical hygiene plan

Medical Consultation and Examinations

Employers must provide employees who work with hazardous chemicals with the opportunity to take medical examinations, including follow-up examinations deemed necessary by the examining physician.

Examinations must be provided under the following circumstances:

- When the employee develops signs and symptoms associated with exposure.
- When monitoring reveals that the employee was exposed routinely above the action level, or in the absence of the action level, the PEL.
- Whenever a spill, leak, or explosion occurs resulting in the likelihood of an exposure. If exposure is due to a spill, leak, or explosion, the employee must be given the opportunity for a medical consultation. The consultation will determine if there is a need for a medical examination.

All medical examinations must be performed by a licensed physician at no cost to the employee and at no loss in pay. The examination must be at a reasonable time and place.

Physician's Information

The physician must be given the identity of the chemical(s) the employee was exposed to; a description of the conditions under which the employee was exposed; and a description of the signs and symptoms of exposure the employee was experiencing, if any.

The physician's written opinion must include the following:

1. Any recommendation for medical follow-up.
2. Results of the examination and tests.
3. Any medical condition that may put the employee at increased risk if exposure to hazardous materials continues.
4. A statement that the employee has been informed of the results of the medical examination or consultation and any medical condition that may require further examination and treatment. The employer cannot be informed of any condition unrelated to the employee's employment.

Hazard Identification

Labels on incoming containers of hazardous materials cannot be removed or defaced.

The MSDSs for incoming materials must be maintained and made available to employees.

Chemical Substances Developed in The Laboratory

If the composition is known, the employer must determine if it is hazardous. If it is, the employer must provide training as required by the standard.

If the chemical produced is a by-product and the composition is not known, the substance must be assumed hazardous and the appropriate standard requirements must be implemented (chemical hygiene plan, exposure control, and so on).

If the chemical is produced for use outside the laboratory, the employer must conform to 29 CFR

1910.1200 Hazard Communication Standard. This includes the preparation of material safety data sheets. This standard is described in Chapter 26.

Respirator Use

Whenever respirators are used in the laboratory, the employer must conform to OSHA 29 CFR 1910.134, which describes the use of respiratory equipment. The respirator standard is described in Chapter 16.

Recordkeeping

Records must be maintained on each employee's monitoring results and the results of any medical examinations, consultations, tests, or written opinions made by physicians.

The records must be kept and made available in accordance with 29 CFR 1910.1020, Access To Employee Exposure and Medical Records. This standard is described in Chapter 5.

CHAPTER REVIEW

True/False

Indicate whether the statement is true or false by circling T or F.

1. T F Chronic exposure refers to exposure that lasts for short periods.

2. T F Employees must be notified of monitoring results within fifteen working days after the employer has received the results.

3. T F Only the material safety data sheet can be used to convey information about the substance to the employee.

4. T F A material safety data sheet need not be generated if the hazardous substance is developed in-house.

5. T F The ACGIH TLVs are legal exposure limits.

Matching

Match the terms in column 1 with the definitions in column 2.

Column 1
6. Hepatotoxin
7. Hematopoietic system
8. Included in training
9. Part of the chemical hygiene plan
10. Neurotoxin

Column 2
a. Provisions made for employee training
b. Methods employees can use to protect themselves
c. Toxic to the liver
d. Blood-making organs
e. Toxic to nerve cells

Short Answer

Briefly but thoroughly answer each statement.

11. Describe the controls and procedures you would use to avoid exposure to extremely hazardous substances.

12. What are some of the reference materials you can use, other than the MSDS, to warn employees of the hazardous substances they are exposed to?

13. What other OSHA standards come into play when enforcing the exposure to laboratory hazardous chemicals standard?

CHAPTER 38

Hazardous Materials

After studying this chapter, you should be able to

➤ Describe the OSHA standards that apply to hazardous materials.

➤ List the various classes of hazardous liquids and how they are defined.

➤ List the terms used to describe the hazards of combustible and flammable liquids.

➤ Describe the safe storage of hazardous liquids.

➤ Identify the requirements of SARA Title III.

OSHA 29 CFR 1910.106 FLAMMABLE LIQUIDS AND COMBUSTIBLE LIQUIDS

The standard covers occupational exposure to flammable and combustible liquids.

Definitions

A **hazardous material** is any substance or material capable of posing unreasonable risk to health, safety, and property. It includes reactive, corrosive, toxic, and ignitable materials.

A **combustible liquid** is any liquid having a flash point at or above 100°F. Combustible liquids are divided into two classes as follows:

1. Class II liquids shall include those with flash points at or above 100°F and below 140°F.

2. Class III liquids shall include those with flash points at or above 140°F.

   — Class IIIA liquids shall include those with flash points at or above 140°F and below 200°F.

   — Class IIIB liquids shall include those with flash points at or above 200°F.

A **flammable liquid** means any liquid having a flash point below 100°F. Flammable liquids are known as Class I liquids. Class I liquids are divided into three classes as follows:

1. Class IA liquids have flash points below 73°F and boiling points below 100°F.

2. Class IB liquids have flash points below 73°F and boiling points at or above 100°F.

3. Class IC liquids have flash points above 73°F and below 100°F.

Flash point means the minimum temperature at which a liquid gives off vapor within a test vessel in sufficient concentration to form an ignitable mixture with air near the surface of the liquid.

Autoignition temperature is the lowest temperature at which a flammable gas or vapor air mixture will ignite from its own heat source or a contacted heated surface without introducing a spark or flame.

Lower explosive limit (LEL) is the lowest temperature in percent of vapor or gas by volume in air that will burn or explode when a source of ignition is introduced. Concentrations below the LEL are too lean to burn.

Upper explosive limit (UEL) is the highest concentration in percent of vapor or gas by volume in air that will burn or explode when a source of ignition is introduced. Concentrations above the UEL are too rich to burn.

Combustible range is the range in percent of vapor or gas by volume in air between the LEL and UEL that defines the combustibility or flammability of the material.

Design and Construction of Tanks. Tanks shall be built of steel, except they may be built of other materials for installation underground or if required by the properties of the liquid stored. Tanks located aboveground or inside buildings must be of noncombustible construction.

Installation of Outside Aboveground Tanks. The distance between any two flammable tanks or combustible storage tanks shall not be less than 3 feet.

Where unstable flammable or combustible liquids are stored, the distance between such tanks shall not be less than one-half the sum of their diameters.

The minimum separation between a liquefied petroleum gas container and a flammable or combustible liquid storage tank shall be 20 feet. Suitable means shall be taken to prevent the accumulation of flammable combustible liquids under adjacent liquefied petroleum gas containers such as by diversion curbs or grading.

Aboveground tanks, low-pressure tanks, and pressure vessels shall be vented.

Tanks and pressure vessels storing Class IA liquids shall be equipped with venting devices that shall be normally closed except when venting under pressure or vacuum conditions.

Tanks and pressure vessels storing Class IB and IC liquids shall be equipped with venting devices that shall be normally closed except when venting under pressure or vacuum conditions, or with approved flame arresters. Flame arresters or venting devices may be omitted if their use may cause tank damage.

Aboveground storage tanks shall have some form of construction or device that will relieve excessive internal pressure caused by exposure to fires.

Where vent pipe outlets for tanks storing Class I liquids are adjacent to buildings or public ways, they shall be located so that the vapors are released at a safe point outside the buildings and not less than 12 feet above adjacent ground level.

Drainage, Dikes, and Walls for Aboveground Tanks. The area surrounding a tank or a group of tanks shall be provided with drainage.

The drainage system shall terminate in vacant land or other area in an impounding basin having a capacity not smaller than that of the largest tank served. The termination area and the route of the drainage system shall be so located that if the flammable or combustible liquids in the drainage system are ignited, the fire will not seriously expose tanks or adjoining property.

The diked area shall not be less than the greatest amount of liquid that can be released from the largest tank within the diked area, assuming a full tank.

Walls of diked areas shall be earth, steel, concrete, or solid masonry designed to be liquid tight.

No loose combustible material, empty or full drum or barrel, shall be permitted within the diked area.

Tank Openings for Other Than Vents for Aboveground Tanks. For Class IB and Class IC liquids other than crude oils, gasolines, and asphalts, the fill pipe shall be so designed and installed as to minimize the possibility of generating static electricity.

Filling and emptying connections shall be located outside of buildings free from any source of ignition and not less than 5 feet from any building opening.

Installation of Underground Tanks. The distance from any part of a tank storing Class I liquids to the nearest wall or pit shall not be less than 1 foot, and to any property line that may be built on, not less than 3 feet. The distance from any part of a tank storing Class II or Class III liquids shall not be less than 1 foot.

Underground tanks shall be set in firm foundations and surrounded with at least 6 inches of noncorrosive, inert materials such as clean sand, earth, or gravel tamped in place. Tanks shall be covered with a minimum of 2 feet of earth, or covered with 1 foot of earth, on top of which shall be placed a slab of concrete not less than 4 inches thick. When underground tanks are subject to traffic, they shall be protected by at least 3 feet of earth, or 18 inches of well-tamped earth, plus 6 inches of reinforced concrete or 8 inches of asphaltic concrete.

Corrosion Protection. Corrosion protection for the tank and its piping shall be provided by one or more of the following:

- Use of protective coatings or wrappings
- Cathodic protection
- Corrosion-resistant materials of construction

Vents. Location and arrangement of vents for Class I liquids shall be so placed that the discharge point is outside buildings, higher than the fill pipe opening, and not less than 12 feet above the adjacent ground level.

Location and arrangement of vents for Class II or Class III liquids shall terminate outside of buildings and higher than the fill pipe opening.

Installation of Tanks Inside Buildings. Tanks shall not be permitted inside buildings except as provided in the standard.

For Class IB and Class IC liquids other than crude oils, gasolines, and asphalts, the fill pipe shall be so designed as to minimize the possibility of generating static electricity.

The inlet fill pipe shall be located outside of buildings at a location free from any source of ignition and not less than 5 feet away from any building opening. The inlet of the fill pipe shall be closed and liquid tight when not in use. The fill connection shall be properly identified.

Tanks inside buildings shall be provided with devices to prevent overflow into the building.

Supports, Foundations, and Anchorage for All Tank Locations. Tank supports shall be installed on firm foundations. Tank supports shall be of masonry, concrete, or protected steel.

Steel supports or exposed pilings shall be protected by materials having a **fire resistive** rating of not less than 2 hours. Fire resistance is the number of hours a material can withstand fire before it fails.

Tanks shall rest on the ground or on foundations made from concrete, masonry, piling, or steel.

Testing. All tanks before they are placed in service must be strength tested in accordance with the procedures established by the American Society of Mechanical Engineers.

All leaks and deformations shall be corrected before the tank is placed in service.

Piping. Piping containing flammable or combustible liquids shall be suitable for working pressures and structural stresses.

Pipe joints must be liquid tight and made from steel, nodular iron, or malleable iron.

Pipes shall be substantially supported.

Pipes must be tested before being put into service.

Container and Portable Tank Storage. These regulations apply to the storage of flammable or combustible liquids in drums or other containers not exceeding 60 gallons individual capacity and those portable tanks not exceeding 660 gallons individual capacity.

Only approved containers and portable tanks can be used.

Each portable tank shall be equipped with one or more venting devices.

Capacity of Storage Cabinets. Not more than 60 gallons of Class I or Class II liquids, nor more than 120 gallons of Class III liquids may be stored in a storage cabinet.

Design and Construction of Inside Storage Rooms. Inside storage rooms shall be constructed to meet the required fire resistive rating for their use. Where an automatic sprinkler is provided, it must be installed in an acceptable manner. Openings to other rooms or buildings shall be provided with noncombustible liquid-tight raised sills or ramps at least 4 inches high. Openings must have approved self-closing fire doors. The room shall be liquid tight where the walls join the floor. In place of a sill or ramp, an open grated trench may be used that drains to a safe location.

Electrical wiring must meet the requirements for hazardous locations.

The inside storage room shall be provided with mechanical or gravity exhaust ventilation that changes room air at least six times per hour.

Inside storage rooms must have one clear aisle at least 3 feet wide.

Storage in inside storage rooms is as follows:

- If the room is fire protected, has a fire resistance rating of 2 hours, and is 500 square feet, it can store 10 gallons per square foot of floor area. If it is not fire protected, it can store 5 gallons per square foot of floor area.
- If it is fire protected, has a fire resistance rating of one hour, and is 150 square feet, it can store 4 gallons per square foot of floor area. If it is not fire protected, it can store 2 gallons per square foot of floor area.

Fire protection systems shall be sprinkler, water spray, carbon dioxide, or other effective system.

Storage Inside Buildings. Flammable or combustible liquids shall not be stored so as to limit use of exits, stairways, or areas normally used for the safe egress of people.

Superfund Amendments and Reauthorization Act Title III (SARA Title III) and Emergency Planning and Community Right-To-Know Act (EPCRA)

The law requires facilities storing and handling extremely hazardous substances (EHSs) to let the surrounding community know that these substances are in their areas. EHSs are defined in the law and are listed as **reportable quantities (RQ)**, which are minimum quantities if released to the environment that must be reported, and **threshold planning quantities (TPQ)**, which are minimum quantities if stored that must be reported.

Section 303 of the law requires owners/operators to provide local emergency planning committees (LEPCs) with the following information upon request:

- The amount, location, and method of storage of any EHS present at the facility
- The routes the facility uses to transport the EHS to and from the facility
- Methods and procedures that facility owners or operators would follow to respond to a release of an EHS
- The designation of a person to act as the facility's emergency coordinator

- Procedures that the facility emergency coordinators would use to provide reliable, effective, and timely notification to the LEPC's emergency coordinator when a release of an EHS occurs
- The facility's method for determining the occurrence of a release
- A description of the emergency equipment at the facility and the name of the person responsible for the equipment

Section 304 of the law requires owners/operators of facilities to make emergency notifications in the event of spills or releases. The emergency notification applies to releases to the environment of SARA Title III extremely hazardous substances or the Comprehensive Environmental Response Compensation and Liability Act (CERCLA) hazardous substances in amounts equaling or exceeding the reportable quantity of the released substance.

Notification must be given to the state emergency response commission (SERC) and the LEPC immediately after release with a written follow-up sent as soon as practicable.

Section 311 of the law requires owners/operators of facilities to prepare or have available material safety data sheets (MSDSs) for hazardous chemicals under the OSHA law. Any facility having present 10,000 pounds of a hazardous chemical must submit a copy of the chemical's MSDS or a list of such chemicals to the local fire department, LEPC, and SERC. If the hazardous chemical is a listed EHS, a lower threshold of 500 pounds of the substance's threshold planning quantity, whichever is lower, applies.

The MSDS or a list must be submitted within three months of the time the hazardous chemical was present at the facility and within three months after discovery of significant new information concerning an aspect of the hazardous chemical.

Section 312 of the law requires owners/operators of facilities that are subject to Section 311 to submit an annual "Emergency and Hazardous Chemical Inventory" form by March 1 of each year to the SERC, LEPC, and local fire department. The form identifies chemicals stored, used, or produced at the facility during the preceding calendar year, the maximum amount and average daily amount present in ranges, and provides information on chemical storage and use.

CHAPTER REVIEW

Multiple Choice

Select the best answer from the choices provided.

1. The lowest temperature at which a liquid gives off an ignitable mixture with air and produces a flame when a source of ignition is present is known as the
   a. lower explosive limit
   b. combustible range
   c. flash point
   d. autoignition temperature

2. When underground tanks are subject to traffic, they must have above them at least
   a. one foot of earth
   b. three feet of earth
   c. two feet of earth
   d. one-half foot of earth

3. Inside storage rooms must have their air changed at least
   a. two times each shift
   b. three times a day
   c. four times a week
   d. six times every hour

4. SARA Title III requires any facility that has EHSs in the workplace that meet the quantity requirement to report this to
   a. the SERC
   b. the LEPC
   c. the local fire department
   d. a, b, and c

5. The minimum distance between a liquefied petroleum tank and a combustible liquid tank must be
   a. 20 feet
   c. 6 feet
   b. 5 feet
   d. 7 feet

True/False

Indicate whether the statement is true or false by circling T or F.

6. T F A combustible liquid has a flash point below 100°F.

7. T F Tanks must be firmly supported.

8. T F Fixed tanks of flammable and combustible materials may be installed inside buildings as long as they are protected.

9. T F Storage cabinets cannot have more than a total of 60 gallons of Class I or II liquids stored in them at any one time.

10. T F Under SARA Title III, an RQ is the maximum quantity of an EHS that must be reported if released into the environment.

Matching

Match the terms in column 1 with the definitions in column 2.

Column 1
11. Combustible range
12. Flammable liquid
13. 660 gallons
14. Requirement for storage tanks
15. Autoignition temperature

Column 2
a. Venting
b. Lowest temperature that will cause ignition without a spark or flame
c. Flash point below 100°F
d. Range in percent of vapor or gas between the LEL and UEL
e. Maximum quantity allowed stored in a portable tank

Short Answer

Briefly but thoroughly answer each statement.

16. Describe some of the other OSHA standards that apply to the combustible and flammable liquids standard.

17. Where in your facility are combustible and hazardous liquids handled and stored? Are the OSHA requirements being met?

18. List the SARA Title III EHSs that may be present in your facility. How would you handle a release into the environment?

19. Describe the protection required for an inside storage room.

20. Describe the protection required for underground storage tanks.

CHAPTER 39

Compressed Gases/ Oxygen Systems

OBJECTIVES

After studying this chapter, you should be able to

➤ State the general requirements for compressed gases.
➤ Discuss the OSHA compressed gas standard.
➤ Discuss the bulk oxygen requirement included in the compressed gas standard.

OSHA 29 CFR 1910.101 COMPRESSED GASES (GENERAL REQUIREMENTS)

OSHA describes general requirements for all compressed gases by referring to the **Compressed Gas Association (CGA)** requirements. OSHA also has requirements for specific gases. Because oxygen is frequently used in health care facilities, this gas is discussed in detail in this chapter.

Inspection of Compressed Gases

Each employer shall determine that compressed gas cylinders under his/her control are in a safe condition to the extent that this can be determined by visual inspection. Visual and other inspections shall be conducted as prescribed in the hazardous materials regulations of the Department of Transportation (49 CFR Parts 171-179 and 14 CFR Part 103). Where those regulations are not applicable, visual and other inspections shall be conducted in accordance with Compressed Gas Association pamphlets C-6-1968 and C-8-1962.

Compressed Gases

The in-plant handling, storage, and utilization of all compressed gases in cylinders, portable tanks, rail tankcars, or motor vehicle cargo tanks shall be in accordance with Compressed Gas Association pamphlet P-1-1965.

Safety Relief Devices for Compressed Gases

Compressed gas cylinders, portable tanks, and cargo tanks shall have pressure relief devices installed and maintained in accordance with Compressed Gas Association pamphlets S-1.1-1963 and 1965 addenda and S-1.2-1963.

OSHA 29 CFR 1910.104 OXYGEN

This standard covers occupational exposure to oxygen, particularly bulk oxygen systems.

Scope

This section applies to the installation of bulk oxygen systems on industrial and institutional consumer premises. This section does not apply to oxygen manufacturing plants or to other establishments operated by the oxygen supplier or his/her agent for the purpose of storing oxygen and refilling portable containers, trailers, mobile supply trucks, or tank cars, nor to systems having capacities less than those stated in the following paragraph.

Bulk Oxygen Systems

A **bulk oxygen system** is an assembly of equipment, such as oxygen storage containers, pressure regulators, safety devices, vaporizers, manifolds, and interconnecting piping, that has a storage capacity of more than 13,000 cubic feet of oxygen at normal temperature and pressure (NTP), connected in service or ready for service. A system is also more than 25,000 cubic feet of oxygen at NTP, including unconnected reserves on hand at the site. NTP is a temperature of 70°F and a pressure of 29.92 inches of Hg (mercury) or 14.7 psi. The bulk oxygen system terminates at the point where oxygen at service pressure first enters the supply line. The oxygen containers may be stationary or movable, and the oxygen may be stored as a gas or liquid.

Location. Bulk oxygen storage systems shall be located aboveground out of doors, or shall be installed in a building of noncombustible construction, adequately vented, and used for that purpose exclusively. The location selected shall be such that containers and associated equipment shall not be exposed by electric power lines, flammable or combustible liquid lines, or flammable gas lines.

Accessibility. The system shall be located so that it is accessible to mobile supply equipment at ground level and to authorized personnel.

Leakage. Where oxygen is stored as a liquid, noncombustible surfacing shall be provided in an area in which any leakage of liquid oxygen might fall during operation of the system and filling of a storage container. Asphaltic or bituminous paving is considered to be combustible.

Elevation. When locating bulk oxygen systems near aboveground flammable or combustible liquid storage, which may be either indoors or outdoors, it is advisable to locate the system on ground higher than the flammable or liquid storage.

Dikes. Where it is necessary to locate a bulk oxygen system on ground lower than adjacent flammable or combustible liquid storage, suitable means shall be taken (such as by diking, diversion curbs, or grading) with respect to the adjacent flammable or combustible liquid storage.

Distance between Systems and Exposures. Systems shall be 50 feet from any combustible structure.

Systems shall be 25 feet from any structures with fire resistive exterior walls or sprinklered buildings of other construction, but not less than one-half the height of the adjacent side wall of the structure.

Systems shall be at least 10 feet from any opening in adjacent side walls of fire resistive structures. Spacing from other structures shall be adequate to permit maintenance, but shall be not less than 1 foot.

Distance of bulk oxygen systems from flammable and combustible liquid storage must be separated as indicated by the following tables.

Flammable Liquid Storage Aboveground

Distance (feet)	Capacity (gallons)
50	0 to 1,000
90	1,001 or more

Flammable Liquid Storage Below Ground

Distance measured horizontally from oxygen storage container to flammable liquid tank (feet)	Distance from oxygen storage container to filling and vent connections or openings to flammable liquid tank (feet)	Capacity (gallons)
15	50	0 to 1,000
30	50	1,001 or more

Combustible Liquid Storage Aboveground

Distance (feet)	Capacity (gallons)
25	0 to 1,000
50	1,001 or more

Combustible Liquid Storage Below Ground

Distance measured horizontally from oxygen storage container to combustible liquid tank (feet)	Distance from oxygen storage container to filling and vent connections or openings to combustible liquid tank (feet)
15	40

Flammable Gas Storage

Distance (feet)	Capacity (cu. ft. NTP)
50	Less than 5,000
90	5,000 or more

Systems must be 50 feet from solid materials that burn rapidly, 25 feet from solid materials that burn slowly (coal and heavy timber), and 25 feet from congested areas such as offices, lunchrooms, locker rooms, time-clock areas, and similar locations where people may congregate.

The distances described in this section do not apply where protective structures such as fire walls of adequate height to safeguard the oxygen storage systems are located between the bulk oxygen storage installation and the exposure. In such cases, the bulk oxygen storage installation may be a minimum distance of 1 foot from the fire wall.

Storage Containers. Permanently installed containers shall be provided with substantial noncombustible supports on firm noncombustible foundations.

Liquid oxygen and high-pressure gaseous storage containers shall be fabricated to meet the American Society of Mechanical Engineers (ASME) boiler and pressure vessel codes for **unfired pressure vessels.** An unfired pressure vessel does not have a flame heating the contents, such as an oil, gas, or coal fired furnace.

Piping, Tubing, and Fittings. Piping, tubing, and fittings shall be suitable for oxygen service and for the pressure and temperatures involved. They must meet the ASME requirements for unfired pressure vessels.

Safety and Relief Devices. Bulk oxygen storage systems, regardless of design pressure, shall be equipped with **safety relief devices** as required by the ASME code or the DOT specifications and regulations. Safety relief devices are valves that relieve excessive temperature and/or pressure.

DOT containers designed in accordance with DOT specifications must be equipped with safety relief devices. ASME-designed bulk storage containers must be constructed in accordance with the ASME code for unfired pressure vessels and be equipped with safety relief devices.

Insulation casings on liquid oxygen containers shall be equipped with suitable safety relief devices.

All safety relief devices shall be so designed or located that moisture cannot collect and freeze in a manner that would interfere with proper operation of the device.

Liquid Oxygen Vaporizers. The vaporizer shall be anchored and its connecting piping sufficiently flexible to provide for expansion and contraction due to temperature changes.

The vaporizer and its piping shall be protected on the oxygen and heating medium sections with safety relief devices.

Heat used in an oxygen vaporizer must be indirectly supplied and be steam, air, water, or water solutions that do not react with oxygen.

If electric heaters are used to heat, the vaporizing system shall be electrically grounded.

Equipment Assembly and Installation. Bulk oxygen systems shall be cleaned in order to remove oil, grease, or other readily oxidizable materials before placing the system in service.

Valves, gauges, regulators, and other accessories shall be suitable for oxygen service.

Installation of bulk oxygen systems shall be supervised by personnel familiar with proper practices with reference to their construction and use.

After installation, all field-erected piping shall be tested and proved gas tight at maximum operating pressure. Testing media must be oil free and nonflammable.

Storage containers, piping, valves, regulating equipment, and other accessories shall be protected against physical damage and tampering.

Any enclosure containing oxygen controls or operating equipment shall be adequately vented.

The bulk oxygen storage location shall be permanently marked to indicate: **"Oxygen—No Smoking—No Open Flames,"** or equivalent warning.

Electrical wiring shall be weatherproof or general purpose depending upon whether the system is installed indoors or outdoors.

Operating Instructions. For installations requiring operation of equipment by the user, legible instructions shall be maintained at operating locations.

Maintenance. The equipment and functioning of each charged bulk oxygen system shall be maintained in a safe operating condition in accordance with the requirements of this section. Wood and long dry grass shall be cut back within 15 feet of any bulk oxygen storage container.

APPENDIX

This appendix describes general safety procedures for compressed gas tanks.

Compressed gases are in the gaseous state in cylinders at normal temperature and pressure (NTP). Normal temperature is 70°F. Normal pressure is 14.7 pounds per square inch. Liquefied gases are in the cylinder in the liquid and gaseous state. Cryogenic gases are liquefied gases in the cylinder at temperatures below –130°F in the liquid and gaseous state.

Liquids become gases as temperature increases or pressure decreases, and gases become liquids as temperature decreases or pressure increases inside the cylinder.

Hints for safe handling of compressed gases:

1. Keep cylinders away from heat.
2. When cylinders are not in use, keep valve caps on.
3. Cylinders must be secured to prevent them from falling over.
4. Only cylinder owners should charge and transfer gases to other containers.
5. Do not mix gases in cylinders.
6. Do not use damaged cylinders. Return them to the supplier or manufacturer.
7. Make sure that safety relief devices are operating properly. Test them.
8. Do not roll or slide cylinders along the floor.
9. Before moving cylinders, remove regulators, close valves, and put valve cap on.
10. Keep oxygen cylinders at least 20 feet from flammable gas cylinders or separate them by a ½-hour fire resistive wall at least 5 feet high.
11. Try to store cylinders in fire resistive, cool, dry, vented places. Do not block egress routes. Do not store where temperatures can exceed 125°F.
12. Check leaks with soap and water.
13. Properly label, showing contents of regular gas cylinders and poison gas cylinders.
14. Use only regulators and other equipment designed specifically for the gas in the cylinder.
15. Thaw valves with warm (not boiling) water.

CHAPTER REVIEW

Multiple Choice

Select the best answer from the choices provided.

1. Bulk oxygen should be stored in what relation to flammable storage tanks?
   a. below
   b. above
   c. same level
   d. doesn't matter

2. Bulk oxygen has to be stored away from areas where people congregate by at least
   a. 10 feet
   b. 50 feet
   c. 25 feet
   d. 100 feet

3. Transfer of gases from large to small cylinders can be done only by
   a. the manufacturer
   b. the owner
   c. the user
   d. a, b, or c

4. Oxygen systems must be set apart from materials that burn rapidly by at least
   a. 10 feet
   b. 20 feet
   c. 30 feet
   d. 50 feet

5. If there is no wall between them at least 5 feet high with ½-hour fire resistance, oxygen cylinders and flammable gas cylinders must be separated by at least
   a. 10 feet
   b. 20 feet
   c. 30 feet
   d. 25 feet

True/False

Indicate whether the statement is true or false by circling T or F.

6. T F OSHA has adopted the CGA requirements for the compressed gas standard.

7. T F Gases may be mixed in cylinders as long as all safety devices are in place.

8. T F Safety relief valves are not required on compressed gas tanks as long as they are in a safe place.

9. T F Cylinder leaks should be checked using the soap-and-water test.

10. T F Visual inspections must be conducted to ensure that compressed gas tanks are safe to use.

Matching

Match the terms in column 1 with the definitions in column 2.

Column 1
11. Normal temperature and pressure
12. Cryogenic gas
13. Relieves excessive pressure
14. Dike
15. 125°F

Column 2
a. Safety valve
b. Contains spillage from a gas tank
c. 70°F and 14.7 psi
d. Gas in cylinder at –130°F
e. Maximum temperature where storing cylinders

Short Answer

Briefly but thoroughly answer each statement.

16. Identify the areas where compressed gases are used and stored at your facility. Do they meet OSHA requirements?

17. Explain how you would safeguard employees who handle and store poisonous gases.

18. Identify the topics you would cover when training employees in the safe handling and storage of compressed gases.

19. What precautions would you take if you discovered a leaking gas cylinder?

20. Explain the precautions you would take when using oxygen in a patient room.

CHAPTER REVIEW ANSWERS

Chapter 1
Multiple Choice:	1. d	2. d	3. b	4. a	5. b
True/False:	6. T	7. F	8. F	9. T	10. F

Chapter 2
Multiple Choice:	1. d	2. b	3. c	4. b	5. b
True/False:	6. F	7. F	8. T	9. F	10. F

Chapter 3
Multiple Choice:	1. a	2. a	3. c	4. a	
True/False:	5. T	6. F	7. F	8. F	9. F

Chapter 4
True/False:	1. T	2. F	3. F	4. T	5. T
Matching:	6. d	7. e	8. a	9. c	10. b

Chapter 5
Multiple Choice:	1. c	2. a	3. d		
True/False:	4. F	5. T	6. F	7. T	8. F
Matching:	9. e	10. d	11. a	12. c	13. b

Chapter 6
True/False:	1. T	2. F	3. F	4. F	5. F

Chapter 7
Multiple Choice:	1. d	2. c	3. c	4. a	5. d
True/False:	6. F	7. F	8. T	9. F	10. T
	11. F	12. F	13. F	14. T	15. T
Matching:	16. e	17. d	18. a	19. c	20. b

Chapter 8
True/False:	1. F	2. T	3. F	4. T	5. F
Matching:	6. e	7. c	8. a	9. b	10. d
Fill-in:	11. permanent				
	12. durable				
	13. I (gases and vapors), II (dusts), III (flyings and filings)				
	14. Warning—High Voltage—Keep Out				
	15. service entrance panel				

Chapter 9

True/False:	1.	F	2.	T	3.	F	4.	T	5.	F

Chapter 10

True/False:	1.	T	2.	F	3.	F	4.	T	5.	F
Matching:	6.	c	7.	e	8.	a	9.	b	10.	d

Chapter 11

Multiple Choice:	1.	d	2.	a	3.	c	4.	b	5.	b

Chapter 12

True/False:	1.	F	2.	T	3.	F	4.	T	5.	T

Chapter 13

True/False:	1.	T	2.	T	3.	F	4.	F	5.	F

Chapter 14

Multiple Choice:	1.	d	2.	b	3.	c	4.	d	5.	a
True/False:	6.	T	7.	F	8.	F	9.	T	10.	F
Matching:	11.	c	12.	e	13.	a	14.	b	15.	d

Chapter 15

True/False:	1.	F	2.	F	3.	T	4.	T	5.	F
Matching:	6.	b	7.	d	8.	e	9.	a	10.	c

Chapter 16

Multiple Choice:	1.	c	2.	a	3.	c	4.	d	5.	b
True/False:	6.	F	7.	T	8.	F	9.	T	10.	F
	11.	F	12.	T	13.	F	14.	T	15.	F
Matching:	16.	c	17.	d	18.	a	19.	b	20.	e

Chapter 17

Multiple Choice:	1.	c	2.	b	3.	c	4.	a	5.	a
True/False:	6.	F	7.	T	8.	T	9.	F	10.	F
Matching:	11.	c	12.	d	13.	e	14.	b	15.	a

Chapter 18

Multiple Choice:	1.	c	2.	c	3.	b	4.	a	5.	a
True/False:	6.	F	7.	T	8.	F	9.	T	10.	F
Matching:	11.	d	12.	c	13.	a	14.	e	15.	b

Chapter 19

Multiple Choice:	1.	d	2.	c	3.	b	4.	d	5.	a
True/False:	6.	F	7.	T	8.	F	9.	T	10.	F
Matching:	11.	c	12.	d	13.	e	14.	a	15.	b

Chapter 20

| True/False: | 1. T | 2. F | 3. F | 4. T | 5. F |

Chapter 21

| Multiple Choice: | 1. c | 2. d | 3. a | 4. c | 5. b |
| True/False: | 6. F | 7. F | 8. T | 9. F | 10. T |

Chapter 22

| Multiple Choice: | 1. b | 2. d | 3. a | 4. b | 5. d |
| True/False: | 6. F | 7. F | 8. T | 9. F | 10. T |

Chapter 23

| True/False: | 1. F | 2. T | 3. F | 4. T | 5. F |

Chapter 24

Multiple Choice:	1. d	2. b	3. c	4. d	5. c
True/False:	6. F	7. F	8. T	9. F	10. F
Matching:	11. d	12. e	13. b	14. c	15. a

Chapter 25

| Multiple Choice: | 1. c | 2. b | 3. c | 4. a | 5. c |
| True/False: | 6. F | 7. T | 8. F | 9. T | 10. F |

Chapter 26

| True/False: | 1. F | 2. F | 3. T | 4. F | 5. T |
| Matching: | 6. d | 7. c | 8. e | 9. a | 10. b |

Chapter 27

Multiple Choice:	1. d	2. d	3. c	4. b	5. a
True/False:	6. F	7. T	8. F	9. T	10. T
Matching:	11. d	12. e	13. a	14. c	15. b

Chapter 28

Multiple Choice:	1. c	2. b	3. a	4. a	5. d
True/False:	6. T	7. F	8. F	9. F	10. F
Matching:	11. d	12. e	13. a	14. b	15. c

Chapter 29

Multiple Choice:	1. d	2. b	3. c	4. c	5. d
True/False:	6. T	7. T	8. F	9. F	10. F
Matching:	11. c	12. d	13. a	14. e	15. b

Chapter 30

Multiple Choice:	1. b	2. d	3. b	4. a	5. c
True/False:	6. F	7. F	8. T	9. F	10. F
Matching:	11. c	12. d	13. e	14. a	15. b

Chapter 31
Multiple Choice:	1.	c	2.	d	3.	b	4.	a	5.	d
True/False:	6.	T	7.	F	8.	F	9.	T	10.	T

Chapter 32
True/False:	1.	T	2.	F	3.	F	4.	F	5.	T
Matching:	6.	e	7.	d	8.	a	9.	c	10.	b

Chapter 33
Multiple Choice:	1.	d	2.	b	3.	d	4.	c	5.	a
True/False:	6.	F	7.	T	8.	F	9.	F	10.	F
Matching:	11.	b	12.	d	13.	e	14.	a	15.	c

Chapter 34
True/False:	1.	F	2.	T	3.	T	4.	T	5.	F
Matching:	6.	b	7.	e	8.	d	9.	a	10.	c

Chapter 35
True/False:	1.	F	2.	T	3.	F	4.	T	5.	T

Chapter 36
Multiple Choice:	1.	b	2.	c	3.	c
True/False:	4.	T	5.	T		

Chapter 37
True/False:	1.	F	2.	T	3.	F	4.	F	5.	F
Matching:	6.	c	7.	d	8.	b	9.	a	10.	e

Chapter 38
Multiple Choice:	1.	c	2.	b	3.	d	4.	d	5.	a
True/False:	6.	F	7.	T	8.	F	9.	T	10.	F
Matching:	11.	d	12.	c	13.	e	14.	a	15.	b

Chapter 39
Multiple Choice:	1.	b	2.	c	3.	a	4.	d	5.	b
True/False:	6.	T	7.	F	8.	F	9.	T	10.	T
Matching:	11.	c	12.	d	13.	a	14.	b	15.	e

APPENDIX B

NATIONAL SAFETY AND HEALTH ORGANIZATIONS

American Conference of Governmental Industrial
    Hygienists
1330 Kemper Meadow Drive
Cincinnati, OH 45240
513-742-2020
comm@acgih.org
Web: http://www.acgih.org/

American Industrial Hygiene Association
2700 Prosperity Avenue
Suite 250
Fairfax, VA 22031-4319
703-849-8888
jmyers@aiha.org
Web: http://www.aiha.org/

American National Red Cross National
    Headquarters
Safety Programs
18th and E Streets, N.W.
Washington, DC 20006
202-737-8300
internet@usa.redcross.org
Web: http://www.redcross.org/

American Society of Safety Engineers
800 E. Oakton Street
Des Plaines, IL 60018
847-699-2929
customerservice@asse.org
Web: http://www.inficad.com/nazasse

Centers for Disease Control and Prevention
1600 Clifton Road N.E.
Atlanta, GA 30333
404-639-3311
netinfo@cdc.gov
Web: http://www.cdc.gov/aboutdc.htm

Department of Labor (OSHA)
Division of Voluntary Programs
200 Constitution Avenue
Room N-3700
Washington, DC 20210
webmaster@www.osha.gov
Web: http://www.osha.gov/

National Center for Environmental Health
    Centers for Disease Control and Prevention
Mail Stop F-29
4770 Buford Highway, N.E.
Atlanta, GA 30341-3724
770-488-7030
Web: http:www.cdc.gov/hceh/ncehhome.htm

National Environmental Health Association
720 S. Colorado Boulevard
South Tower
Suite 970
Denver, CO 80222
303-756-9090

National Environmental Training Association
3020 E. Camelback Road
Suite 399
Phoenix, AZ 85016
602-956-6099
Web: http://www.envirotraining.org/ calendar.htm

National Institute for Occupational Safety and
    Health
U.S. Department of Health and Human Services
4676 Columbia Parkway
Cincinnati, OH 45226
513-533-8287
pubstaff@cdc.gov
Web: http://www.cdc.gov/niosh/homepage.html

National Safety Council
1121 Spring Lake Drive
Itasca, IL 60143-3201
630-285-1121
webmaster@nsc.org
Web: http://www.nsc.org/

OSHA Publications Office
U.S. Department of Labor
200 Constitution Avenue
Room N3101
Washington, DC 20210
202-219-4800
Web: http://www.osha.gov/oshpubs/

World Safety Organization
305 East Market Street
P.O. Box 518
Warrensburg, MO 64093
816-747-3132
wsodrz@semo.net
Web: http://www.worldsafety.org

A

abatement certification. A certification signed by the employer to OSHA that citations noted by a compliance health and safety officer (CHSO) have been corrected. The certification must be submitted to OSHA within ten calendar days of the date of the citation.

abatement documentation. A written document sent to OSHA notifying them that citations noted by a compliance health and safety officer have been corrected. This is required for any willful or repeat violations, or specific serious violations.

abatement plan. A plan that must be submitted to OSHA to indicate how any citation with an abatement date of ninety days or more, or for specific citations indicated by OSHA, will be corrected.

accident prevention tag. A tag that contains a single word and major message, such as **"Danger,"** **"Caution,"** or **"Biohazard,"** or the biohazard symbol. The message must clearly define the hazard and be placed as close to the hazard as possible.

acid fast bacilli (AFB). Bacilli that retain certain stains or dyes when washed with acid and alcohol. The bacilli retain the dye, but surrounding tissue becomes decolorized.

action level. The level of airborne contaminant of a substance, indicated by OSHA, that mandates employee training, medical surveillance, monitoring, and/or use of personal protective equipment. It is generally one-half the time weighted average.

active TB. The stage of tuberculosis where the TB bacilli have infected the person. This stage is highly contagious and the bacilli can be easily transmitted to other people.

acute exposure. An exposure to a toxic substance that lasts for a short period of time. The time of exposure is usually measured in minutes or hours.

aerosolized pentamidine. A therapy process for tuberculosis patients that involves the use of aerosol pentamidine.

aerosolized treatment. A therapy process for patients with pulmonary disorders that involves the use of aerosolized medications.

air changes per hour (ACH). The number of times per hour the air is completely changed in a space or room.

air purifying respirator. A respirator that draws in outside air through a filter upon inhalation and purifies the air before it reaches the breathing zone of the wearer. Air is under negative pressure in the respirator compared to outside air.

alpha radiation. A positively electrically charged particle comprised of two neutrons and two protons that is released by various radioactive substances.

alternating current (AC). Current that travels back and forth in a circuit. This back and forth movement is sixty times a second.

American Conference of Governmental Industrial Hygienists (ACGIH). Private organization that has governmental industrial hygienists as its members. They are responsible for establishing the threshold limit values (TLVs) of toxic substances and making recommendations concerning industrial hygiene in the workplace.

ampere. A measure of the current in a circuit. Current is the result of a voltage applying a force on electrons in the circuit.

anesthetic. Drug that causes partial or complete loss of sensation.

annual summary. The calendar year's total of reportable injuries and illness that the employer must indicate on the OSHA 200 log. The summary of the previous years totals must be posted by February 1 of the next year and remain posted until at least March 1.

antibiotics. A variety of natural and synthetic substances that retard or destroy the growth of microorganisms.

antineoplastic drugs. Drugs that inhibit or prevent the growth of malignant cells.

antiviral drugs. Drugs that inhibit viruses.

asbestos. A hydrated magnesium silicate in the form of a fiber.

asbestos-containing materials (ACM). Materials known to contain at least 1% asbestos and, if disturbed, may release airborne asbestos fibers into the air.

as-built construction drawings. Construction drawings, revised and prepared after the building is completed, that reflects all the changes made to the building and its systems.

assembly occupancy. Occupancies where fifty or more people gather for various events. The fire codes are more restrictive concerning these occupancies because of the number of people involved.

atmosphere supplying respirator. A respirator that supplies air to the wearer other than outside air. Air is supplied by either an air compressor or compressed air cylinder.

attendant. Person designated by the employer who is responsible for monitoring an authorized entrant inside a permit required confined space (PRCS). The attendant must be outside the PRCS and be ready to summon help in the event of an emergency. He/she must remain at the space while the authorized entrant is in it.

authorized entrant. Person, by virtue of training and experience, who has been designated by the employer to enter a permit required confined space.

autoignition temperature. The lowest temperature at which a flammable gas or vapor/air mixture ignites from its own heat source or a heated surface it contacts without the introduction of a spark or flame.

B

back belt. Device worn that is comprised of elastic material to help support the back during lifting activities.

backflow (backsiphonage) device. Device used in plumbing systems to prevent contaminated water from getting into potable water. Backflow preventers and vacuum breakers are such devices. Backflow devices (flame arresters) are also used to prevent welding gases from getting back into the cylinder during welding.

bacteria. One-celled microorganisms that lack chlorophyll.

benzene. A solvent derived from coal or petroleum. It is a member of the aromatic family of hydrocarbons. Formula: C_6H_6.

beta radiation. A negatively electrically charged particle identical to an electron. It is emitted from various radioactive materials.

biohazard. A combination of the words biological hazard that indicates organisms that pose a risk to people. These organisms can be bacteria, fungi, viruses, and the like.

biological hazard sign. A sign that identifies a presence or potential presence of a biological hazard and identifies equipment, rooms, containers, and experimental animals or combinations thereof that contain or are contaminated with hazardous biological agents.

biological hazard tag. A tag that identifies the actual or potential presence of biological hazards and identifies equipment rooms, containers, and experimental animals or combinations thereof that contain or are contaminated with hazardous biological agents.

bronchoscopy. Visual examination of the interior of the bronchus (windpipe).

bulk oxygen system. Oxygen systems that have an assembly of equipment including interconnecting piping that has a storage capacity of more than 13,000 cubic feet at normal temperature and pressure

(NTP) connected in service or ready for service. It is also more than 25,000 cubic feet at NTP, including unconnected reserves on hand at the site.

C

carcinogen. Cancer causing agent.

carpal tunnel syndrome (CTS). Disorder that occurs when the median nerve in the wrist is squeezed or compressed by the carpal bones or strong carpal ligament. It occurs in people who put their wrist and hands in awkward positions for long periods, such as when using a keyboard.

caution sign. Signs that warn employees of potential hazards or unsafe practices.

caution tag. Tag put on equipment or its controls to warn employees of a potential hazard with the equipment or control.

ceiling limit (C). OSHA permissible exposure limit that mandates that employees cannot be exposed above that limit for any period.

chronic exposure. Exposure to a toxic substance that is prolonged or repeated. Usually measured in days, weeks, or months.

combination air purifying and supplied air respirator. Respirator that uses the supplied air type respirator for primary protection and an auxiliary air purifying respirator for emergency purposes.

combustible liquid. A liquid that has a flash point at or above 100°F.

combustible range. The range of the concentration of a gas or vapor by percentage of volume in air between the lower and upper explosive limit that ignites when a source of ignition is present.

compressed gas. A gas under compression that exists in a cylinder in the gaseous state at normal temperature and pressure (NTP). Liquefied gases under compression exist in the cylinder in partly the liquid and gaseous state at NTP. Cryogenic gases are liquefied gases below –130°F in partly the liquid and gaseous state at NTP.

Compressed Gas Association (CGA). Association that describes the requirements for the handling and storage of compressed gases. OSHA has adopted the CGA recommendations as a requirement in their standard for compressed gases. The CGA requirement is a national consensus standard.

conductive hearing loss. A hearing loss because of a disorder in the outer or middle ear that prevents sound from reaching the inner ear.

confined space (CS). A space that is large enough for a worker to enter and perform assigned tasks, has limited or restricted means for entry and exit, and is not designated for continuous occupancy.

cube tap. A device at the end of an extension cord that allows for more than one electrical connection. It is also a device that is plugged into a receptacle, allowing for multiple flexible cords to be plugged into it.

cumulative trauma disorder (CTD). An injury to the musculoskeletal system because of the added effect of repeated aggravation to the system.

cumulative trauma syndrome (CTS). A group of signs and symptoms that indicate cumulative trauma disorder.

cytotoxic drugs. Drugs that destroy cells.

D

danger sign. A sign that is used to indicate an immediate hazard that can cause death or serious injury.

danger tag. A tag that is used to indicate an immediate hazard that can cause death or serious injury.

dBA. Decibel or sound level reading obtained on the A scale of a sound level meter.

decibel (dB). A measure of sound levels.

deet. A liquid soluble in water, alcohol, and ether. It is used as an insect repellent. It can be an irritant to the eyes and mucous membranes and can cause central nervous system disturbances. Chemical name: n,n-diethyl-m-toluamide; formula: $C_{12}H_{17}NO$.

density. The ratio of mass to volume. Material densities are usually compared to air, which has a density of 1. Material with densities of less than 1 are lighter than air and therefore rise; those with more than 1 are heavier than air and gravitate to the floor.

differential cell count. Determination of the number of each variety of cell in one milliliter of blood.

diluent. A substance that dilutes.

dilution ventilation. Ventilation that brings in fresh air to dilute contaminated air to safe levels.

direct current (DC). Current in a circuit that moves in one direction in contrast to alternating current (AC). Direct current limits the voltage that can be applied in the circuit.

dust. Solid particles generated by the handling, crushing, grinding, rapid impact, detonation, and decrepitation of organic or inorganic materials, such as rock, ore, metal, coal, wood, and grain.

E

electrical hazardous location. A location that contains hazardous airborne levels of gases, vapors, or particulates that could ignite if an electrical spark or arc was introduced.

emergency lighting. Lighting that is designed to operate when there is an outage of normal lighting. It illuminates stairwells, corridors, critical rooms, areas of assembly, and below exit discharge spaces of certain sizes.

endotracheal intubation. The process of providing an airway through the trachea by inserting a tube.

engineering controls. A method used to eliminate hazards by modifying the source of the hazard or by reducing the levels of contaminants that become airborne. A ventilation system and providing a container for sharps are examples of engineering controls.

entry supervisor. This is an employee, by virtue of training and experience and designated by the employer, who determines if entry into a permit required confined space can be done safely. He/she oversees entry procedures and terminates entry when it is required by regulations.

Environmental Protection Agency (EPA). Federal agency that is responsible for enforcing the nation's environmental laws.

ergonomics. The process of dealing with the disciplines that involve the interaction between the worker and his/her total working environment. Its goal is to have the work environment adapt to the worker rather than the reverse.

erythrocytes. Mature red blood cells or corpuscles.

erythrocyte indices. Reference points for medical evaluation of the red blood cells.

ethylene oxide (EtO). A sterilizing agent used in hospitals. Formula: C_2H_4O.

excursion limit. The maximum concentration of a contaminant that is allowed for fifteen or thirty minutes as averaged over a fifteen- or thirty-minute sampling period. The particular OSHA standard defines the period of the excursion limit.

exhaust ventilation. Ventilation that removes the airborne contaminant to a safe location.

exposure record. A written record that includes the level of a toxic substance or harmful physical agent to which the worker was or is exposed. It also includes calculations that determine exposure and the results of biological monitoring.

F

face velocity. The average velocity across the face of a duct or fume hood. It is usually measured in feet per minute (fpm).

Factory Mutual (FM). Private agency that certifies and approves various safety protective items, such as safety cans, flammable storage cabinets, and so on.

fire brigade. An organized group of employees who are knowledgeable, trained, and skilled in at least basic fire-fighting operations.

fire classes. Categories of fires that are determined by the material involved in the fire. There are four classes of fire: A, B, C, and D.

fire detector. Device installed in a fire alarm circuit that detects different stages of fires. The basic detectors are heat, smoke, ionization, and flame.

fire rated. This pertains to the number of hours a particular assembly or material can withstand a fire before it fails. If a door and frame are rated "2 hours," it means that it should withstand a fire for that period.

fire resistive. This is a general term indicating that a particular assembly or material has some degree of being able to withstand a fire.

fire watch. A term used in welding that requires an employee to stand guard during a welding operation to make sure that no materials are ignited by sparks or flame.

fit factor. A quantitative estimate of the fit of a particular respirator to a specific individual. It estimates the ratio of the concentration of a substance in ambient air to its concentration inside the respirator when worn.

fixed equipment. Equipment that has a relatively stationary position and location. It may or may not be secured to the floor.

fixed extinguishing system. A system to extinguish fires that is comprised of pipes, actuating devices, detectors, spray nozzles, and compressed gas tanks.

flammable liquid. A liquid that has a flash point below 100°F.

flash point. The lowest temperature at which a liquid gives off sufficient vapor to form an ignitable mixture with air to produce a flame when a source of ignition is present.

forced expiratory flow (FEF). A method to determine the condition of the lungs by measuring the expulsion of air when it is forcibly breathed out.

forced expiratory volume in one second (FEV-1). The volume of air forcibly expelled from the lungs in one second.

forced vital capacity (FVC). The volume of air that can be expelled following full inspiration.

formaldehyde. A chemical used to preserve tissue. Because of its tendency to polymerize, it is mixed with varying amounts of methanol and is used as an aqueous solution. Formula: HCHO

fume. Particulate that becomes airborne. It is formed by the evaporation of solid matter.

fungi. Plantlike organisms that include molds and yeasts.

G

gamma radiation. Electromagnetic wave radiation that has great penetrating power because of its extremely high frequency and short wavelength.

gas. Material that has low density and viscosity. It takes the shape of the container it is in because it uniformly distributes itself throughout the container. A gas can go from the liquid to the solid state or vice versa by changing temperatures and pressures. It also expands and contracts with changes in temperature and pressure.

general duty clause. Section 5(a)(1) of the OSH Act that is used by OSHA to cite for workplace violations that do not come under a specific OSHA standard. In order to cite under this clause, several conditions must be met.

general exhaust. An exhaust system that is designed to exhaust contaminated air in a room to safe levels. Also known as general ventilation.

general exhaust ventilation. A ventilation system designed to dilute contaminated air. It uses outside air (OA) to dilute contaminants. It is also known as dilution ventilation.

glutaraldehyde. A constituent of cold sterilents. Formula: $C_5H_8O_2$.

grade D breathing air. Air approved by OSHA that is to be used in situations where air is supplied to the worker as in respiratory protection.

grounding. A system in an electrical circuit that directs current to a safe location to prevent shock or electrocution.

ground fault circuit interrupter (GFCI). A device put in an electrical circuit that cuts off the power in approximately 1/40 second to prevent shock or electrocution when there is a ground fault.

H

halothane. Gas used as an anesthetic.

hand shield. Shield held over a welder's face to protect the eyes and face from sparks and arcs.

hazardous locations. Locations that pose fire or explosion hazards because of flammable or combustible gases, vapors, or particulate matter that is airborne or could become airborne because of an unintentional release.

hazardous material. Any material or substance capable of posing unreasonable risk to health, safety, and property. It includes toxic, reactive, corrosive, and ignitable materials.

hazardous waste. Any solid, liquid, or contained gaseous material no longer used. It is to be recycled, discarded, or stored until treated or disposed of. It is capable of posing an unreasonable risk to safety, health, and property.

hearing conservation program. A program that the employer must put into effect when employee sound level exposure exceeds 85 dBA. It consists of monitoring, audiometric testing, audiogram evaluation, hearing protection, training, and recordkeeping.

heating, ventilating, and air-conditioning system (HVAC). Building systems that comprise the heating system and the ventilation and air-conditioning system that maintains air quality and comfort.

hematocrit. An evaluation of the iron-containing pigment of the red blood cells by using a centrifuge to separate the solids from the plasma in the blood.

It is also the volume of erythrocytes packed by centrifugation in a given volume of blood.

hematopoietic system. System that involves the production and development of blood cells.

hematopoietic toxin. A toxin that attacks the blood cells.

hemoglobin. Iron-containing pigment of the red blood cells.

hepatotoxin. An antibody or toxin that attacks liver cells.

hertz. Term used to denote cycles per second.

high-efficiency particulate air (HEPA) filter. Filter capable of trapping 99.97 percent of particles 0.3 microns or larger.

high-level critical items. Items that constitute a risk of infection that is high if not properly disinfected. These are items that penetrate the body.

high-level disinfection. The highest method of disinfection and sanitation that must be used on items because of their use.

hydrostatic testing. Pressure testing given to fire extinguishers at required intervals to ensure that the extinguisher shell is capable of withstanding required internal pressure.

I

immediately dangerous to life or health (IDLH). An atmosphere that poses an immediate threat to life, would cause irreversible adverse health effects, or would impair an individual's ability to escape from a dangerous atmosphere.

indoor air quality (IAQ). The quality of air in the building as it relates to airborne pollutants. The pollutants can come into the air from outside or from within the building.

intermediate-level critical items. Items that require a disinfection level that is high because they contact mucous membranes and openings in the skin.

intermediate-level disinfection. The method of disinfection that destroys most bacteria except tuberculosis bacilli.

iodophors. A general antiseptic that is comprised of iodine and a solubizing agent that liberates iodine from the solution.

ionizing radiation. Radiation that has the ability to release electrons from neutral atoms.

isolating means. The process whereby energy sources are controlled to ensure that the sources do not reactivate while an employee is working on the equipment.

L

lead poisoning. A poisoning of the body due to the inhalation or ingestion of lead or lead compounds.

leukocyte count. A count of the white blood corpuscles.

level A. Clothing selected when the highest level of skin, respiratory, and eye protection is required.

level B. Highest level of respiratory protection worn but a lesser level of skin protection.

level C. Clothing worn when concentrations of hazardous substances are known and the criteria for wearing air purifying respirators are met.

level D. A work uniform when minimal protection is needed.

Life Safety Code (LSC) 101. National consensus standard of the National Fire Protection Association (NFPA) that describes fire safety requirements in public buildings.

lifting formula. A formula devised by the National Institute for Occupational Safety and Health (NIOSH) that calculates the recommended weight limit (RWL) for a healthy person over an eight-hour period.

local exhaust ventilation. Exhaust system that captures the contaminant near its source. The system is comprised of a hood, duct system, fan, and filter.

local hazard. This refers to a substance that affects one part of the body. A skin sensitizer is a local hazard.

log of injuries and illnesses. The OSHA 200 log that employers must maintain. This log individually lists the injuries and illnesses for the calendar year and is maintained during the year as the incidents occur.

lower explosive limit (LEL). The lowest percentage by volume of an ignitable gas or vapor in air that causes the gas or vapor to ignite or explode when a flame is introduced.

low-level disinfection. The method that is the lowest level of disinfection. It is permitted on those items that are catagorized as noncritical. It destroys bacteria (except TB bacilli), and a few viruses and fungi.

M

makeup air. Air that is brought into a room to replace the air being exhausted from the room. The volume of makeup air should equal the volume of air that is being exhausted.

manifold. A system of compressed gas tanks, including the pipes, valves, safety appurtenances, and the like, connected together to ensure a long-term supply of the gas.

material safety data sheet (MSDS). Written or printed material concerning a hazardous chemical that describes the information as required by OSHA's hazard communication standard.

mechanical lifting device. Device used to lift material and people to prevent musculoskeletal injuries. An example of a lifting device is a patient lift used in nursing homes.

mechanical ventilation. Ventilation system that uses fans to move air.

medical record. A record that describes the employee's health status and that is made or maintained by a physician, nurse, or other health care personnel.

medical removal. The temporary removal of an employee from a hazardous exposure in order to reduce the exposure when other methods cannot.

medical surveillance. A medical examination that includes a work and medical history for employees who are exposed to hazardous substances above the action level (AL), time weighted average (TWA), or excursion limit.

methyl methacrylate. A constituent of bone cement. Formula: $CH_2C(CH_3)COOCH_3$.

micron. A unit of length equal to 10^{-4} centimeters. Also called a micrometer.

microorganism. Minute living organism that cannot be seen by the naked eye.

milliampere. 1/1,000 ampere. An ampere is a unit of current.

millirem. 1/1,000 rem (roentgen equivalent man). A millirem is a unit of radioactive dose.

Mine Safety and Health Administration (MSHA). Federal agency responsible for safety in the nation's mines. It also certifies and approves respirators.

mist. Suspended liquid droplets generated by the condensation of matter from the gaseous to liquid state or by the breaking up of a liquid into a dispersed state by splashing, foaming, or atomizing.

musculoskeletal. Refers to the muscle and skeletal system.

mutagen. Agent that causes genetic mutations.

N

National Institute for Occupational Safety and Health (NIOSH). Federal agency that is responsible for conducting research and making recommendations for the prevention of work-related injuries and illnesses. It is also the investigative and experimental arm of OSHA and sets standards for respiratory protection. The agency certifies respiratory protection.

natural ventilation. Ventilation that makes use of openings in the building, such as windows and doors, to move air. This is in contrast to mechanical ventilation, which uses fans.

nephrotoxin. A toxin that attacks kidney cells.

neurotoxin. A toxin that attacks nerve cells.

neutron radiation. Radiation that consists of neutrons formed when certain radioactive materials decay. It is a form of particulate radiation.

nitrous oxide. A colorless gas used as an anesthetic. Formula: N_2O.

noncritical items. Items that can have the lowest level of disinfection because their contact is restricted to intact skin and not mucous membranes.

non-ionizing radiation. Electromagnetic radiation at the lower end of the electromagnetic spectrum. It has much lower frequencies and longer wavelengths than gamma or X radiation. It has the ability to heat up body tissue.

normal temperature and pressure (NTP). A temperature of 70°F and a pressure of 29.92 inches of Hg (mercury) or 14.7 psi. Gases are usually referred to as existing in the liquid or gaseous state at NTP.

noise reduction rating (NRR). This is the rating given to hearing protectors based on their ability to reduce sound levels by a specified decibel number.

O

Occupational Safety and Health Administration (OSHA). Federal agency responsible for enforcing the occupational safety and health standards.

octopus connection. An electrical connection that has several plugs connected to it.

ohms. A measure of electrical resistance.

OSHA referenced methods (ORM). Methods required by OSHA to correct hazardous conditions.

outside air (OA). Air brought in from the outside through the fresh air intakes that mixes with the recirculating inside air. It is also the air brought into a space by wall fans during general exhaust (dilution) ventilation.

oxygen deficient. An atmosphere that has less than 19.5% oxygen by volume.

P

particulate. A particle of a solid or liquid whose size is measured in microns.

PbB test. A test that measures the level of lead in the blood. When levels exceed 40 µg (micrograms) per 100 grams of whole blood, workers must be notified.

performance standard. An OSHA standard that is written to give the employer flexibility in how to meet requirements.

permissible exposure limit (PEL). The maximum concentration of a toxic substance that employees can be exposed to over a designated period of time. It can be a time weighted average (TWA), a short-term exposure limit (STEL), or a ceiling limit (C).

permit required confined space (PRCS). A space that contains—or has the potential to contain—a hazardous atmosphere; or contains a material that can engulf an employee; or has an internal configuration that can cause an employee to be trapped or asphyxiated by inwardly converging walls or by a floor that slopes downward and tapers to a small cross section; or contains any other recognized serious safety or health hazard.

permit system. A written permit that allows designated employees to enter the PRCS.

personal protective equipment (PPE). Equipment worn by the employee that protects against particular hazards, both actual and potential.

physician or other licensed health care professional (PLHCP). A physician or other licensed health care professional whose legally permitted scope of practice (that is by license, regulation, or certification) allows him or her to independently provide, or be delegated the responsibility to provide, some or all of the health care services required by the respirator standard.

plug strip. Multioutlet receptacle tap that allows several items to be plugged into it.

polarization. Term used to denote the proper connection of hot, neutral, and ground wires.

polymerization. Term used when two or more molecules in a substance form a larger chain of molecules that contain the structure of the original molecules. This causes the substance to become unstable and release energy.

portable equipment. Equipment that is easily moved from place to place. It refers to hand-held and movable equipment.

portable fire extinguisher. A fire-fighting device that can be handled by a person that is used to extinguish small or incipient stage fires. The extinguishing agent is in a shell under pressure. Extinguishers are rated for various types of fires.

portable tank. A tank small enough to be easily transported to different locations. It can be carried or easily transported on wheels or on materials-handling equipment.

presumed asbestos-containing materials (PACM). Materials that are presumed to contain more than 1% asbestos.

priming. Procedure preparing drug administration sets for use.

Q

qualitative fit test. A pass/fail test that assess the adequacy of a respirator fit. It relies on the person's response to a test agent such as banana oil, irritant smoke, or a sugar aerosol.

quantitative fit test. A test that numerically assesses the adequacy of a respirator by measuring the amount of leakage in the face piece.

quantitative thrombocyte count. A count of blood platelets. Platelets are found in the blood but do not contain hemoglobin. They are important to blood coagulation.

R

radiation absorbed dose (rad). A measure of radioactive dose. It is the amount of energy absorbed per unit of mass.

radon. A colorless and odorless gas that is created when radium in soil and rock breaks down into smaller particles (radon daughters).

reactivity. A substance's ability to undergo a chemical reaction that may produce another substance that could be corrosive, be toxic, explode, or burn.

recommended exposure limit (REL). A limit of exposure for a toxic substance that is recommended based on studies of the substance. A recommended limit implies that there are no OSHA PELs for the material. Some anesthetic gases have RELs.

recordable injury or illness. The injury or illness that must be reported on the OSHA 200 Log because it meets the criteria for being reportable.

regulated area. An area that has required controls because exposure to hazardous substances are or may be above mandated limits.

regulated medical waste (RMW). Medical waste that is soiled with blood and other bodily fluids.

reentrainment. The process whereby exhausted airborne contaminants get back into a building.

relative biological effectiveness (RBE). The relative effectiveness of the same absorbed dose when comparing two different ionizing radiations that produce a measurable biological response.

repetitive strain injury (RSI). Injury to the musculoskeletal system because of repeated trauma.

reportable quantity (RQ). The minimum quantity of an extremely hazardous substance (EHS) that must be reported to designated federal, state, and local agencies if there is a release into the environment.

reproductive toxin. A poison or toxic material injurious to tissue of the reproductive system.

Resource Conservation and Recovery Act (RCRA). Act that describes the requirements for the generation, treatment, storage, disposal, and transportation of hazardous waste.

reversed polarity. The condition when wires are connected incorrectly in an electrical circuit. An example would be when a "hot" wire is connected to a "neutral" wire.

roentgen equivalent man (rem). A radioactive dose that equals rads times the appropriate value of the relative biological effectiveness (RBE) for that particular radiation.

S

safety instruction sign. Sign used to convey general safety instructions and suggestions.

safety relief valve. Valve installed in systems under internal pressure. The valve relieves excessive temperature and/or pressure.

sensorineural hearing loss. Loss of hearing due to damage to the inner ear or to the fibers of the eighth nerve.

service entrance panel (SEP). The electrical panel that receives the incoming power from the street lines and distributes power to building circuits. It also terminates the building grounding system.

short-term exposure limit (STEL). OSHA limit of exposure to a toxic substance that cannot be exceeded as averaged over any fifteen-minute period.

smoke doors. Nonrated doors that are installed in corridors in specified locations. They are designed to keep smoke out of circulation areas.

smoke vents. Vents installed usually in stairwell roofs to vent smoke and flame that are in the stairwell. They should operate manually, mechanically, and electrically.

soil gas. Gas found in the soil as a result of decaying matter, leakage, or spills. A common soil gas is methane. Formula: CH_4.

specific gravity. The ratio of the mass of a unit volume of a substance to the mass of the same volume of water. If the substance has a specific gravity of less than 1, it floats. If its specific gravity is more than 1, it sinks in water.

sprinkler system. A system of pipes, valves, sprinkler heads, annunciation, and detection devices that conveys water to the fire area.

sputum induction. The process of inducing a cough in order to expel sputum for evaluation of microorganisms.

standard threshold shift (STS). The loss of hearing in either ear of 10 decibels or more at certain frequencies.

standpipe hose system. Hose systems installed on the floors of buildings. These systems are designed for use by trained building occupants and/or the fire department.

static pressure (SP). Pressure produced by a fan. It is exerted in all directions as it goes through a duct. It is also the algebraic difference of the total pressure and the velocity pressure in the duct. SP is negative upstream and positive downstream of the fan.

systemic poison. A poison that affects many parts of the body. When toxic substances get into the bloodstream, they can affect several body organs.

T

TB infection. The stage of tuberculosis where the TB bacilli are present in the body but have not become active. This stage of TB cannot be transmitted to other persons.

threshold limit value (TLV). The maximum allowable concentration of toxic substances as recommended by the American Conference of Governmental Industrial Hygiensts (ACGIH). In most cases the ACGIH TLVs are the same as the OSHA TWAs or PELs. Unlike the OSHA PELs, the TLVs are not legal limits.

threshold planning quantity (TPQ). The minimum amount of a toxic substance regulated under SARA Title III that, if stored at a facility, must be reported to designated federal, state, and local agencies.

time weighted average (TWA). The concentration of a toxic substance, as averaged over an eight-hour day, that cannot be exceeded.

total pressure (TP). The algebraic sum of the static pressure and velocity pressure as it goes through the duct. TP is negative upstream of the fan and positive downstream of the fan.

transport velocity. The velocity of the air in a duct system needed to convey contaminants. It is measured in feet per minute (fpm).

U

Underwriters Laboratory (UL). Private agency responsible for testing and certifying the safety of various products.

unfired pressure vessel. Vessel that contains a gas under pressure that does not have a flame heating the contents, such as in an oil, gas, or coal fired furnace.

universal precautions. The assumption that all infectious materials are hazardous unless proven otherwise.

upper explosive limit. The highest percentage by volume of an ignitable gas or vapor in air that causes the gas or vapor to ignite or explode when a flame is introduced.

V

vapor. The gaseous form of a substance that is normally in the solid or liquid state at normal temperature and pressure. It can be changed back to the solid or liquid state by increasing pressure or decreasing temperature.

velocity pressure (VP). Pressure due to the velocity of the air as it travels through the duct. It is exerted in the direction of air flow. It is also the algebraic difference between the total pressure and the static pressure. VP is positive both upstream and downstream of the fan.

velocity pressure method. A method used to design a local exhaust system. It determines system losses that determine airflow, the size and shape of the hood, duct size, fan size, and stack.

virus. Microorganism not visible under a microscope that relies on the nutrients inside cells for its survival.

volatile organic compounds (VOC). Organic liquid compounds that have the ability to vaporize very rapidly.

voltage. Electromotive force that causes current to flow in a circuit by creating a potential difference.

W

warning tag. A tag used to denote a hazard level between danger and caution. It must contain the word "**Warning.**"

waste minimization. The process of reducing the volume and toxicity of hazardous substances, particularly hazardous waste.

watt. A unit of power. It is the amperage times the voltage. It is also the load a device puts on a circuit.

work practice controls. Supervisory or administrative controls used to control or eliminate hazards. Examples of work practice controls are reducing the time workers are in a hazardous location to make sure no one person is exposed to a toxic substance above the OSHA PEL or mandating that all ladders must be inspected before they are used.

worksite analysis. An evaluation of the work area to identify unsafe conditions and/or acts in order to correct them.

written authorization. The documentation in writing that allows a designated representative of the employee access to exposure and medical records.

written compliance program. A program written by the employer that indicates the methods and procedures used to comply with certain OSHA standards. Written programs are required in the respirator standard and the bloodborne pathogens standard, among others.

X

X radiation. High-speed electrons moving in wave form. When the electrons strike an object, they become X rays.

Z

zinc protoporphyrin test (ZPP). A test that determines the effects of lead on the body.

Z tables. The Z-1, Z-2, and Z-3 OSHA tables are described in 29 CFR 1910.1000. The Z-1 table describes the TWAs and ceiling limits of chemical substances; the Z-2 table describes the TWAs, ceiling limits, and acceptable peak above the acceptable ceiling concentration for an eight-hour shift; the Z-3 table describes the TWA of mineral dusts.

INDEX